P9-DYB-078

THE
GREAT SECRET

THE
GREAT SECRET

THE CLASSIFIED
WORLD WAR II DISASTER THAT
LAUNCHED THE WAR ON CANCER

———•◆•———

JENNET CONANT

W. W. NORTON & COMPANY
Independent Publishers Since 1923

For information about permission to reproduce selections from this book, write to
Permissions, W. W. Norton & Company, Inc., 500 Fifth Avenue, New York, NY 10110

For information about special discounts for bulk purchases, please contact
W. W. Norton Special Sales at specialsales@wwnorton.com or 800-233-4830

Manufacturing by LSC Communications, Harrisonburg
Book design by Michelle McMillian
Production manager: Beth Steidle

Library of Congress Cataloging-in-Publication Data

Names: Conant, Jennet, author.
Title: The great secret : the classified World War II disaster that
launched the war on cancer / Jennet Conant.
Description: First edition. | New York : W. W. Norton & Company, 2020. |
Includes bibliographical references and index.
Identifiers: LCCN 2020016332 | ISBN 9781324002505 (hardcover) | ISBN
9781324002512 (epub)
Subjects: LCSH: Chemotherapy. | Cancer—Treatment. | Cancer—Research. |
Mustard gas—Toxicology.
Classification: LCC RM260 .C63 2020 | DDC 615.5/8—dc23
LC record available at https://lccn.loc.gov/2020016332

W. W. Norton & Company, Inc., 500 Fifth Avenue, New York, N.Y. 10110
www.wwnorton.com

W. W. Norton & Company Ltd., 15 Carlisle Street, London W1D 3BS

1 2 3 4 5 6 7 8 9 0

In wartime, truth is so precious that she should
always be attended by a bodyguard of lies.

—WINSTON CHURCHILL

The real war will never get in the books.

—WALT WHITMAN

Contents

"Little Pearl Harbor"

When the two *Time-Life* war correspondents arrived in the old port town of Bari on Italy's Adriatic coast on Thursday, December 2, 1943, they were delighted to find the bars and restaurants open and doing a booming business. Will Lang, a twenty-nine-year-old veteran American combat reporter, and George Rodger, a trailblazing English photojournalist six years his senior, grabbed the first empty table in the Albergo Oriente, a glass-fronted hotel on a wide, tree-lined boulevard in the new part of the city. Exhausted, they collapsed onto the rickety chairs and grinned at each other. By some stroke of luck, they had a two-day layover and planned to take a little break and over-indulge in the local wines before returning to the grind.

Even though the front lay only 150 miles to the north, Bari seemed not to have a care in the world. The British had taken the capital of Puglia unopposed in September, and the citizens had celebrated in the streets, relieved and grateful to fall under Allied protection. The shop windows were full of fruit, cakes, and bread, along with other delicacies not seen since before the war. Waiting customers happily gossiped, argued, and haggled. Young couples strolled arm in arm, as they had for centuries. Even the ice cream vendors were doing a brisk winter trade, an incongruous sight for the journalists after having passed lines of women and children begging for black-market food only a few miles outside of town. After witnessing the chaos and misery in one village after another flattened by German bombs, the men were amazed that the medieval city, with its massive cliffs cradling the sea, had escaped the fighting almost unscathed. Its famous landmark, the gleaming white Basilica di San Nicola, home to the crypt of St. Nicholas, appeared intact. It was good to know that in the midst of this terrible war, at least the bones of Father Christmas still rested in peace.

No doubt High Command had ordered that the splendid harbor be spared. Bari was a crucial Mediterranean service hub, supplying both the American Fifth and the British Eighth Armies, which comprised the better part of the half-million Allied troops engaged in driving the Germans out of Italy. The grand buildings along the waterfront were the newly designated headquarters of the Fifteenth Air Force, under the command of General James H. "Jimmy" Doolittle, leader of the daring raid on Tokyo. He had arrived on December first and was busy trying to locate his personnel and get his organization, based seventy-five miles away at the Foggia airfields, off the ground as quickly as possible. Much to Doolittle's chagrin, he was only there in a supporting role. The liberating Tommies had already chased the Nazis from the skies over Italy, and his long-range B-17 "Flying Fortresses," B-24s, and fighter groups were being brought in to help mop up and expand the strategic bombing campaign against Germany.

The British, who controlled the port, were so confident they had won the air war that, earlier that afternoon, Air Marshal Sir Arthur Coningham had arranged a press conference to announce that Bari was all but immune from attack. Radiating an irritating self-satisfaction, he assured the gathered reporters that the RAF had "knocked out" the Axis forces in the Mediterranean, adding, "I would regard it as a personal affront and insult if the Luftwaffe should attempt any significant action in this area."

The port was teeming with activity. Some thirty Allied ships—British, Dutch, Norwegian, and Polish—were crammed into the harbor, taking up every available spot within the breakwater. Four days earlier, the American Liberty ship *John Harvey* had pulled in with a convoy of nine other merchantmen. The vessels were tightly packed against the seawall and all along the pier, moored so closely they were virtually hull to hull. The dockyards were working around the clock to unload the supplies for the next big push—the advance on Rome. Allied strategy hinged on making steady progress up the rugged mountainous Italian peninsula, culminating in a proposed amphibious attack at Anzio, about thirty-two miles south of the capital. The success of the advance depended on the long supply line sustaining the march northward. Because of the urgency to keep the incoming stream of war matériel moving to where it was needed most, the usual blackout orders were suspended, and the lights blazed in Bari Harbor all night.

Lang knew the ships' holds were laden with tons of vital cargo—everything from food, blankets, and medical gear for hospitals and field aid stations to corrugated steel for landing strips, engines, and fifty-gallon drums of aviation fuel for Doolittle's bombers. Visible on the upper decks were vehicles of every kind—tanks, armored personnel carriers, jeeps, and ambulances—full of gas and ready to roll. A procession of tarp-covered trucks lumbered into town, hogging the roads. On the quayside berths, which were all occupied, bright lights winked atop huge cranes that continually hoisted baled equipment up and out. A veritable mountain ridge of boxed ammunition and shells lined the long, broad stone mole, a sign of the heavy fighting that lay ahead.

The American-led campaign to free Italy, now in its sixth month, had not gone as planned. The invasion of Sicily, code-named Operation Husky, which commenced on July 10, 1943, secured the island after only thirty-eight days of fighting, but the Germans exacted a bloody toll in retreat. The British followed up on September 3 with Operation Baytown, the initial assault on the Italian mainland—and the first invasion of the European continent. General Bernard "Monty" Montgomery's Eighth Army crossed the Strait of Messina and occupied the "toe" of Italy's "boot," while Royal Navy battleships and other forces converged on Calabria. It was a cover operation, intended as a diversion, and on September 8, the Americans launched Operation Avalanche, with General Mark Clark's Fifth Army and the British X Corps landing south of Naples at Salerno at 3:30 a.m. There was a furious battle for the beachhead, but by daylight the worst was over. Hitler's army headed for the hills.

In what could only be described as lousy timing, on the eve of the Salerno assault, General Dwight D. Eisenhower, Supreme Commander of the Allied Expeditionary Force of the North African Theater, took to the airwaves to announce that Italy had accepted an armistice. That night, the American soldiers, having heard the dramatic news over the ships' loudspeakers, were so busy whooping it up that they almost forgot why they were there, and it dulled their fighting edge. The Italian government surrendered unconditionally, leaving behind a confused olive-green-clad army without orders or leadership. The stunned Italian soldiers were now expected to fight alongside their former enemies, the Americans and the British, and against their former allies, the Germans. Defeated and divided, unsure whether they wanted to redeem their honor by helping to eject the Nazis from their land, they were of little use in the ensuing conflict.

Victory was not all it was cracked up to be. Lang and Rodger spent the fall covering the slow, hill-by-hill drive as the Fifth Army climbed and clawed the steep slopes of rock and sparse scrub that offered scant protection from the Wehrmacht pillboxes and mauling artillery fire that blocked the route to Rome. Monty's troops inched their way through orchards and vineyards, and across treacherous ridge tops, grappling with heavy rains, swollen rivers, and the resolute German infantry. Lang's *Time* dispatches told a depressing tale: The combined American, British, New Zealand, Canadian, and Indian forces were suffering greater than expected losses while making a "snail's progress." The record rainfall transformed the roads into impassable bogs, rendering their vehicles useless and forcing them to use mules to haul their food, water, and weapons. The weather grew colder by the day. Morale was low, and no one relished slogging up the spine of the muddy Italian boot in winter, a task that Scripps Howard's intrepid correspondent, Ernie Pyle, dubbed "the misery march."

Gen. Clark had boasted that he would capture Rome by mid-October, but that deadline had come and gone, and their objective seemed farther away than ever. After the fall of Naples, the Germans had left the city booby-trapped with time bombs, killing hundreds—mostly civilians. The butchery taught Clark and his American forces to take nothing for granted: "There are no holds barred in this war," he wrote. "It is a dirty game." The latest latrine rumors had it that questions were being raised at Allied High Command about how far to push the inglorious Italian campaign.

As dusk fell, drinks in hand, Lang and Rodger were morosely contemplating what little choice they had in their wartime assignments when the air-raid siren sounded. It was 7:35 p.m. The lights quickly went out in the Albergo Oriente. There was a blinding flash, followed by a terrific bang, and then here and there an artillery barrage, which they realized was the ancient port's one and only antiaircraft battery opening fire on the intruders. The enemy planes were not getting the angry reception from Bari's defenses they had anticipated. An American officer newly arrived from North Africa cocked his head and observed dryly, "They don't seem to have many ack-ack guns around this town."

Suddenly an earsplitting explosion hurled them to the ground, shattering the hotel's front windows and littering the tile floor with splinters of glass. Then came the sound of another explosion, and another. A large formation of German Junkers Ju-88s flew in low over the town, dropping the first few bombs short of the harbor among the narrow, winding streets and white stucco buildings in the old part of the city. Plumes of smoke and flame rose from the five sites that had been hit.

Pandemonium broke out in the hotel. Terrified customers cowered under tables and huddled in corners. In the cacophony of voices, Lang heard the American officer calling to his friends. A chambermaid, crying, ran up and down the stairs. Outside, hysterical civilians stampeded down the road and poured into the town's few shelters, trampling anyone who fell in their path. Wide-eyed, white-faced Italians dug through the rubble searching for bodies, wailing, *"Madonna, Madonna mia."*

The lead pathfinders dropped *Düppel*, or "Window," foil strips designed to confuse Allied radar, achieving almost complete surprise. The cloud of thin aluminum strips hung in the air, slowly twirling and floating to earth, reflecting the strings of chandelier flares and streams of tracer bullets in a ghostly, flickering light. As the incendiaries began to rain down on the harbor, they turned night into day, lighting up the sky like a brilliant fireworks display. German bombs were screaming into the harbor. Gunners aboard the anchored ships scrambled into position and tried desperately to shoot down the enemy—too late. Opposition was virtually nonexistent. The attacking airplanes pulled away and into the night, unchallenged by patrolling Allied fighters. Although the raid lasted less than twenty minutes, the results were devastating.

By 8 p.m., Lang and Rodger were crunching along debris-strewn streets as they ran toward the docks. Ambulances blared as they raced by, adding to the deafening crack and crash of the Bofors that filled the night. The noise was overpowering, unbearable, and relentless. A great red glow silhouetted the building tops between them and the burning ships. Just as the men reached the port fence, where they hoped to have an unobstructed view of the stricken harbor, there was a tremendous roar from an explosion that blotted out everything for several seconds.

The blast wave knocked Lang to the ground. He could feel a flash of heat like that of a volcanic eruption on his face. Looking up, he saw a huge rolling mass of flames rising a thousand feet high. Three hundred yards away, the tanker disintegrated before their eyes and disappeared in a pall of smoke. "There goes Monty's ammunition," cracked Rodger, whose back was pinned against a stone wall as he fumbled for his camera and shot picture after picture.

Hearing the clatter of hobnail boots on asphalt, Lang saw the British soldiers on the quay abandon their rescue efforts and begin running from the water's edge. Tied up close inshore, right in front of them, was another tanker. It looked like it was about to blow. He shouted, "Let's get out of here."

They dashed to the comparative shelter of a nearby building and climbed out onto the rooftop. Squatting there in frightened fascination, Lang later cabled *Time*, they surveyed the "fiery panorama":

```
Through the smoke we counted eight ships already burning
fiercely. One ammunition ship was already settling at the bow
shooting out fresh geysers of fire as stores exploded flinging
red, green and white flares into high pathetic parabolas. A
mile out to sea another ship, apparently towed or steamed
there after being hit, burned by itself. The entire center of
the harbor was covered with burning oil....
```

A bomb ruptured the bulk-fuel pipeline on the petroleum quay, sending thousands of gallons gushing into the harbor, where it ignited into a gigantic sheet of flame, engulfing the entire north side of the port. Like a prairie fire, the tongues of flame spread rapidly across the surface of the water, leaping from ship to ship, so even vessels that had survived the bombing with only slight damage were soon consumed. Crews worked frantically to save their ships, struggling to free them from the cable shackles and shift them out of harm's way before the raging, uncontrollable fires forced them to jump overboard and swim for it. Every now and then, in the brief lulls between explosions, they could hear the faint cries of "Help, help!" coming from the direction of the inferno. "There are a lot of poor wretches dying out there," Rodger muttered under his breath as he continued to document the carnage.

They had witnessed one of the worst naval catastrophes of the war, but there was no way to get their big scoop into print. A gag order was in effect. News of the night raid on Bari was being held up by the military censors. Eisenhower's December fourth air communiqué from Algiers released only a few details and stated that "damage was done." The *New York Times* ran a short item on the bombing, but it was a hazy account and full of errors. In the end, the *Washington Post* broke the story on December 16, describing the severe blow to Allied shipping as the costliest "sneak attack" since Pearl Harbor, with an estimated thousand casualties. More than thirty-one thousand tons of valuable cargo was completely destroyed. It would be weeks before the port could be cleared and resume normal operations, seriously disrupting the Allied advance. Adding insult to injury, the first account of the air raid had actually come from the Germans themselves. A Berlin propaganda broadcast on December 5 gloated over the mission's spectacular success, claiming the congested harbor was so poorly protected their bombers were able to pick off the Allied ships like sitting ducks. More than 105 Ju-88s had taken part in the surprise attack, and all but two returned safely to base.

At his weekly press conference in Washington, DC, on December 16, a visibly irate Secretary of War Henry L. Stimson confirmed the *Washington Post* story and reluctantly revealed that the toll was of considerably greater magnitude than first reported. The Nazis had sunk a total of seventeen Allied ships, including two ammunition ships and five American merchantmen, with additional vessels hit or partially damaged. Loss of life among Naval Armed Guard personnel and American seamen was heavy.

Angry that the Bari story had leaked hours earlier, Stimson gave only a sketchy account of the raid and refused to identify the nationality of the ammunition ship that had magnified the conflagration or to furnish any other details. His wrath at the premature publication of the story struck many as out of character. When one correspondent inquired whether he would comment on the report that the well-planned, boldly executed German raid had caught the Allies "napping," Stimson cut him off midsentence and snapped, "No! I will not comment on this thing!" Abruptly ending the question-and-answer session, he stalked out of the room.

Lang's eyewitness account of the deadly Luftwaffe strike finally ran in the December 27 issue of *Time*. Rodger's dramatic images were never published. The magazine's editors included a companion piece covering the "belated and patently embarrassed" administration tally of the disaster, along with a blunt appraisal of the news delay, which seemed to endow the story with even greater significance. "The news of Bari was bad," they wrote. "What was even worse was the skittishness in Washington (or London) about telling the facts."

Whatever happened at Bari, all indications were that this was no ordinary affair. Rumors abounded that the losses were greater than those disclosed by the War Department. There was some speculation that the strict censorship pointed to the involvement of a German secret weapon, possibly the new rocket-driven glide bomb, which might have been used with appalling effectiveness against the nautical targets. Walter Logan, the United Press correspondent on the scene, hinted as much in dispatches. "Bari had all the makings of a hot spot," observed Robert Casey, a veteran *Chicago Daily News* correspondent who was also present. One glance at the line of merchant ships stretching into the distance and even he had known the port would be "marked with a large red tack on the German operational maps." The pool reporters did not let Coningham forget his unqualified boast of the day before the attack, adding to the RAF's embarrassment. The US Navy was criticized for putting so many valuable eggs in one small basket, resulting in such a dividend of destruction, particularly when installations within range of enemy bases just across the narrow Adriatic were known to be vulnerable. Congressional concern over the debacle was underscored by the announcement that Eisenhower had asked a special Senate committee to look into the painful setback.

All told, the Bari bombing, which a skeptical and aggrieved press corps called "a little Pearl Harbor," was a great tragedy. It shook the complacency of the Allied forces, who had been convinced of their overwhelming air superiority in Italy and overconfident of continued victories. They had once again underestimated a dangerous foe and had paid for it dearly. It was a lesson they would not soon forget. As a clearly disturbed Rear Admiral Emory Scott Land, the war shipping administrator responsible for the US merchant marine fleet across seven seas, told *Time*: "You're going to hear more about that raid before you hear less." But that was the last official word on the matter, and the incident remained shrouded in mystery.

The day after filing their story, Lang and Rodger rejoined the Fifth Army as they pressed the combat line northward to Monte Cassino. They never dreamed it would be almost thirty years before the world would learn the truth about what took place on that fatal night. Or that while they had stood there helplessly watching the ships burn and hundreds of sailors brave the oily waters, another tragedy was in the making. One that was rendered far worse by wartime secrecy, and the determined efforts of both the American and British governments to cover up the incident so as not to endanger the preparations for the most important operation of the war, Overlord, the Allied invasion of German-occupied France planned for the spring.

THE
GREAT SECRET

——— ◆ ———

CHAPTER ONE

"A Regiment of Wizards"

The summons came in the middle of the night. He was awake at the first harsh jangle of the telephone. The next insistent ring had him on his feet. It was second nature to him. Always a light sleeper, Lieutenant Colonel Stewart Francis Alexander attributed the trait to his father, an old-fashioned family practitioner whose response to every late-night distress call was to reach automatically for his raincoat and medical bag. A doctor's son through and through, he was dressed and ready to go in under ten minutes.

The clipped voice on the other end of the line ordered him to report at once to his boss, Brigadier General Frederick A. Blesse, chief surgeon for the Fifth Army and the North African Theater of Operations at Algiers. The briefing was cursory, amounting to little more than the recitation of a handful of facts. There appeared to be a developing medical situation in Bari following the December 2 air strike. Too many men were dying, too quickly, of unexplained causes. The symptoms were unlike anything the physicians in the local military hospitals had seen before, and they had begun to suspect the Germans had used some new, unknown poison gas. When the number of mysterious deaths increased rapidly with each successive day, the British placed a "red light" call alerting Allied Force Headquarters (AFHQ) at Algiers. There was an urgent request for assistance. "Expert advice" was the way Blesse had put it. Fortunately, they had just the man for the job. Alexander, a twenty-nine-year-old medical officer attached to Eisenhower's staff, had received special training in chemical warfare. He was being dispatched immediately to the scene of the disaster.

Alexander looked young for a combat doctor. Five feet eight, skinny, with close-cropped fair hair and hazel eyes, he had the kind of open, honest face that people invariably described as earnest. The dimple in his chin added to his choirboy appearance, and it was only the fact that his hair had started to thin at the temples that lent him any air of authority. Gentle and soft-spoken, he was popular with the troops, though some patients kidded him that his bedside manner was better suited to a pediatrician than someone who had by choice seen more than his fair share of war. But he had come over with Operation Torch under the command of no less a figure than Major General George S. Patton, and he had been through the brutal invasion assault on North Africa. Despite his quiet modesty, Alexander had proven himself to be confident, determined, and resourceful. He had a good head on his shoulders and knew how to handle himself.

The day after the attack on Bari, Eisenhower's headquarters had been buzzing with the news that the Luftwaffe's hit-and-run raid had pummeled the unsuspecting harbor. The first reports described a scene of utter devastation. Parts of the town and port were still on fire. The carcasses of burned-out ships, their towering masts and funnels smashed, were smoldering and belching black smoke. The basin was so crowded with sunken wrecks that the rescue tugs could hardly work their way around the length of the seawall to search for survivors. Casualties were said to be enormous. Grotesquely charred and bloated bodies bobbed to the surface and were fished out of the water in nets. The grisly remains were laid out on the dock in full view—arms, legs, and torsos, already nibbled by crabs. Most of the sailors and merchant seamen who perished would never be found. There would be no way to identify the dead. No way to give them a proper burial.

SITTING IN HIS SUNBAKED OFFICE in the medical department at AFHQ, Alexander shuddered to think how the overstretched hospitals in Bari would cope with the masses of injured men. From the reports stacked on his desk, he knew that every Allied facility in the region—British, New Zealand, Indian, and Italian—was already loaded with wounded from the months of continuous combat and operating far beyond normal capacity. His mind flashed back over familiar scenes from battalion aid stations following a major assault: litter bearers, moving with swift efficiency, carrying in the wounded; surgeons in blood-spattered coveralls patching torn flesh and binding shattered limbs for further procedures once they had been evacuated; nurses hooking up copious bottles of plasma to sustain failing bodies; then clearing the decks as quickly as possible to make room for the next round of incoming. At Bari, they would be doing all that and more, only the numbers would be staggering.

But that had been just one of his concerns. He had been dismayed to learn that among the tons of lost cargo was the long-overdue equipment to outfit five planned American field hospitals, one of them a thousand-bed unit. All of the medical supplies had been aboard the Liberty ship *Samuel J. Tilden,* which was destroyed in the enemy attack. The newly arrived personnel were all safe, having bivouacked some distance from town, but everything they needed to provide assistance in the emergency, from bandages to syringes and morphine, was at the bottom of the harbor. Under the circumstances, the American 26th General Hospital had scrambled to open on December 4 to care for some of the bombing victims, assembling a medical wing and borrowing a hundred beds, plus linens and pajamas, from the Italians. A few surgical instruments and small amounts of dressings were scrounged from an Air Force storage depot. Complicating matters, the town's communication system, which was knocked out in the attack, was still down, making the relief effort that much more difficult. The grim reality was that the shortage of medical supplies was going to compound the tragedy. Alexander's initial orders had been clear. One way or another, Blesse had told him, they were going to have to find a way to replace the lost inventory in one hell of a hurry.

Now, he realized, that might turn out to be the least of their worries.

The white city of Algiers, shimmering in the soft morning light, seemed far from the ravages of war. The half-moon harbor below looked like a picture postcard, with boats of every size and shape nestled along the bay. Alexander hastened to the waiting jeep that would whisk him to Maison Blanche Airfield on the outskirts of town. Arrangements were being made for a plane to take him to Bari. He was the expert and he was going alone, without staff.

ALEXANDER'S PRESENCE IN ALGIERS was no accident. It was fortuitous, a result of Gen. Eisenhower's foresight and his own willfulness. When he later looked back on the sequence of events that led to his being there, it always seemed to him to be more than mere coincidence, one of those serendipitous events in which it is impossible not to see the hand of fate.

Quiet and scholarly by nature, he could have sat out the war in a stateside hospital or research laboratory. At the start of the conflict, it was easy enough for a doctor to claim he could not be spared from his civilian occupation. He had heard of more than one colleague who had been categorized as "essential" and exempted from conscription. From the first, however, Alexander felt that this was a war in which he had to participate, and he had enlisted early of his own initiative.

The desire to serve ran deep. He was from self-made, self-reliant immigrant stock, part of the wave of Eastern European Jews who had journeyed to the United States in the 1880s, fleeing famine, unemployment, and political and religious persecution. His grandfather came from Bratislava in the Austro-Hungarian Empire, now the Czech Republic, as a boy without a penny to his name. He struggled to earn the passage funds for each of his siblings and parents, bringing them over one by one. He put his hand to dozens of odd jobs, determined to prosper and provide his family with a better life. Poor but proud, he embraced all things American, especially baseball, which he played with gusto and without a glove, despite breaking several fingers. He inculcated in his eight children a profound sense of obligation to the new land that had given them so much. Samuel, the oldest son, began working at the age of five, selling newspapers. By dint of hard work, long hours, and night classes, he put himself through college and medical school. He eventually rose from a humble small-town doctor to become a pillar of the community in Park Ridge, New Jersey, building a large obstetric practice and delivering hundreds of babies over four decades, as well as founding the state's first county hospital. He became president of the state medical society, president of the local bank, and served several terms as mayor.

Having spent his childhood going on rounds with his boundlessly energetic and gregarious father, conspicuous in the neighborhood as the doc's bright boy, Stewart Alexander had only one ambition: to follow in his father's footsteps. Born on August 30, 1914, in a small stone house that also served as his father's office and surgery, he raced along the path set out for him. His mother, a teacher, recognized that her boy was a fast learner when he refused to go to kindergarten, declaring it a waste of time. Always the youngest and smallest in his class, he skipped several grades at the public school across the street and consistently earned top marks. In need of a greater challenge, and perhaps a bit of toughening up, he was packed off to the Staunton Military Academy in Virginia for his last two years of high school. He entered Dartmouth College at the age of fifteen, excelled at his scientific studies, and was allowed to advance directly to medical school at the start of his senior year, graduating at the top of his class in 1935. As Dartmouth only had a two-year program, he went on to earn his MD from Columbia University College of Physicians and Surgeons in New York and then did postgraduate work in chest diseases and neurology at Bellevue Hospital. He declined an offer to stay on—the big city held little allure for him. After completing his internship and residency training, he returned to Park Ridge and proudly hung out his shingle next to his father's.

He had only a few months to enjoy their shared dream of practicing medicine together. By the spring of 1940, Germany was on the march, conquering France, Belgium, Luxembourg, and the Netherlands. Any real hope of avoiding the conflict evaporated as President Franklin D. Roosevelt began to urge the country toward a new, more serious phase of preparedness. Alexander, who had joined the Reserve Officer Training Corps the day he finished medical school, notified the draft board he was "available any time." He was called up in November and inducted into the Army Medical Corps as a first lieutenant. Despite his disappointment, his father would not have had it any other way. During World War I, he had tried in vain to volunteer for the Army Medical Corps, but, to his everlasting shame and regret, he was repeatedly rejected because of a deviated septum, even after undergoing an operation to correct it. Dedication and duty—to his patients, community, and country—were the animating principles of his life. He had always taught his son: "We must do those things we ought to do." The young Dr. Alexander absorbed the lesson, and, conscious of his old man's thwarted efforts to serve, felt all the more compelled to do his part.

His bags were packed, good-byes said and done, when he went for the routine physical, only to be told he had flunked the exam. Like father, like son. He, too, was deemed ineligible because of a minor hereditary defect—in his case, compound myopia, or nearsightedness. In truth, he was almost blind without glasses. While the Army physician was explaining that his vision was 20/100 and "well below the minimum standard," Alexander, looking over his shoulder at the eye chart, quickly committed the lines of random letters to memory. Insisting there must be some mistake, he removed his glasses again and demanded to be retested. This time, he passed with flying colors and was duly accepted into the service. It was a trivial incident, and the episode would have soon been forgotten had it not given rise to a new concern about whether his impaired vision would be a handicap at the front. Almost as quickly, it set him thinking about what could be done to help soldiers like himself headed for combat.

He continued to mull over the problem during the first few months he spent in the medical detachment of the 16th Infantry Regiment, First Division, at Gunpowder Creek, near Edgewood Arsenal in Maryland. Green and jittery, the new recruits were naturally apprehensive about what they would encounter in the field. The barracks were rife with rumors that sooner or later the enemy would resort to chemical warfare. Poison gas had been Germany's weapon of choice in World War I, and it was widely believed that if the war went badly and Hitler's back was to the wall, he would retaliate by unleashing a chemical attack, even though the use of chemical and biological weapons had been banned by the 1925 Geneva Protocol. They had all read about the agonizing deaths caused by artillery shells packed with toxins, and asphyxiating gases that smothered soldiers in the trenches before they could escape. The fear was real and pervasive.

Faced with this familiar threat, it struck Alexander that if the men were confident there were good safeguards in place to counter the gas menace, they might be less nervous. He had his own misgivings, dating back to his days as a reserve officer. During routine gas drills, he had discovered that the gas mask supplied by the Army did not fit over the metal frames of his spectacles, forcing him to go without them. His poor performance on the eye exam had only exacerbated his anxieties, reminding him of the not-inconsiderable risk of having to choose breathing over seeing in the event of a gas attack. Moreover, as a doctor, he felt it was his responsibility to make sure that none of the soldiers in his care were sent into battle with anything less than complete protection. He decided to write to the Chemical Warfare Service about the problem and proposed a solution, sending along several sketches. His letter so impressed the CWS's technical team that he was invited to make a presentation at their research and development center at Edgewood. After further correspondence, and a number of modifications, Alexander succeeded in devising a new form of spectacles that could be worn within the molded facepiece of the mask. He was granted a patent on his design, but he turned over all the rights to the Army. The new glasses soon became standard service issue.

Not long afterward, he was contacted by Colonel William D. Fleming, chief of the Medical Research Division of the Chemical Warfare Service, who inquired into his background and then, apparently satisfied with his CV, announced, "I really think you belong here with us." It took several months for Fleming to disentangle him from the First Division, but, in the fall of 1941, Alexander was transferred to the CWS at Edgewood Arsenal. After a soggy year of amphibious landing exercises that had taken his regiment from the freezing waters of Maryland to the wilting heat of Puerto Rico and Martinique, and had most recently put them ashore in the Carolinas, he was not sorry to be moving on. He hoped, at least, that he had gained a better understanding of some of the hazards of combat, including possibly the biggest hazard—bullheaded officers who tried to drown half their company in the name of training. The mulishness of one battalion major determined to "harden" the men despite subzero temperatures inspired special fury. Alexander had not joined the Army to treat needless and debilitating bouts of bronchitis and pneumonia. With half the men sick, the executive officer, Colonel Charles Van Way, had advised him to intervene.

"Won't I get into trouble for doing that?" Alexander asked, taken aback.

"Maybe," he replied, "but there isn't anyone else who can do it."

Alexander promptly placed the entire battalion under quarantine, suspended the training exercises, and wrote a memorandum to the Surgeon General of the Army, explaining that if the cold did not kill the men, the major would. The medical inspector who reviewed the case agreed and closed down the operation.

When the wire came through with his travel orders to Edgewood, Alexander was more than ready to go. Told he could leave that day, he did. He knew almost nothing about chemical weapons, only that the chance to be part of a classified program to defend against toxic agents sounded "exciting."

The Chemical Warfare Service—created in 1918 to organize the production of poison gas and defensive equipment during World War I—built a vast complex of munitions works on the grounds of Edgewood Arsenal. Congress made it a permanent part of the US Army in 1920, with duties to continue the "investigation, development, manufacture or procurement and supply of all smoke and incendiary materials, all toxic gases, and all gas defense appliances." The unit later received approval for its distinctive insignia, a green dragon breathing flames, and its motto—*Elementis Regamus Proelium*—"Let Us Rule the Battle by Means of the Elements." Over the next two decades, despite almost continuous debate about its peacetime preparations, the CWS focused on refining its production of lethal compounds and creating better delivery systems. Primarily, the service was expected to maintain what Roosevelt, with evident distaste, called the "defensive necessities" of the United States—in other words, maintain a state of readiness for chemical warfare.

Although bordered by beautiful woods and a sparkling river, the Edgewood facility was a somewhat uninviting place where, in the words of Major General William N. Porter, chief of the CWS, "every living soul must stay within five minutes of his gas mask." The acrid smell that permanently hung in the air around the manufacturing plants was enough to make anyone nervous. Assigned to the Medical Research Laboratory, Alexander quickly became proficient in the field of poison gases. With characteristic drive and intensity of purpose, he spent weeks educating himself in the library. He read everything he could find about the principal killing agents: chlorine (a powerful irritant that damaged the eyes, nose, and throat), phosgene (cheap and deadly, it attacked the lungs with no effective treatment after prolonged exposure), and sulfur mustard (a liquid that vaporized, and lethal in both forms). The cornerstone of Germany's chemical arsenal, mustard gas—the so-called king of battle gases—killed more than a hundred thousand men in World War I and badly injured a million more. The most potent gas, lewisite, developed at the end of the last war, was a new type of blister agent, or severe vesicant, that quickly penetrated the body.

He learned to identify the different toxins by their telltale odors—the pungent aroma of an indoor pool (chlorine), the fragrant but pernicious smell of newly mown hay (phosgene), the nose-tickling bouquet of garlic (mustard gas), and the faint, sickly sweet scent of geraniums (lewisite). There was no practical method of detecting most gases other than via the sense of smell, but it was a hazardous and uncertain business. Soldiers needed a quick, foolproof test. When Alexander first arrived, the lab was in the process of perfecting a new detector kit, essentially a miniature portable chemistry set for identifying gases in the field. Every soldier was issued a chart listing the main chemical warfare agents and told to memorize the odors that might be the harbinger of a deadly attack.

(Gunner Nice.)

CHEMICAL WARFARE AGENTS

REFERENCE AND TRAINING CHART — Prepared by Lt.-Col. Walter P. Burn, C.W. Res.

SYMBOL	NICKNAME	NAME	FORM	BANDS COLOR	LOADING	ODOR	TACTICAL CLASS	PHYSIOLOGICAL EFFECT	PROTECTION	FIRST AID	COLOR & STATE LOADED / RELEASED	PERSISTENCE	TACTICAL USES	FIELD NEUTRALIZATION
HS	Hot Stuff	MUSTARD	Gas			Garlic Horseradish Mustard		Burns skin or membrane. No immediate effect		Remove clothing. Wash affected parts to body with plenty water. Do not bandage	HEAVY DARK OILY LIQUID / Liquid Slowly evaporates	Open 1 Day / about 1 Wk	To neutralize areas. Counter-Battery. Attack on Personnel	Cover with water. Chlorinated earth. 2% soln of NO_2SO_3
MI	Mustard Imitator	LEWISITE	Gas			Geraniums		Irritates nasal passages. Later thin burns, pain		Wash with oil, hot water, soap. Cut heat small amt of flesh. Apply Anti NaOH. Apply Ferri Hydrate paste	DARK GREEN OILY LIQUID / Slowly evaporates	Open 1Day / 1 Week	Similar to Mustard.	Wash down with water. Caustic soda earth. Blasted. NaOH Spray
ED	Enemy's Delight	ETHYLDI-CHLORARSINE	Gas			Biting Stinging		Causes blisters, sores; paralysis of hands		Wash with gasoline, hot water and soap	/	1 HOUR	Counter-Battery Preparation fire. Harassing fire	Cover with earth, caustic, NaOH solution
PS	Puking Stuff	CHLORPICRIN	Gas	+CG CN		Fly paper Anise		Causes severe coughing, crying, vomiting		Wash eyes, keep quiet and warm. Do not use bandages	YELLOW OILY LIQUID / Colorless Gas	3 Days More 12 Hours	Harassing fire	Na_2SO_3. Sodium Sulfite in alcohol solution.
DP	Di-Phos	DIPHOSGENE	Gas			Ensilage Acrid		Causes coughing, breathing hurt. eyes water, tears		Keep quiet and warm. Give coffee as a stimulant.	COLORLESS LIQUID / Colorless Gas	30 MIN.	Harassing fire	Alkali
CG	Choky-Gas	PHOSGENE	Gas			Musty hay Green corn		Keep quiet and warm. Give coffee as a stimulant.		Keep quiet and warm. Give coffee as a stimulant.	COLORLESS LIQUID / Colorless Gas	10 to 30 MINUTES	Surprise attacks, projectiles. Gas cloud release. For quick physical effect.	Alkali
CN (CNS)	Cry Now	CLORACETO-PHENONE	Gas / Solution			Apple blossoms		Makes eyes smart, shut tight; tears flow. Temporary		Wash eyes with water or boric acid. Do not rub or bandage. Stove, NaCO, soln.	BROWN CRYSTALLINE POWDER / Cloud of small solid particles	10 MIN.	Training. Mob control. CNS used in counter-battery to force mask wear.	
CA	Cry Always	BROMBENZYL-CYANIDE	Gas			Sour fruit		Eyes smart, shut tears flow. Effect lasts some time		Wash eyes with boric acid. Do not bandage.	DARK BROWN OILY LIQUID / Slowly evaporates	SEVERAL DAYS (more in Winter)	To neutralize areas. Counter-battery.	Alcoholic Soda or Hydromole spray
DM	Dirty Mixture	ADAMSITE	Gas		Bock	Coal Smoke		Causes sneezing, sick, depressed feeling		Remove to pure air and keep warm and quiet	YELLOW-GREEN GRANULAR SOLID / Yellow Smoke	10 MIN.	Gas Cloud Attacks. Mob control.	Bleaching Powder Solution
DS	Dirty Smoke	SNEEZE GAS	Smoke			Shoe polish		Causes sneezing, flow of tears		Remove to pure air and keep warm and quiet.	BLACK VISCOUS MASS / Grey Smoke	5 MIN.	Harassing and screening.	None needed
HC	Harmless Cloud	HC MIXTURE	Smoke			Sharp-acrid	NONE	Harmless		Produces no effect requiring treatment	GREY SOLID / Grey Smoke	WHILE BURNING	To screen small operation in own lines and for training purposes.	None needed
FS	Fuming Spray	SULPHUR TRIOXIDE	Smoke			Burning matches		Causes prickling of skin, flow of tears.		Wash with Soda solution	CLEAR LIQUID / Dense white Smoke	5-10 MIN.	Airplane spray for screen on broad front.	Alkaline Solution
FM	Floating Mantle	TITANIUM TETRACHLORIDE	Smoke			Acrid	NONE	Harmless		Produces no effect requiring treatment	YELLOWISH LIQUID / White Smoke	10 MIN.	Screening operations	None needed
DA	Dopey Ache	DIPHENYL-CHLORARSINE	Smoke			Not pronounced		Causes sick feeling and headache		Remove to pure air, keep quiet. Sniff chlorine. Use bleaching powder bottle	/ Summer 10 MIN.		Harassing fire	Bleaching Powder Solution
WP	White Phos.	WHITE PHOSPHORUS	Smoke			Burning Matches	NONE AVAILABLE	Burning pieces adhere to skin, clothing		Plunge in mud to smother	PALE YELLOW SOLID / Burns to white smoke in Air	10 MIN.	To screen advancing troops. Cause incendiary effects, losses. Harass enemy columns.	Burns out
TH	The Heat	THERMIT	Incendiary					5000 degree heat ignites materials	Cover with earth, sand	Treat for severe burn.	/	5 MIN.	Destruction of Materiel.	Quickly cover with earth or sand
CL	Chlorine	CHLORINE	Gas	+ PS + CG		Highly Pungent		Lung Irritant		Remove from gassed area. Keep quiet and warm. Coffee as stimulant.	YELLOW LIQUID / Yellow-green gas	10 MIN.	Surprise attacks (cloud)	Alkaline Solution

This reference chart, prepared by Lt. Col. Walter P. Burns, lists the main poison gases used during World War I. It was used to train troops at the beginning of World War II on the different methods of delivery, telltale odors, physiological effects, and first aid to be administered in the event of exposure. (William Frederick Nice Collection [AFC/2001 /001/01339], Veterans History Project, American Folklife Center, Library of Congress)

The history of gas warfare was one of steadily increasing toxicity, matched by a quickly evolving array of defensive measures. By the end of World War I, it had become a kind of technological chess match, with military strategists and scientists devising ways to check each new offensive threat. The Medical Research Laboratory was still focused on preventions and procedures to care for chemical casualties. Work was in progress on improving protection against toxic agents, including new, adjustable gas masks and antigas-impregnated uniforms, including underwear, socks, hoods, gloves, and leggings. While all of this lifesaving equipment vastly reduced the destructive capacity of most poison gases, it had its limits. Nothing was 100 percent reliable. The new gas masks were still hot and heavy, could cause claustrophobia, and were so bulky and inconvenient to carry that troops had a habit of leaving them behind on combat maneuvers. And there was only so much that could be done to mitigate human error in donning the protective gear in those panicked seconds prior to an attack. "It's the natural fear of asphyxiation," a CWS officer explained with resignation. "The average sergeant will run from a stink and walk straight into a machine-gun nest."

When Alexander first arrived, the lab's top priority was to find a means of protecting vulnerable skin from corrosive chemical agents. He and his colleagues developed a chlorine-based ointment to neutralize mustard residue on the skin before it began to destroy cells and tissue, but it had to be modified many times before it was proven to be safe and effective. The Army finally approved it and ordered millions of tubes to be manufactured and sent to the front. Lewisite remained a troublesome agent, as it contained arsenic to produce systemic poisoning. They tackled the problem by conducting a series of experiments on ways to counter arsenic and heavy-metal poisoning. After postulating that since the skin was an active and rapid absorption organ for toxic agents, then perhaps it could be equally efficient in absorbing therapeutic agents, they were on their way to creating a transdermal drug. Several months later, the threat from arsenicals was downgraded, thanks to three Oxford University researchers who had discovered an antidote, known as British Anti-Lewisite, or BAL. By the following year, soldiers were issued M5 gas treatment kits containing four tubes of the protective skin ointment and, tucked under the tin's lid, one tiny tube of BAL eye ointment.

Intrigued by the work, Alexander explored every poison suspected of being of interest to the enemy and every known or conjectured aspect of gas casualty aid. He wrote detailed memoranda, consulted specialists, and set up experiments on animals to evaluate different toxic agents and forms of treatment. He tested medications, administering them in various ways—topically, ingested, and inhaled—following up on even the most obscure references he found in the existing literature. Given license to improvise, he tried anything and everything he could think of to improve the current methods of dealing with chemical injuries, minimizing the effects of exposure, and protecting military personnel, civilians, and food and water supplies. He even familiarized himself with the lab's veterinary section, an entire research apparatus devoted to the preservation of animals—and, more to the point, the country's meat resources. All of these classified research projects were going on simultaneously. Alexander found it fascinating. He had certainly never dreamed of pursuing such a morbid subject as a career, but it was without a doubt the most important and stimulating work he had ever done. And when he was able to notch some clinical progress, and make a contribution to medicine, it was also the most rewarding.

The December 7, 1941, attack on Pearl Harbor greatly accelerated his activities. While the military divisions of the CWS provided the supply, support, and training for combat operations, the medical division's mission took on new urgency. The push was on for the lab to complete the field tests and get new antigas protective equipment in the hands of troops as rapidly as possible. When the chemical rearmament program was launched in late 1941, Congress turned on the taps and the money began flowing. The CWS budget soared from a mere $2 million in 1940 to $60 million the following year, and an astounding $1 billion in 1942. More than a dozen planned chemical warfare plants—from a new, fifteen-thousand-acre site at Pine Bluff Arsenal in Arkansas that opened five days before Pearl Harbor to an even larger one under construction at Rocky Mountain Arsenal near Denver—spurred the CWS hiring spree. The staff swelled from five thousand Army personnel to sixty thousand in 1942. The shortage of qualified CWS officers meant there was a tremendous increase in programs to train medical personnel in the handling of chemical casualties, care procedures, and decontamination methods. A major training center was erected at Carlisle Barracks in Pennsylvania. Alexander helped to organize the course and write the manuals and then delivered the initial series of lectures.

He also served as the point person for coordinating their efforts with the National Defense Research Committee (NDRC), as well as large chemical corporations engaged in defense work and universities that had been awarded classified military research projects. This brought him into regular contact with what the CWS described as "the Supreme Court of chemical brains," represented by such scientific luminaries as Dr. James Bryant Conant, the president of Harvard University and the head of the NDRC; Dr. Roger Adams, head of the University of Illinois's chemistry department, who helped develop adamsite, an arsenical used as a vomiting agent or sneeze gas; and Dr. Milton Charles Winternitz, former dean of the Yale School of Medicine and chairman of the Committee on the Treatment of War Gas Casualties of the National Research Council.

Alexander traveled all over the country, attending conferences and observing spectacular exhibitions of new chemical warfare weapons. They ranged from magnesium, oil, and thermite incendiaries, which could be dropped from planes and could burn through steel tanks, to new smoke bombs and smoke screens that fogged the enemy's vision, making them extremely valuable in combat. The Germans had cracked the Maginot Line in May 1940 in part by blinding the French with smoke bombs and then sending soldiers forward to put TNT and flamethrowers through the embrasures in the turrets above the concrete fortifications. Colonel E. P. Gempel, training director of the CWS School, expressed his pride at the great strides it had made in smoke generators, stating, "Smoke saves blood—your blood."

When the director of the laboratory was transferred, Col. Fleming asked Alexander to take over and threw in a promotion, telling him, "It will look better to have a major in charge of the medical division." It was a wholly unexpected boost up the ladder, not only in rank but also in responsibility. All of twenty-seven at the time, with limited preparation for a job of such magnitude, he suddenly found himself in charge of a large department staffed by brilliant scientists and physicians, along with twenty researchers with advanced degrees in biology and organic chemistry, all of whom were older and more experienced. The rapid expansion of the whole organization meant that everybody was being advanced and asked to do the work of two people. If Alexander had had only minimal knowledge of poison gas when he arrived at Edgewood, he had undergone a crash course over the previous ten months and was now a member of an elite group of chemical warfare experts. It was, he later recalled, "a very heady time."

IN THE FALL OF 1942, the Combined Chiefs of Staff turned their attention to the problem of chemical warfare, with the result that a United States policy, in addition to a broader Allied policy, began to be formulated. It called for a cooperative American and British effort at achieving the "defensive preparedness" of all United Nations troops, and for the accumulation of sufficient toxic munitions to make "immediate retaliation possible should the enemy initiate gas warfare anywhere in the world." For Eisenhower, recently promoted to lieutenant general and named head of Operation Torch, the Allied invasion of French North Africa, this development was not the least bit reassuring. Raising more questions in his mind than it answered, the still-vague, ill-defined policy on gas warfare left him with some scenarios for which there seemed to be no possible good outcome.

Although the universal outrage and revulsion that followed World

War I had led the Axis and Allied powers to sign the 1925 Geneva Protocol, which banned the *use*, but not the *possession*, of chemical and biological weapons, neither side trusted the other. Neither side believed the bargain would be upheld. More to the point, there was no ban on the research and development of a fearsome array of new offensive poisons. Despite Hitler's reaffirmed promise in September 1939 not to conduct chemical warfare—he claimed to despise poison gas after being temporarily blinded by a mustard shell as a cadet—Allied intelligence had obtained evidence that the Wehrmacht was secretly overseeing the production and stockpiling of a variety of chemical agents. Numerous laboratories in Germany—in Berlin and the Ruhr—had been identified as possibly developing poison gas, with three more experimental plants said to exist near Münster, Wünsdorf, and List auf Sylt.

The Japanese not only were researching poison gas but also were actively employing it in their war against China. In October 1941, Japan, which had never ratified the Geneva Protocol, released clouds of gas at Yichang, in the Yangtze Valley, reportedly killing six hundred Chinese soldiers and wounding more than a thousand. The Japanese were known to be aggressively developing offensive gases; from 1937 onward, there had been repeated reports that they had used mustard and lewisite against the Chinese to drive them from caves and tunnels into the open, where they would be slaughtered by waiting troops. Both Prime Minister Winston Churchill and President Roosevelt immediately condemned the Yichang attack and vowed to take action if Japan did not desist. Photographs of the atrocities were published in American newspapers, fanning the public's fears about Japan's barbaric methods and monstrous chemical arsenal.

While the CWS maintained that there were no "authenticated reports" of the tactical use of poison gas on the European battlefield, a sizable haul of enemy literature and instruction manuals related to gas warfare had been seized. Army experts were of the opinion the pamphlets were more of the usual Nazi "horror propaganda," and military officials assured the public they remained alert to the ever-present danger. CWS chief Maj. Gen. Porter confidently asserted that the Axis powers would never catch America asleep at the wheel when it came to poison gas. "The best defense against poison gas," he told the *New York Times*, "is to be ready. We are ready." Every report of a gas incident was thoroughly investigated. Every threat, regardless of how imprecise or improbable, was taken seriously.

Churchill took the threat very seriously. A staunch advocate of poison gas in World War I, he never missed an opportunity to remind his countrymen of the danger posed by what he called Germany's "perverted science." His philosophy on chemical warfare remained unaltered since his speech to the House of Commons a decade earlier, when he stated that "the attitude of the British government had always been to abhor the employment of poison gas," but in the same breath he urged continued research and development so as not to be at a "hopeless disadvantage" if it were used against them. His sense of foreboding was fueled by frequent, if unsubstantiated, intelligence reports of Axis offensive action with chemical weapons. In a radio broadcast on May 10, 1942, responding to rumors of an alleged Nazi gas attack in Crimea, Churchill went further, bluntly stating that if the enemy used it first, he would be compelled to use it in return. "I wish now to make plain that we shall treat the unprovoked use of poison gas against our Russian ally exactly as if it were used against ourselves," he warned. "And if we are satisfied that this new outrage has been committed by Hitler, we will use our great and growing air superiority in the West to carry gas warfare on the largest possible scale far and wide against military objectives in Germany."

Completely dedicated to winning the war, Churchill was a difficult man to disagree with when conviction compelled his views. Like most American military leaders, Eisenhower was not as gung-ho when it came to using poison gas. He preferred Roosevelt's restraint and moral reservations. But then the United States had not come out of the previous war with the same searing memories of German industrialized death that marked every British man or woman over the age of forty. Some differences in military doctrine were to be expected. As the European theater commander, Eisenhower dreaded the possibility of gas warfare but understood the need to plan for every contingency. He also knew Churchill could be excessively oratorical—Ike once observed that the prime minister "drew on everything from the Greek classics to Donald Duck for quotation, cliché, and forceful slang to support his position"—but his logic was inescapable. No Allied commander could be sanguine that the Germans were not poised for chemical combat.

The close partnership between the two countries regarding chemical warfare actually predated America's entry into the war by a year. In a secret deal, negotiated in the winter of 1940, the United States began supplying Britain with two hundred tons of phosgene a month, just in case they found themselves in a tight spot and had to repel an invading German army. "To preserve the image of neutrality," according to historians Robert Harris and Jeremy Paxman, "the gas was manufactured in private U.S. plants (which were financed by the British) and then carefully shipped to Europe in foreign-registered vessels; technically the American government's only official connection was the granting of export licenses." The clandestine arrangement, which could have backfired terribly if the Germans had fathomed the true state of affairs, was typical of the Allied tendency to cloak all matters pertaining to chemical warfare agents in a mantle of secrecy that would evade notice and permit subsequent deniability.

Although the CWS leaders believed that the Axis powers were unlikely to conduct gas warfare in the North African Theater, where tactical and logistical difficulties blunted its utility, the possibility was sufficiently real that the Allied forces at least had to be prepared. In the spring of 1942, the Operations Division concurred, approving the rapid overhaul of the North Africa campaign's capacity for chemical warfare. All theaters immediately began to implement the necessary defensive measures. As time was short, the top CWS officers all pitched into the job of forming the chemical battalions and providing the protection kits and detection devices, along with the trained personnel to handle them. With the large buildup of American troops on the continent, and in the midst of planning offensive actions, Eisenhower could not take any chances. He sent a cable from Norfolk House in London, where he had set up his temporary headquarters, to Army Chief of Staff General George Marshall, requesting that a medical officer well versed in chemical warfare be assigned to his staff.

Once Eisenhower's request reached Col. Fleming at the CWS base at Edgewood, he passed it on to Alexander, with instructions to pluck a suitably trained man from one of his courses to ship overseas. After reading the cable a number of times, however, Alexander decided on impulse to put his own name forward. Frustrated after a promising study on the physiochemical properties of mustard gas was shelved because it did not directly benefit the war effort, he had had enough of laboratory research. He wanted to return to the field and practice medicine where it might do the most good. Fleming refused to even consider it. He could not afford to lose one of his main instructors at the very moment when there was an increased demand for their services. Alexander persisted, arguing he was by far the best qualified, and, being young and able-bodied, he did not want to spend the entirety of the war behind a desk. In the end, he got his way. In August 1942, Alexander received orders that he was being sent to England.

The next thing he knew, his orders were canceled. Alexander found himself stuck in Indiantown Gap, Pennsylvania, sitting on his tail and wondering where the Army would ship him next, when he received a call from Col. Van Way. One of the finest officers he had served under in his time with the 16th Infantry, Van Way was now with the War Department, and apparently important enough that he did not have to go through the usual channels. He informed Alexander that he had been selected to serve as the Consultant in Chemical Warfare Medicine to the Western Task Force under Gen. Patton. As part of Torch, the Western Task Force would travel three thousand miles across the Atlantic and attack the coast of Morocco, the first time US ground forces would be put into action against the Germans and other European Axis armies. Van Way assured him no chemical warfare activity was expected, it was just a precautionary measure, and his duties would "evolve as needed." Colonel Maurice E. Barker, former head of the CWS and newly appointed chief chemical officer for the Western Task Force, joked that Patton would have included "a regiment of wizards" with his assault force if he thought it would promise victory on the far shore.

Alexander embarked from Hampton Roads, Virginia, with the first part of the Western Task Force on the afternoon of October 23, 1942. It was an immense invasion force—thirty-five thousand troops in a convoy of more than a hundred ships. As Alexander stood at the rails of his transport ship, the sight of the large armada left him gasping. Several days out, they rendezvoused with another huge convoy, consisting of innumerable battleships, heavy cruisers, destroyers, and aircraft carriers, as well as a flotilla of seagoing tugs, subchasers, mine sweepers, mine layers, and repair ships. It was, Patton told them more than once, the greatest amphibious operation of its kind ever attempted. Far out at sea, the enormous US Navy war fleet looked to Alexander like a floating city on the horizon, gray and ominous in the distance.

It was not an easy crossing. He was part of a small group of specialists from Patton's headquarters—including a counterintelligence officer, several Signal Corps radio operators, and a handful of others skilled in ordnance—traveling under the code 1848D to disguise their classified missions. Before departing, they had been carefully instructed that under no circumstances were they to indicate who or what they were to any of their fellow passengers. Although it was never spelled out, Alexander surmised that if they were captured, the War Department did not want the nature of their wizardry known. In a typical bureaucratic snafu, however, the ship's commanding officer, a big, red-faced Navy man, took offense at being left out of the loop. He demanded to know the meaning of their 1848D designation. When Alexander and his comrades refused to divulge their secret orders, he became visibly annoyed and declared, "Well, I'll fix you gentlemen."

All eight of them were then assigned to menial labor: half to latrine detail, half to mess duty. Ordinarily, the jobs should have gone to more junior personnel, but the group's protests were overruled. Since Alexander did not know the first thing about cooking, let alone feeding the crew of an entire ship, he said, "Yes, Sir, I have very little knowledge in this field, Sir." It earned him a sharp rebuke—"Don't answer me back"—and no reprieve. He spent the rest of the journey as a mess officer below decks in a boiling galley, attempting to help feed five thousand men two meals a day.

The Western Task Force swarmed Morocco's western coast at dawn on November 8, going ashore at three points—Safi, Fédala, and Mehdia—along more than two hundred miles of coastline. By the time Alexander's ship put in at Casablanca three days later, the naval battle was over and Patton's forces had seized the port, but they had encountered the most determined opposition of the three task forces. It was immediately apparent that the planners of Torch had underestimated the toll of the mass offensive. Making matters worse, the weather turned treacherous. A storm moved in, lashing the harbor with huge waves, wind, and rain. Many of the plywood landing craft were smashed to pieces by the rough surf and rocks, hurling men, weapons, and equipment into the water. Dozens drowned. Wounded soldiers struggled up from the landing beaches, hundreds of them, but there was no medical support to speak of—no hospital ships, no field hospitals, nothing.

Alexander and a handful of other battalion doctors did what they could with their meager supplies. That first night, they had little medicine or food. They scraped the barrel, Alexander recalled, and what they administered in the way of care was "very haphazard." Flashlights furnished the only illumination. Abandoned buildings, squalid huts, and beach casinos were hastily converted into aid stations, the stretchers laid end to end. When ambulances managed to get through to the beaches, they bogged down in the sand and became easy targets for the enemy. For days they worked around the clock, fighting confusion and exhaustion, and slept when they could on the floor. Many of the more severely injured were lost. Although Alexander had a hardy constitution, the grueling ordeal brought him to the limits of his stamina. Past the point of weariness, he succumbed to a fever. By then, the 48th Surgical Hospital had arrived and he became one of its first patients.

He remained at Patton's headquarters, confined to light duty, until late December, when he was selected for another classified assignment. Brigadier General Alfred Gruenther, deputy chief of staff for AFHQ under Eisenhower, informed him they were in the process of setting up the Casablanca Conference, scheduled to take place January 14 to 24, 1943. It would be a top secret meeting of the Allied leaders to coordinate military strategy for the next phase of the war. In attendance would be FDR, Churchill, the representatives of the Free French Forces, Charles de Gaulle and Henri Giraud, and a slew of Allied generals, one more indispensable than the next. Alexander would be the attending physician, responsible for the welfare of probably the most important group of patients ever entrusted to a doctor. It was the first time the US president would be venturing to a foreign land since the start of the war. His health and security were paramount.

As part of the advance planning, Alexander was instructed to look out for any "potential hazards" posed by the selected site. He had to resist the temptation to point out that Casablanca, so recently conquered, was a less than ideal location. There had been several air raids in the area in recent weeks, and they regularly had to douse the lights and wait out the passing bombers. Possibly the planners had hoped that Soviet Premier Joseph Stalin might be induced to come that far, but he was reportedly focused on the fighting in Stalingrad and declined the invitation. Still, there was no disputing the fact that the site in question, the Anfa Hotel and surrounding villas, situated on a promontory high above the city, was one of the most beautiful spots he had ever seen. The four-story art deco hotel looked like a grounded luxury liner, its curved white façade commanding a view of the wide Atlantic. Security was tight. The whole compound was ringed with barbed wire, not once but three times, and very heavily guarded. MPs with dogs patrolled the perimeter and the lush gardens lined with orange and lemon trees and gaudy thickets of pink and purple bougainvillea.

Alexander scouted the property and tried to anticipate every lurking danger. He scrutinized the rooms and kitchens, checked for vermin, and had the water tested, though a special bottled supply was being flown in for the president all the way from Washington. He requisitioned ambulances and arranged to have three medical officers on duty at all times. As an added precaution, he had another twenty-seven men from the Army Medical Corps standing by. Because the conference was to remain under wraps until the talks were concluded, the preparations required extreme subterfuge. Alexander went to great lengths to conceal the true nature of his assignment, with the result that all his special demands and meticulously crafted cover stories were greeted with a mixture of disbelief and outrage. Intractable delegation deputies returned scowling after consulting their superiors, and they grudgingly granted his requests while leaving him in no doubt that they could not wait to see the back of him in Casablanca.

Just when he thought he had everything squared away, it suddenly occurred to him that there was nothing to keep an enemy submarine from surfacing and tossing a few shells their way. Gen. Gruenther paled at the suggestion and immediately arranged for a covering group of destroyers to patrol the surrounding waters. The threat of an air raid remained omnipresent. It was a constant source of anxiety, as was the problem—with such a daunting list of VIPs—of how to prioritize his patients should casualties occur. If he treated a British admiral before an American general, it would not go unnoticed. He became adept at identifying planes, and the appearance of one in the distance always spurred a silent prayer that it was friendly.

The ten-day conference went off without a hitch. The generals were overworked and overtired, but their ailments were minor. He gave Gen. Marshall his inoculations for India and cured General Hastings Ismay, Churchill's chief military assistant, of a nasty cough. Both the prime minister and the president brought their own private physicians, leaving Alexander free to relax and enjoy the distinguished company. No great admirer of Roosevelt's politics—he had never voted for him—Alexander was nonetheless surprised by how impressive the man was in person. FDR had remarkable presence and managed to be very imposing and dynamic in spite of his wheelchair. Roosevelt was eager to see the scene of the great battle in Casablanca Harbor, but the Combined Chiefs of Staff vetoed anything that would expose him to unnecessary danger. Nonetheless, he insisted on inspecting the troops in the combat zone, the first American president since Abraham Lincoln to do so.

The trip to Rabat to review Patton's troops required a demanding performance. Watching as Roosevelt was carefully lifted into the Daimler while a fifteen-car convoy waited, flanked by jeeps carrying Secret Service agents, and trailed overhead by a fighter escort, Alexander could not help but come away with a new respect for him as a leader. When they drew close to Rabat, Roosevelt was transferred to a jeep, with Gen. Clark, looking impossibly boyish and brash, like central casting's idea of a commanding officer, seated behind him. The whole thing was beautifully staged. Seeing Roosevelt riding high like a conquering hero, the familiar gray fedora set at a jaunty angle atop his noble head, did a world of good for the GIs. Alexander had to admit that the visit boosted morale—it was just the "shot in the arm" the men needed after two tough months on a hostile shore.

Although the Casablanca adventure was quite a thrill, Alexander was too conscientious to enjoy the cushy assignment for long. On Sunday, January 24, 1943, Anfa camp ended with a public display of unity. Churchill, Roosevelt, and the two French generals met with fifty reporters on the hotel lawn to discuss their secret deliberations, and FDR stunned one and all by announcing they would demand the "unconditional surrender" of their Axis enemies. If Churchill looked momentarily discomfited, it was only because he had not expected the president to blurt out the terms for ending the war then and there, in the glare of the hot North African sun.

Now that it was common knowledge, Alexander dashed off a brief note to his family, letting them know he had been present at the historic summit. While he was still wondering how a "small potato" like him got asked to look after so many of the big shots running the war, part of him was itching to get back to the front. "I don't know how much good I do, but I sure do get around," he wrote. "I'm almost getting a little lonesome to take care of some sick and wounded." He was flabbergasted when, two weeks later, he received an unexpected commendation from Roosevelt for his diligent work at the conference, along with a letter praising the "splendid manner in which he performed his varied and arduous tasks."

After a wasted detour eastward to Gen. Mark Clark's base in Oujda, which was empty now that the garrison was gone, the Army finally got around to sending him where he was supposed to go in the first place. On January 29, Alexander flew to Algiers and joined Eisenhower's staff as a consultant in chemical warfare. He had yet to meet his new boss, as the busy theater commander had spent only a day at the conference before hurrying back to headquarters to deal with the snarled military operations in North Africa.

His first encounter with Eisenhower, who had just been awarded the fourth star of a full general, made a lasting impression. After warmly welcoming Alexander, along with a new group of officers, Eisenhower told them that he did not want anyone on his staff at AFHQ thinking of themselves as either American or British, but only as one unified Allied force. In the early days, he recalled that officers of the two nationalities were apt to conduct business with the attitude of "a bulldog meeting a tomcat," but he added that a mutual respect had developed over time. Then, addressing his remarks directly to the US personnel, his voice turning stern, he emphasized that he would not under any circumstances tolerate anti-British comments or sentiments. Teamwork, coordinated action, and complete "unity of purpose" were necessary if they were to be effective. If he perceived any mindset insufficiently aligned with the Allied partnership, he would personally see to it that that officer was sent back to the United States, preferably on a slow freighter. As the Atlantic was infested with submarines, this was not a happy prospect. Alexander heeded the warning and made a point of getting along with his British colleagues.

He was detailed to the theater medical section run by Major General Albert Kenner, deputy chief surgeon at AFHQ and Eisenhower's personal front-line emissary, and his deputy, Colonel Earle Standlee, an intelligent, thoughtful officer who Alexander sensed could become a friend. Predictably, Standlee informed him that they had no need of a chemical warfare specialist at the moment, but he added cheerfully, "I'm rather glad to have you here in case we do."

Alexander was told he would have a dual function: As the chemical warfare consultant to the surgeon for the North African Theater of Operations, he would advise on all matters that might affect the care and treatment of casualties from chemical action from both the Amer-

ican and the British forces; he would also serve as a technical aide to
the chief of the Chemical Warfare Section. One of the main challenges
of his job would be to maintain an adequate level of preparedness for a
gas attack in the absence of any overt action by the enemy. The emphasis would be on directing a continuous chemical defense training program, maintaining the troops' vigilance and alertness to the threat, and
keeping all the units supplied with antigas kits, equipment, and first aid
facilities. He would also be expected to stay on top of new treatments
for chemical injuries and the latest developments in toxic agents and
their dispersal.

Alexander joined a team of truly extraordinary pioneering physicians. His bunkmate was Colonel Perrin H. Long, head of the Department of Preventive Medicine at Johns Hopkins University Medical
School. He had been awarded the Croix de Guerre for his service in
the Army Ambulance Corps in World War I and was credited with
helping to introduce one of the greatest advances in wartime medicine,
an antibacterial drug known as sulfanilamide, the forerunner of anti-
biotics. Ten days after the Japanese attack on Pearl Harbor, he flew to
Hawaii and wrote a decisive report about the first use of sulfonamides
en masse in a military setting. Equally brilliant and beloved, Colonel
Edward D. Churchill, a Harvard Medical School professor who served
as chief surgical consultant in the Mediterranean Theater, was dedicated to improving the quality of wound care in forward hospitals.
During his first tour of the North African battlefields, he discovered
that the reliance on plasma, a blood substitute, was costing lives and
was not a substitute for whole-blood transfusions. While whole blood
was more complicated and cumbersome—it had to be transported in
refrigerated trucks and had a limited shelf life—he insisted it was worth
the effort. He first sent a highly critical report to the Army surgeon
general. When that did not get results, he drew attention to the problem in the press, succeeding in pushing through reforms that made

whole-blood transfusions at the front a reality and greatly increasing the survival rates of casualties.

Thrilled to be in such awe-inspiring company, Alexander offered to put himself at their disposal and pitch in any way he could. There was plenty to do. Perrin Long had arrived to find the Army Medical Corps in complete disarray and the policies "all at loose ends." Alexander put his CWS duties aside for the time being and got to work helping their small Anglo-American staff ride herd on a number of vexing problems—ranging from the dire shortage of doctors (they had permission to "steal" them from any Allied planes and ships entering Algiers) and the lack of fixed hospital beds to the ongoing medical supply problem afflicting the North African Theater.

He spent the first few months trying to evacuate the casualties from the Tunisian battlefronts, where the Americans were fighting the Axis troops, back to the North African Theater, where the Allied forces were now solidly established. The original idea was for patients to be moved in a constant flow by train to Oran, in Algeria, or still farther back to Casablanca, the main Mediterranean support bases where they were in the process of setting up large hospitals. It was a relatively simple plan that proved exceptionally difficult to execute. To begin with, whichever backroom genius conceived of the plan had obviously never seen the train. It was an old, rickety narrow-gauge railroad that slowly threaded its way through Algeria, crossed the steep Atlas Mountains before reaching Oran, and then lurched another thousand miles to Casablanca. Much of the infrastructure had been destroyed. Locomotives and track had to be requisitioned, ordinary rolling stock converted into ambulance cars, and endless repairs made in the North African outback. Distances were so great that an injured man could spend a day and a night on a train before receiving treatment. The widespread fighting and rough terrain were a challenge for a medical system whose lack of mobility was better suited to the static fronts of World War I than the era of mechanized war.

As the wounded began to pile up in Tunis and Bizerte, it became apparent that they needed to find a more efficient means of transportation. It took a lot of persuading to convince the Air Force to pick up the casualties in the forward areas, where the pilots and their crews had no desire to hang around under fire a moment longer than necessary. After protracted negotiations, they reached a compromise, giving the ground surgeons a maximum of twenty minutes to load the casualties on the C-47s before they took off again.

It was a real circus act, with everyone racing around, but they made it work. To help streamline the process, Alexander devised a method of placing hooks inside the transport planes so the wounded could be loaded in their litters, which could then be secured in place. Eventually the transports would be equipped with metal racks that allowed them to stack eighteen stretchers at a time, with room for attendants. Evacuations sometimes totaled as many as 350 in a twenty-four-hour period. Once the plan got going, the air ambulances delivered the injured to hospitals in a matter of hours rather than days, which made all the difference in the number of lives saved.

Alexander was still in Tunisia when the First Armored Division suffered a terrible defeat at the hands of Field Marshal Erwin Rommel at the Kasserine Pass in February 1943. After months of fighting in the desert, the Afrika Korps and the 10th and 21st Panzer Divisions had become a seasoned fighting force and proved a far more dangerous opponent than expected. Because of faulty intelligence, they plowed through the defensive line and quickly overran the unprepared Americans. While more than six hundred wounded men filled the evacuation hospital, orders came to "pack and run" on a frigid, snowy night. British artillery and tanks rushed in; with the help of US reinforcements, they stalled Rommel's progress. In the weeks that followed, the Allies regrouped. In March, Eisenhower put Patton in command of II Corps, which had been shaken by the Kasserine debacle. Whatever else might be said of Patton, he was a fighting commander, and the troops soon rallied and resumed their advance. The mobile medical units prepared for their beds to fill again. Ultimately, the Germans ran out of fuel and supplies. On May 7, Tunis fell. So many German and Italian soldiers surrendered—more than two hundred fifty thousand—that the Army was not prepared to feed and detain them, creating a whole new set of headaches for AFHQ.

Before his old medical detachment pulled up stakes, Alexander went out and took photos of Hill 609, which had been hard won. It was a "bleak, difficult place." American losses exceeded seven thousand men—dead, wounded, missing, or captured. Capturing the high ground had cost more lives than any other objective in the Tunisian campaign. "The sooner they give this country back to the natives," he wrote home, "the happier I'll be."

AT CASABLANCA, THE ALLIED LEADERS had agreed that as soon as North Africa was cleared of the enemy, they would press on to Sicily as a prelude to the invasion of the Italian peninsula. With the massive assault on the European mainland underway, the war was entering a critical stage. Germany was on the defensive. Axis divisions, however, continued to pour into Italy to carry on the battle. The enemy seemed to be gathering strength to make one last major effort to repel the Allies' invasion force. British fears of chemical warfare were once again heightened by intelligence, albeit vague and fragmentary, that seemed to suggest the German High Command might be preparing to use poison gas in the near future. A classified Chemical Warfare Service memorandum confirmed that the Germans were well trained, well equipped, and "capable of initiating the employment of toxic chemicals at any time on a major scale." However, the Joint Chiefs of Staff concluded that the danger of chemical warfare remained slight, given Allied air superiority, and advised Churchill that the chances, "though less remote than hitherto, are still small." But they could not rule it out absolutely: "Hitler, faced with imminent military disaster might order it introduced."

Convinced the Germans would strike first at the Eastern Front, Churchill issued an almost unprecedented public statement shortly before midnight on April 21, 1943, reiterating Great Britain's intention of retaliating immediately if the recent reports of Germany's chemical weapons rearmament proved correct. Vowing that any use of gas would trigger a massive response in kind, Churchill added ominously: "British resources and scale of delivery have greatly increased."

The following morning, UP published a story revealing that the prime minister's unexpected declaration stemmed from his "increasing unease" that Hitler had become more disposed to the use of gas. Unnamed British "military sources" contended that "The Germans are like the Japs—they know no rules. Germany carries complete gas equipment into the field in containers marked 'To be used only on orders from the Fuehrer.'" The *New York Times* published a similar story, claiming the Nazis were "likely to employ lethal fumes," and reprinted comments by British Minister of Information Brendan Bracken, speculating that Hitler, like the biblical figure Samson, might go to his end "pulling down the pillars of civilization with him." When asked at a Washington press conference later that same day whether the Americans would follow the British example and retaliate if the Nazis used gas, Under Secretary of War Robert P. Patterson seemed nonplussed, saying there had been no discussions on the point, and he referred reporters to FDR's earlier statement to the Japanese.

In June, alarmed by reports indicating the Axis powers were "making significant preparations" to use poison gas to stop the Allied landings in Italy, Roosevelt renewed his warning to the Germans not to employ these "inhumane devices of war." After categorically stating that the United States "shall under no circumstances resort to the use of such weapons unless they are first used by our enemies," he went on to outline a poison-gas policy that paralleled Great Britain's. There was no question the Allies would reciprocate. But then the president put Berlin on notice, issuing an explicit threat: "We promise to any perpetrators of such crimes full and swift retaliation in kind. . . . Any use of gas by any Axis power will immediately be followed by the fullest possible retaliation upon munition centers, seaports, and other military installations through the whole extent of the territory of such Axis country."

Despite these strongly worded cautionary messages, concerns about gas warfare still persisted. Germany responded to the repeated threats with similar rhetoric, boasting that its army was infinitely better equipped for gas warfare and had "made the most minute preparations." As American and British troops slowly and painfully drove back the Germans, Eisenhower grew increasingly apprehensive that Hitler, in a last desperate move, might launch a gas attack. Even a limited attack would stall the already bogged-down offensive. It would further disrupt their supply routes, to say nothing of the demoralizing effect on the men.

Based on Italian intelligence, Eisenhower warned Gen. Marshall in late August that Berlin, infuriated that their former ally was colluding with the Allies, had "threatened that if Italy turned against Germany gas would be used against the country and the most terrible vengeance would be exacted." The Nazis use of gas would also send a powerful message to other weak-kneed Axis countries that betrayal would be met with stiff punishment. The situation was precarious. Churchill raised the possibility of "gas reprisals" in a memo to Roosevelt, based on what he was hearing from his generals about Nazi efforts to stiffen Italian resistance. On September 8, the day before the invasion of the Italian mainland, the Joint Chiefs of Staff instructed Eisenhower to warn Berlin that any use of gas against the Italians would "call forth immediate retaliation upon Germany with gas, using to the full the Allied air superiority."

At AFHQ, Alexander, now newly promoted to lieutenant colonel, turned his attention to the chemical threat in Italy. By the fall of 1943, he was hearing with increasing frequency, from a variety of sources, reports of evidence of intensified enemy preparations. Fifth Army interrogators reported that German prisoners of war, in private conversations overheard by their captors, whispered, "Adolf will turn to gas when there is no other way out." A recent Enigma decrypt indicated the German army was about to have all its respirators upgraded. Rumors circulated of new, far more powerful toxins.

As part of his remit, Alexander was charged with reviewing and interpreting all the chemical intelligence gathered. He had to be able to furnish Eisenhower with advice, recognize any suspicious developments, and decide when to begin taking defensive measures—all on very short notice. But Italy's past reliance on chemical warfare complicated matters, making the risk harder to assess and raising unsettling questions about the country's hidden chemical resources. US military intelligence (G-2) issued a series of reports, entitled *Tentative Lessons Bulletins*, that detailed the Italians' extensive use of mustard gas against the Ethiopians in the Abyssinian campaign of 1935–36 and drew attention to the fact that they had maintained chemical-storage facilities in Libya throughout that conflict. There was also the large Seronio chemical factory in Foggia, which produced phosgene and mustard and had been under tight German control since 1941.

In the course of reviewing the raw intelligence data from the landings in Sicily, Alexander made another unsettling discovery. In a memorandum to Colonel Cornelius P. Rhoads, chief of the new, expanded Medical Division of the Chemical Warfare Service, Alexander reported that significant stores of an unknown vesicant had been captured. "It is probably a mixture of fifty percent Mustard and fifty percent phenyldichlorarsine," he wrote, adding that it would be analyzed to confirm its composition. "This mixture is probably of Italian manufacture, and we have known for some time that the Italians were partial to mixtures. I have no definite information as yet as to whether the Germans are preparing this mixture or perhaps some other mixture. There is no doubt that the Nitrogen Mustards are well known to them and have been carefully considered for some time."

By the end of September, the British took Foggia without firing a shot, but the departing Germans blew up the chemical plant and dumped their hoard of mustard bombs in the harbor, depriving the Allies of the spoils of conquest. German ships also discarded mustard bombs and other war matériel outside the port of Manfredonia, aware the submerged munitions would render the shallow waters unsafe and require a costly and time-consuming salvage operation, thus sabotaging another key supply channel. It was strict Wehrmacht policy to leave no chemical weapons behind to prevent their capture in case of retreat, and thus to deny the Allies any pretext to respond in kind. One thing was certain either way: There was no shortage of poison gas in Puglia, the southern region of Italy where the war was being bitterly contested.

The intelligence reports, compiled from all over Europe, did not make pleasant reading. Not only could Alexander see that mustard gas and other chemical agents were being produced in large quantities by Germany and other Axis countries, it was horrifyingly clear to him that they could be used to annihilate Jews and other defenseless civilians. "The development of the concentration camps were well reported and authenticated in these reports," he later recalled. At the time, the methods of execution were thought to be by shooting, electrocution, and in some cases asphyxiation via carbon monoxide inhalation. (Gas chambers and the systematic extermination of prisoners using a formulation of hydrogen cyanide known as Zyklon B were a cruelty yet to be discovered.) But he worried about the implications of what he read. He worried about the scope of the Nazis' murderous activities inside Germany. Above all, he worried about his friends in the First Division.

They were the first line of defense. If and when the enemy unleashed a gas attack, they would be "among the first to be exposed."

From the first days of the war, Churchill and Roosevelt had feared and expected that the Germans would use poison gas. They had hoped their strong and repeated warnings would deter the enemy from such an attack and thus avert the need for retaliation. But events had overtaken their cautious strategy. Now they had no choice but to prepare for the worst. To ensure the capacity for prompt retaliation, the War Department secretly authorized the stockpiling of a forty-five-day supply of chemical warfare munitions in the Mediterranean. In October 1943, AFHQ complied and began taking steps to have one-third of those supplies, equivalent to a fifteen-day cache, progressively built up in Italy over the next three months. Depots storing bulk mustard and other chemical weapons had already been established in Oran and elsewhere in North Africa, well camouflaged so the Axis forces would not learn of their existence. Every theater was being fully equipped to defend against a possible surprise attack. From then on, Eisenhower recalled, "We were always forced to carry [mustard gas] with us because of the uncertainty of German intentions in the use of the weapon."

That fall, the Allies began to move stocks of poison gas to Italy to be held in readiness, securing them in special ammunition dumps close to their front lines. After careful consideration, the White House signed off on a large-scale shipment to be stored in a forward cache at Foggia. It was a calculated risk. They knew that if their secret reserves were discovered, the enemy could use that as an excuse to initiate an all-out chemical war.

—— • ◆ • ——

CHAPTER TWO

"The Die Is Cast"

When his plane touched down on the Bari airfield at 5 p.m. on December 7, Stewart Alexander could tell at once from the strained expressions on the faces of the British officials hurrying across the tarmac to greet him that something was very wrong. They explained that the plane on which he was reported to be flying had crashed on landing moments earlier, killing everyone aboard. This information had only just been relayed to AFHQ at Algiers, causing considerable consternation. Although the fighter he was aboard turned up all of five minutes later, his safe arrival clearly came as a relief. He was warmly received by Colonel Joseph H. Bayley, the senior Royal Army Medical Corps officer for the district, and a group of British hospital directors, but they could not hide their impatience for him to begin his investigation into the sudden, inexplicable deaths of so many of their young naval men. "Their agitation was immediately apparent," Alexander recalled, "and I was taken to the hospital at once."

As they drove through Bari, the city seemed strangely empty. Only five bombs had fallen among the buildings in the oldest part of town, but the local limestone in the cramped medieval quarter was soft and could not withstand the violent reverberations caused by all the explosions. In places, the destruction was nothing short of apocalyptic. Roofs caved in, foundations collapsed, and walls crumbled into mounds of dust. It seemed as if every pane of glass within a seven-mile radius of the port lay in the street. Where one bomb hit, two whole blocks had been reduced to rubble. The ancient cathedral, pockmarked by shrapnel, had sustained several near misses, but the homes directly adjacent had been decimated. Hundreds of local inhabitants had been killed outright. Tragically, many women and children died in a shelter flooded by a burst pipe and blocked by the heaving mass of humanity at the entrance pushing to get in. Hearing their frantic cries of *"Acqua, acqua,"* a fireman had turned his hose on the narrow opening, unaware the trapped inhabitants were trying to escape the rising water.

In the aftermath of the attack, Bari had been reduced to medieval living conditions. The situation had quickly become dire. Drinking water was hard to find and food was scarce. With the cracked sewers overflowing, and no one to fix them, rats and mice were taking over. Disease had already begun to set in. Everyone who was able had packed up their families and the few belongings they could carry and had headed out of town. For days after the raid, the roads leading out of Bari were clogged with civilians fleeing the city.

By some miracle, the 98th British General Hospital, located in a large, unfinished complex of some twenty brick buildings fifteen minutes from the harbor, had been spared. Built on the monumental scale beloved by the Fascists, and expropriated by the Allies in October, the Bari Polyclinic, as it was known, housed sizable medical wards, a surgical block, laboratories, an X-ray department, a chapel, administrative offices, residential wings, and various unfinished structures. Also contained within its high walls were several smaller field hospitals, including the 14th Combined General Hospital, the 3 New Zealand General Hospital, and the 30 Indian General Hospital. The main group of buildings was arranged in a horseshoe pattern, bifurcated by a long road that ushered the ambulances through the outer layers of sentry huts and guard stations straight into the heart of the hospital compound.

As the 98th General was only a short distance from the docks, the staff on duty the night of December 2 heard the gunfire and intense antiaircraft barrage coming from the harbor. Some of the nurses and orderlies even paused to watch the fearful spectacle until an enormous explosion forced them to dive for cover. For a few seconds, they thought they were all going to be blown to kingdom come. "With every fresh explosion, the building creaked and rattled, rocking like a ship in a storm," recalled E. M. Somers Cocks, a nurse with the 3 New Zealand. "Doors were wrenched off hinges, windows were shattered, and the bricked-up windows scattered their bricks like hail." With an appalling crash, the concussion blast knocked out the power, plunging them into darkness. The nurses ran to their wards, relieved to find none of the patients had been hit by glass or falling debris. They hastily dragged the beds to the centers of the rooms and cleared away broken furniture that had been hurled in the corners and cluttered-up passageways. They tried tacking makeshift coverings over the vacant windows, but it did not stop the bitter December wind from whipping through the halls. They were still sweeping up glass and lighting hurricane lamps when the first influx of wounded began arriving.

By all accounts, it was a nightmarish scene, as an unending line of casualties made its way up the drive, hundreds upon hundreds of bloodied and bedraggled sailors and merchant seamen. The walking wounded staggered in unaided, suffering from shock, burns, and exposure after having been in the cold water for hours before being rescued. Others had to be supported, as they cradled fractured arms in improvised slings or dragged mangled limbs. They stood huddled together, shivering and shaking, their faces smeared with soot, uniforms in tatters and drenched in filthy, reeking seawater. Almost all of them were covered in thick, black crude oil. The litter-bearers brought up the rear, carrying the more grievously injured. These were sailors who had been pulled out of the water by rescue launches, treated at a casualty clearing station hastily set up on the HMS *Vienna*, and later taken to the hospital in the backs of jeeps, trucks, delivery vans—anything with wheels. Many had jumped from blazing ships, or swum through pools of flaming oil, and were horribly burned. Their agonized pleas could be heard above the cacophony of voices, shouted commands of the doctors, and frightened cries of men, some little more than boys, calling for their mothers in a multitude of accents and languages.

The main reception area was already full, occupied by a large group of soldiers waiting for a morning flight to England, with the result that the hallways were soon overflowing. Every passageway was lined with oil-slicked men lying on stretchers, camp beds, mattresses, and, more often than not, greatcoats. It would be many, many hours before they could all be attended to. The stink of burning petrol filled the air. Overwhelmed by the number of patients, the hospital abandoned its normal admittance procedures. The orderlies brought in torn bodies and put them wherever they could find room, often leaving them in the aisles, and then dashed off to get another load. When they ran out of space, they put stretchers in an unfinished building, even though it had no light or water or facilities of any kind. Many men died along the way or were beyond help by the time they arrived. In the remorseless calculus of triage, these inert figures were discreetly taken to a back room referred to as the "death ward," where the hope was that unconsciousness had eased their end.

With so many patients needing urgent attention, there was no time to get the sailors out of their soiled clothes, washed, and changed into hospital gowns—not that they had anywhere near enough on hand—so the ward matrons did what they could to make them comfortable. As a major forward hospital, they had long experience with disaster victims, but even the chief of the surgical division, Lieutenant Colonel

Alphonsus L. "Pon" d'Abreu, acknowledged being "considerably puzzled by the extremely shocked condition of the patients with negligible surgical injuries." He made sure all the "immersion" cases were given the prescribed emergency treatment: a shot of morphine, blankets to keep them warm, and strong, hot, sweet tea. Then they were left to rest. Those capable of speaking mentioned "smarting eyes" and stinging burns, but that was attributed to the large fires and fuel-oil contamination and thus discounted at the time. Most just lay there quietly. A few murmured their thanks and apologized for being "such a nuisance." It was understood that surgical cases were given priority.

The sheer volume of casualties—more than 440 were admitted to hospitals that first night—put an enormous strain on the medics and made it impossible to pay close attention to everyone. There was so much to be done that any convalescent who was not a complete "cot case" gave up his bed to a bombing victim and tried to help out in any way he could. Run ragged, the staff struggled to tend the crush of wounded under extraordinarily difficult conditions. A British nurse, Gwladys Rees, remembered at one point trying to fix an intravenous line by the light of a single match held by an orderly in front of a screen to prevent the wind from blowing it out. "We worked by the dim glow of hurricane lamps," she recalled. "Long into the night and early morning. Intravenous bottles were dripping from every third bed and the corridors were crammed with patients for whom we could find no accommodation. We were soon receiving patients via the operating theatre, patients with bilateral amputation of legs still wearing their life belts."

The first indication of anything "unusual," the doctors informed Alexander, was noted that evening in the resuscitation wards. Casualties thought to be suffering from shock, immersion, and burns did not fit the usual picture and did not respond in the typical manner. Upon admission, the patients were pale and lethargic, with a thready pulse and low blood pressure, yet they did not appear to be in clinical shock. Instead of exhibiting restlessness, anxiety, or distress, these patients were apathetic and their extremities were warm rather than cold. They had no shallow rapid respirations, and only a moderately rapid heartbeat. Given the tremendous violence of the explosions, it had been assumed many blast injuries would be admitted, but those diagnosed as blast cases did not present chest pain, injured eardrums, or blood-tinged sputum. When asked how they were, however, they would sit up in bed and say they felt "rather well"—even at times when their pulse was barely palpable and their systolic pressure perhaps as low as 50!

Even more notable was the lack of response to the standard resuscitation measures. Plasma infusions, at best, produced only a small, temporary rise of blood pressure. Most cases showed no response to the plasma, or to such typical therapies as external heat, morphine, or stimulants such as adrenaline and Coramine. They could be roused, but only fleetingly. "No treatment that we had to offer amounted to a darn," admitted one doctor.

It was not until a few hours after dawn that the nurses noticed something "odd" was happening to their patients. First, a few of the men complained of being thirsty, even though the orderlies had just gone around with the drinks cart. Then suddenly there were so many clamoring for water and getting up and going in search of taps that the whole ward was in an uproar, and it was difficult to keep the men under control. They were yelling about the intense heat, tearing off their gowns, and, in their growing frenzy, even trying desperately to rip off their dressings and bandages.

By morning, as the light began to filter in, the nurses saw that the majority of the immersion cases had red and inflamed skin. Lying stripped on their hospital bunks, these patients looked like they had bad sunburns, while others appeared very tanned or were reddish-brown in coloration. Overnight, Rees recalled, they had developed blisters on their bodies "as big as balloons and heavy with fluid." In cases where the blisters clustered around the face and neck, they differed from the usual flash burns caused by exploding ordnance in that there was no singeing of the eyebrows or hair. Those with extensive lesions in covered parts of the body—notably in the underarm, pelvic, and groin regions—were diagnosed with some kind of "chemical burns." This, together with the presence of nausea and vomiting common to nearly all the patients, led the doctors to guess they might be dealing with victims of poisonous fumes, possibly from the fuel oil and explosives, but probably from something even more toxic. That was when Rees started to worry whether the staff was at risk: "We began to realize that most of our patients had been contaminated by something beyond all imagination."

The first report of eye problems came from the surgeons. With the operating theaters going full tilt throughout the night, they found themselves repeatedly troubled by streaming eyes. The theater nurses also spoke of red, sore eyes. Six hours after the attack, patients who had managed to get some sleep awoke with painful eye symptoms. They said their eyes felt "gritty, as though sand particles had gotten in." Soon their eyes were burning, extremely sensitive to light, and weeping uncontrollably. Within twenty-four hours of the attack, the wards were full of men with eyes swollen shut. Their lids were clamped down so tightly they could not see. Many believed they had been permanently blinded and became distraught. In order to reassure them, the doctors explained, it was necessary to "force them to open their eyes to prove that vision was still possible." Extra nurses had to be recruited and round-the-clock "eye teams" organized to care for more than 140 incapacitated patients needing urgent treatment, including copious saline eye washes and the regular application of atropine drops. Forced to make do with what they had, the doctors issued all the eye patients temporary handmade shades consisting of a flap of cloth to wear during the daylight hours to help them cope with their intense photophobia.

Throughout the morning and over the course of the day, patients with acute eye problems continued to arrive. It soon emerged that not all the corneal lesions could be due to thermal burns caused by the explosions, as first presumed, because many of them had not experienced any discomfort until hours after the incident. At that point, Dr. Bernard Gluck, an ophthalmologist with the 98th General, began to think in terms of some form of chemical irritant, "as rumors were heard during the morning, more or less confirmed by noon, that mustard gas had escaped." By midday on Friday, December 3, the situation appeared to be "very serious," he reported. "The hospital was overfilled with several hundred cases from the incident, nearly all with involvement of the eyes and one could not foresee the probable course, as it was not known whether the noxious agent was indeed mustard gas or some other vesicant vapor with, to us, unknown action."

As the staff's unease deepened, notification came from headquarters that there was a "possibility of blister gas exposure" among the casualties. The hundreds of burn patients with unusual symptomology were to be classified "Dermatitis N.Y.D."—not yet diagnosed—pending further instructions.

Meanwhile, with the Eighth Army in the middle of an ongoing offensive, a continuous stream of new battle casualties poured into the area hospitals. "Among the battle casualties were some German POWs," recalled nurse Cocks. "They looked as pleased as punch and gabbed away excitedly to one another. They were lucky we didn't knock their blocks off, but I suppose we would have felt the same had the boot been on the other foot."

With the surge in patients, the medical staff had no time to deliberate about what might be poisoning the Bari victims. Adding to the chaos, many nonurgent cases that could not be admitted the first night because the hospital was swamped with traumatic injuries had started to develop symptoms. A large group of patients—who had appeared in reasonably "good condition" several hours after the attack and were sent to the Auxiliary Seamen's Home still wearing their wet uniforms—returned the following morning, all doing poorly and needing to be admitted.

Placed at the bottom of the triage list, men without obvious injuries were still sitting around in damp, grimy clothes streaked with the purple dye of burn unguent. Whenever the nurses could find a spare moment, they got busy cleaning them up, but the black scum clung to their skin and proved difficult to remove. They had to scrub them with kerosene, which was tricky because of the multiple burns, and then bathe them in warm, soapy water. When the last of their garments were removed, the brown and red patches beneath were pronounced. The reaction in the vulnerable genital region was especially severe and painful, causing "much mental anguish." The penis in some cases was swollen to three or four times its normal size, the scrotum was enlarged, and sepsis had set in. Keeping the lesions clean and dry, whether bandaged in Vaseline and sterile gauze or simply dusted with sulfanilamide powder, was a full-time job, but even with doctors, nurses, and corpsmen working in relays, they lacked the necessary hands to tend all the burn cases.

The hospital staff still had received no definite information about the presence of mustard gas in the harbor, but that did not stop the rumors. "With what little knowledge we had, our first thought was that these boys were suffering from mustard gas burns," recounted Rees. "The medical officers tried to get through to the War Office in London for information, advice, and an antidote, but none was forthcoming. We were all furious. And yet, if the war office couldn't release the information, it must be a military secret, and if that was the case, we were certain we were witnessing the effects of a poison gas."

Unsure what they were dealing with, the nurses worried about what might be in the clear amber fluid that leaked from the ruptured blisters. They asked whether they should be taking protective measures such as wearing gloves and masks but received no instructions. They tried to get tests done on the fluid but were never informed of the results. Despite the heroic efforts of Rees and her nursing colleagues, patients who had been expected to improve suddenly took a turn for the worse and died. So many were in pitiable condition. The futility of their ministrations frayed Rees's reserve. "We did everything humanly possible, but it was no good," she added reproachfully. "It was horrible to see these boys, so young and in so much obvious pain. We couldn't even give them strong sedatives, since we weren't quite sure how they would react with whatever had poisoned them."

What made it so awful was that most of the men were conscious throughout their ordeal and expressed confusion about their injuries. Warren Brandenstein, a young gunner aboard the American Liberty ship *John Bascom*, could not understand why his vision was becoming more and more blurry with each passing day. "That's when the rumors started to spread this was poison gas," he recalled. Through a conjunctival haze, he watched an official-looking group come through the hospital and collect all the patients' belongings, including his. "They came with big tarpaper bags and they took all our clothing," he said. "They took *all our clothing*," he repeated, his voice quavering with emotion, "and shoved them in this bag." Everything went—the oil-covered blankets, shirts, pants, even belts and shoes. That created a panic among the survivors, who thought their fates were surely sealed.

As the men grew weaker, they grew more afraid. "Their eyes asked us questions we couldn't answer," recalled Rees, who held their hands as they quietly slipped away. "I think they knew we were doing our best to save them. We tried to make their last hours as painless as possible."

The first unexplained death occurred eighteen hours after the attack. Several more occurred at twenty-four hours. There were fourteen within the first forty-eight hours.

Without warning, and for no apparent medical reason, patients were dying. This type of "early death," the doctors told Alexander, was most impressive to anyone who witnessed it, and it became the focus of special attention, as each was "as dramatic as it was unpredictable." In case after case, the physicians described the same startling downward spiral. "Individuals that appeared in rather good condition," they reported, "in a matter of minutes would become moribund and die." There was, for example, the case of Seaman Phillip Henry Stone, age eighteen: admitted on Thursday, December 2, cold and shocked, coated in oil, but without visible injuries, he developed blisters the following day, and by nine o'clock Saturday morning was unconscious, "cyanosed and respirations gasping." An intravenous plasma drip was started. At 3:30 p.m., he regained consciousness, asked for a drink, and "abruptly died" seconds after he finished speaking.

What disturbed the doctors most, Alexander noted, was that there were "no prognostic signs of this possibility." Some patients just rapidly went downhill, became cold, and the heart stopped beating. They had never seen anything like it. And they could not explain it.

Shock, first clearly identified in World War I, was still a problematic and inadequately understood condition. There were numerous forms of shock, from the loss of blood to infection. In the case of so-called wound shock, the symptoms included low blood pressure, cold extremities, elevated pulse rate, and feelings of anxiety that could take strange forms and often led to strange dying requests. A young man in deep shock could have the metabolic rate of an old man, and if doctors were not careful, repeated doses of morphine could further depress his respiration. The condition could herald the beginning of a series of destructive changes in the body, and data piling up in forward hospitals in North Africa and Italy increasingly pointed to shock as a primary cause of battle casualty deaths. Even though they had seen men brought out of shock by transfusion suddenly relapse and die, the surgeons felt sure something more was at work here, clouding the medical picture.

While some of the British doctors believed that mustard gas might be responsible for the sudden deaths, many of the physical findings did not correspond to the World War I case histories described in the medical books and Chemical Warfare Service manuals, leaving them mystified. If it was mustard vapor, then respiratory complications should have been more prominent, along with marked cyanosis (bluish tinge to the skin due to lack of oxygenation), blood-tinged sputum, parenchymal sounds (rattling caused by excessive fluid), and pneumonitis. But the hearts, lungs, abdomens, and central nervous system showed "no or only very minimal findings." Then, several days later, a number of patients with no previous respiratory problems began to get sick. They became hoarse and congested and developed very sore throats, making it hard to swallow. This was followed by a cough. These symptoms rapidly progressed and the patients became desperately ill and died—not as a result of broncho-pneumonia, as might have been expected, but from serious cardio-circulatory failure.

D'Abreu had seen enough. As head of the surgical division, and a medical bureaucrat of rare skill, he was determined to find out what was afflicting the Bari casualties. On Sunday, December 5, three days after the air raid, he sent a report to Colonel Wellington J. Laird, the commanding officer of the 98th General Hospital, outlining the growing medical crisis and asking for outside help. The patients' dermatitis and rapidly deteriorating condition did "not conform to any previously described for mustard poisoning," or, for that matter, to anything in the "official manual." The peculiar symptoms left the doctors confused and at a loss as to how to proceed. D'Abreu concluded his report with the stark declaration that he did not know if and when any of the hundreds of disaster victims would be stable enough to be moved: "At the moment of writing, few are fit for evacuation since it must be stated that deaths are occurring quite unexpectedly in patients with minimal lesions."

With the death toll continuing to escalate, alarm had begun to spread among the medical teams that perhaps they were dealing with a new, unknown German toxin. Down a short flight of stairs from the wards, the hospital basement had been turned into a temporary morgue. The hundreds of bodies already accumulated were deposited everywhere on the earthen floor. The town had already run out of caskets. In a small side room, a local Italian carpenter was banging together rough pine coffins as fast as he could. By the week's end, another six young men had expired for unfathomable reasons, and that number was expected to more than double.

D'Abreu had made his point. After being apprised that members of the staff of the 98th General had expressed "considerable anxiety" about the prognoses of their patients, Col. Bayley sent the signal to AFHQ requesting the presence of a chemical warfare physician in Bari.

STEWART ALEXANDER ASSESSED all this as he walked the crowded wards, jammed to the rafters with row after row of maimed and critically wounded men. He listened to the doctors' and nurses' accounts of the "strange deaths," the unusual symptomology, and the widespread eye and skin lesions. He examined the patients, gently lifting the blankets to study their wounds and then patting the cotton spreads neatly back into place. With extraordinary delicacy, he probed the strange patches of thickened red skin. He spoke with each in turn, asking where they had been when the bombing started and how they had come by their injuries. Leaning in close, so the men did not have to raise their voices, he slowly took them through their experiences on that harrowing night. Which ship were they on? How did they come to be rescued? Did they receive any first aid at the docks? What about when they got to the hospital? One sailor after another told of being caught in the firestorm, of the pandemonium that followed, and of somehow making it to the hospital. There they had waited, bundled in blankets, for as long as twelve and even twenty-four hours before receiving treatment.

Drawing back the covers from another patient, Alexander studied the distribution of the burns on the otherwise healthy, well-muscled body. The sailor told him he had been aboard a PT boat in the harbor when the first wave of German bombers came over. He had heard the loud boom as a nearby ship blew up, and he was hightailing it back to shore when he felt a spray of oily liquid land on his neck and run down his chest and back. He stated that he had not received any first aid.

Alexander observed the sharply defined outline of the raw, raised skin, shiny with ointment, delineating where the liquid had come into contact with his body. It was almost as if the splash had been imprinted on his flesh in red. The burns Alexander had seen on the other victims were quite varied, but already he could distinguish between chemical and thermal burns, and "certain patterns were present depending on how the individual had been exposed." It appeared that sailors who had been thrown overboard and completely immersed in the oily cauldron in the harbor were burned extensively, while those in boats who had just been sprayed had comparatively superficial burns wherever the toxic soup had hit them. Several men who had sat in the solution, possibly in lifeboats, had only local burns of the buttocks and groin. The soles of the feet and the palms of the hands were consistently free from burns, reflecting the thickness of the epidermal layers of skin in these areas. A few lucky souls who took it upon themselves to wipe off the oily mixture that first night sustained only minor injuries. He wondered whether they realized that the simple instinct for cleanliness had probably saved their lives.

Some of the men had skin lesions that he deduced were from mustard vapor. These patients fit into two groups: those directly exposed sustained relatively mild burns to uncovered skin and especially the face; the other group consisted of those who had small amounts of the chemical on their clothing, which allowed a certain amount of vapor to penetrate the axillary and inguinal skin folds.

The three most common blister agents were sulfur mustard, lewisite, and nitrogen mustard. Although generally referred to as "gas," all three chemical agents were liquids at room temperature. All three were vesicants that produced skin injuries resembling burns and serious eye injuries. On inhalation, they could affect the respiratory tract as well as the lungs, causing pulmonary edema. Particularly worrying was the new, pure-grade nitrogen mustard developed by the Germans. Its effects on the body were reportedly more rapid as compared to sulfur mustard, and it could penetrate intact skin and cause systemic poisoning. Practically colorless and odorless, apart from a faint fishy smell, it was not easily detected in the field. Alexander had received G-2 memos warning that the Axis forces had stores of the new blister agent on hand. Since lewisite and nitrogen mustard had never before been used in combat, he and the British doctors were bound to have difficulty recognizing their local effects. The Germans were also known to use mixtures of vesicants, so any combination of the three agents was a real possibility.

Another point of consideration was that, judging by the number of patients with superficial burns, the chemical agent in the harbor did not seem to have been terribly strong. In Alexander's experience, liquid mustard or lewisite burns would have been far worse. Mustard was 1.3 times heavier than water. Thrown onto seawater, it would form a slight surface film that would quickly hydrolyze into a harmless compound, while the bulk would sink to the bottom and would be slowly hydrolyzed by the action of the water. Mustard, however, was highly soluble in petrol. Based on his research at Edgewood Arsenal, Alexander knew mustard could form a true solution in oil up to 20 percent, but even this concentration was much too strong to have caused the body surface burns he had observed on the ward.

On the whole, the majority of the burns were remarkably mild in degree: Most could be characterized as first or second degree, affecting the outermost layers of skin, with only a handful deep enough to qualify as third degree and permeating the dermis to the underlying tissue. In many cases, the burns were so extensive that the small fluid-filled sacs or vesicles were diffuse in nature. These were not of the "textbook" variety associated with liquid mustard, which produced more severe, circumscribed lesions surrounded by the telltale halo of erythema, or angry reddened skin. Equally significant was the long delay before the first sign of symptoms. According to the doctors, the lesions on the Bari victims did not appear until "twelve to fourteen hours later." In addition, some lesions did not even make their appearance until several days after exposure.

Alexander knew that the interval between the exposure to the agent and the onset of the first symptoms was an important clue. Some chemical agents acted faster than others. With mustard, for example, which acts as a cell irritant and then as a cell poison on all exposed tissue, blisters usually took four to six hours to appear. Lewisite, an arsenical, produced lesions much more rapidly. Mixtures of the two could result in immediate pain and eye spasms. As a rule, the higher the concentration of the agent, the shorter the interval between exposure and the manifestation of the first symptoms. The time lapse could vary—depending on the duration of the exposure and whether the solution was diluted. But such a long latent period was not typical. The fact that only a few of the doctors, nurses, and attendants handling the Bari victims sustained any injuries, and those were mostly limited to their hands or mild eye lesions, also pointed to the solution being "rather dilute." The logical conclusion was that the chemical agent had become mixed in with the oily harbor water.

Aware of the multiple factors that could influence the effects of any vesicant, Alexander knew there was only so much he could extrapolate from the lesions themselves. He again noted the generalized edema, or swelling, of the skin, which had impressed him early on as being of a "strikingly brawny character." The skin was thickened and not of normal texture. The pigmentation was also unusual, having deepened into a distinctive bronze hue characteristic of mustard gas exposure. In some of the immersion cases, the exposed area covered 80 to 90 percent of the body surface. Whole layers of the outer skin had come loose and were stripped off by movement, often taking the hair with it. The question that troubled him was how a diluted form of mustard could have done so much damage. Then there was the unusual progression of the injuries, and their ultimate severity, which included a shock syndrome with low blood pressure, apathy, and systemic effects. When he had had a chance to appraise all the case histories, and review the pathological findings, he hoped to have a better idea of how these myriad symptoms fit together.

As he made his rounds, Alexander filled out dozens of medical case sheets listing the injuries: burns, blisters, dermatitis, breathing difficulties, blurred vision, vomiting, and acute pain due to elephantiasis of the genitals. These were, without question, all symptoms of contamination. While it was immediately apparent to him that most of these patients had been exposed to some kind of chemical agent, there were a number of anomalies that were baffling. Some of the burns were due to vapor exposure alone because the men had not been in the water, but, in his opinion, the large majority of lesions could not have been incurred this way. How to explain it? What was the method of delivery?

If it was a hostile chemical attack, was the poison gas dispersed as an aerosol by the German planes, or as a liquid in chemical bombs? Why did some of the victims have much more serious burns than the others? Did it indicate that they were in different parts of the harbor, or perhaps were indirectly exposed? His instincts told him the intensity of the symptom development lay in the mode of exposure. But there were too many contradictory pieces of information, and he did not yet have a clear picture of what had happened.

He was now faced with two problems. Before he could prescribe proper treatment, he first needed to identify the chemical agent—and he needed to do it quickly. It had been five days since the initial exposure to the toxin, and he feared it was already too late for some of these "unfortunate souls." If there was any chance of saving the hundreds of other victims lying in hospitals all over Bari, and countless hundreds of Italian civilians who might be suffering the same symptoms and be completely ignorant of the danger, he would need to act swiftly and decisively. Immediate decontamination would be required to limit further injury. There might still be time to contain some of the destructive effects of the poison, prevent possibly lethal secondary infections, and promote healing. Then he would have to determine how the toxin was deployed, and by which side. That part of the inquiry might prove both militarily and politically sensitive and have grave implications. Had the Germans carried out their threat to use gas against Italian targets? But he was getting ahead of himself. The one "almost absolute correlation" he had established at this point was between the men who came into direct contact with the oily harbor waters and their subsequent lesions. He would have to start his investigation there and see where it led.

All the while he was examining the patients, Alexander had been bothered by something he had noticed upon entering the hospital. Almost from the first, he had been struck by the peculiar smell that permeated the corridors. It stood out from the usual cloying mix of sweat, urine, and disinfectant common to all hospitals. Turning to one of the British medical officials accompanying him, he asked, "What is that odor?"

Col. Laird, the head of the 98th General, explained that most of the bombing victims had been covered in crude oil when they were brought in, and the mucky stuff had gotten all over the walls and floors of the hallways where they lay. Hard-pressed to keep up with all the casualties, the staff had not had time to mop the wards. Alexander accepted the explanation without comment. But he had spent too many hours doing research at the Edgewood laboratory to forget that deadly scent: "Traces of an odor implanted in my mind said mustard gas."

Mustard was by far the best all-around battle gas—persistent, easily handled, with a high vapor pressure, and known to cause local and systemic effects. It was colorless and painless on contact, which often precluded early decontamination if the victim was oblivious to it. Furthermore, there was no antidote. Although he suspected mustard, the medical evidence did not completely support this explanation. There were also different forms of delivery, which affected how the chemical was deposited on tissue. He felt uneasy. He disliked theorizing ahead of the facts and could ill afford to waste precious time by going off half-cocked in the wrong direction.

He decided to put the question directly to Laird. "I feel these men may have been exposed to mustard in some manner, Colonel," Alexander stated tentatively. "Do you have any idea how this might have happened?"

"None," came the concise retort.

Aware that it was not only the Germans who had mustard shells in their arsenal, and that the Allies had also been secretly stockpiling chemical munitions in Italy, Alexander tried to tactfully inquire whether there was any way the poison gas could have found its way into Bari Harbor on the night of December 2. "Have you checked with the port authorities?" he asked. "Could the ships in the harbor have been carrying mustard?"

Laird replied, "I have and they tell me they have no such information available."

It sounded like a classic dodge. Was the information really unavailable or was the man just being evasive? It was entirely possible, of course, that the British port authorities did not have all the manifests of the Allied ships in the crowded harbor that night, or that some had been lost or misplaced in the chaotic aftermath of the attack. It was equally possible the British officials did possess the classified information about the origin of the poison gas but were intent on blocking his investigation—whether for reasons of military security, propaganda concerns, or political repercussions. As chemical warfare consultant to

AFHQ, Alexander was cleared to the "highest degree." By all rights, he should have been granted immediate access to the relevant documents. But he had learned the hard way that the British were a tight-lipped bunch. Secrecy was their default mode. He sensed there was much his hosts did not want to disclose. He was not getting the full story, or their full cooperation.

Alexander realized then that if he was going to establish the lethal agent as mustard gas, the burden of proof rested with him. He would have to collect a great deal more data in order to identify the unknown toxin in Bari Harbor. He immediately took charge, ordering a series of tests for the patients who were still alive. Then he insisted that "careful and complete autopsies" be performed on all the patients who had died under mysterious circumstances, and where there were clearly no other conventional injuries. While the bulk of the casualties had been taken to the 98th General, Alexander asked that autopsies also be done on those sent to the other Allied hospitals in Bari: the 14th Combined General Hospital (Indian), 3rd New Zealand, 70th General Hospital (British), and the 84th General Hospital (British). Under "great protest," the British officials agreed, with much grumbling—"Did he not know there was a war on!"—and complaining that medical personnel were in short supply and under enormous pressure.

Alexander had no recourse but to depend on the British, since they controlled the port. Moreover, there were no American hospitals on the entire Adriatic coast to turn to for assistance. All the equipment for five new US field hospitals had been destroyed in the bombing. After a flurry of calls, Alexander arranged through his good friend Major James Flynn, stationed at the Foggia Air Base, to temporarily borrow pathologists and personnel from the displaced hospital units to assist in the gathering of data, laboratory studies on tissue samples, and histopathological reports. The British accepted the offer of a few extra pair of hands, but Alexander fretted that the lack of equipment would still handicap their work. "Certain of the scientific investigations and laboratory studies desired," he lamented, "were utterly impossible to have accomplished."

Advised that shortly before his arrival another group of patients had started to fail, Alexander carefully reviewed their charts. He saw that while they had showed no signs of respiratory distress in the first thirty-six hours, by the fifth day they began to develop severe coughs and diminution of breath and were bringing up blood-tinged sputum. It sounded symptomatic of lower respiratory-tract infections, and he asked that X-rays be taken immediately. They might be suffering from blast injuries to their lungs, but he was willing to bet they had breathed in the toxic mustard vapor or aspirated contaminated harbor water and sustained burns to their trachea, larynx, and bronchi. Whatever chemical was involved, he was increasingly convinced it had been present in the water. He ordered samples of the harbor waters to be collected and analyzed posthaste. Because of the risk of pneumonia, he decided not to wait for the results. He instituted doses of oral sulfadiazine for all patients at the first signs of fever and lower respiratory involvement.

Alexander then proceeded to question the medical staff and patients about whether they had heard anything about the presence of mustard gas in the harbor the night of the air raid. To him, it seemed "remarkable that no general alarm of gas was raised that evening." Was it possible no gas fumes were detected in the hours following the attack? Then again, the heavy clouds of acrid smoke from the explosions and burning petrol could have masked the smell down by the docks. By the time the men reached the hospital, they might have been too numb to heed much of anything going on around them. It was hardly surprising they did not register its significance. On direct questioning, however, a few survivors remembered identifying the characteristic peppery odor. "Some of the survivors spoke of commenting earlier on a 'garlicky odor,' " he noted. "Some even had joked about the odor during the evening, attributing it to the quantities of garlic consumed by the Italians." The doctors drew a blank. "In the hustle and rush of work," they told him, "no odors were detected."

Alexander was curious to know where all the rumors of gas had come from if the hospitals had received no notification. Where did they originate? He came away with the impression that most people had heard one or more of the rumors but in all the excitement and commotion could not remember who told them, and they could only cite vague or anonymous sources. Word had it that a Royal Navy surgeon who was helping at the docks "picked up a rumor that gas was in the port" and passed it on to hospital personnel before midnight, when he came through with a load of casualties. Yet, unaccountably, he was told that rumor was soon refuted.

Stunned by this, Alexander made a careful note for his preliminary report: "A rumor had been heard at one hospital of this possibility, but it was authoritatively(?) denied by an unknown naval officer." Another rumor, or another version of the same rumor, had it that a phone call placed by the 98th British General Hospital to Navy House, the admiralty's local headquarters, on the morning of December 3 could "obtain no verification of the presence of mustard gas in the harbor." Navy House, which was thought to be a target of the raid, was damaged in the bombing and was in a state of disarray. In any event, the rumor could not be confirmed, so the matter was dropped.

This was a profoundly depressing discovery. Had information of the possible risk of mustard gas exposure been communicated to the hospitals that evening or even the next morning, lives could have been saved. Many of the men had become contaminated while swimming, hanging from life rafts, or pulling their shipmates into rescue launches. If the physicians and first-aid teams had been warned, the survivors could have been hosed down and given fresh clothes and a fair chance at recovery. It was only natural for them to assume the victims were coated solely in crude oil because the medics had treated thousands of sailors rescued from the sea after their ships were struck, and they had no reason to suspect these casualties were any different. As a result, men mistakenly believed to be suffering from immersion had been wrapped in blankets while still in their oil-soaked uniforms, fed warm tea, and left to marinate in mustard—measures guaranteed to aggravate the condition. It was tantamount to a death sentence.

Alexander felt a surge of anger. Writing up his notes later that night, he emphasized: "No attempt was made to decontaminate or wash them. Their oil contaminated clothing was not removed." How could this have happened? How could no one have known? "It must be repeated," he wrote, "that rescue squads at the port and hospital personnel had no idea or information that the casualties were, or had been, exposed to mustard." All remained unaware of the peril.

The time factor in the treatment of injuries was always crucial. In the case of chemical injuries, it was decisive. The first point every chemical warfare manual emphasized was the need for immediate intervention to minimize the absorption of the poison. How many CWS memoranda, bulletins, and circulars had he written that all began with the same instruction: "The speed with which first aid is instituted is the greatest single factor in its effectiveness." Chemical damage began in the first one to two minutes. The worst damage had all been done within a relatively short window—probably within the first four to six hours. By the next day, whatever remedial action was taken was largely ineffectual. By then, as any chemical warfare expert knew, "The die is cast, and death follows."

At Alexander's insistence, Col. Bayley escorted him that same evening to the disheveled Navy House, so he could confront the British authorities with what he had learned. It did not help matters that Captain John Oliver Campbell, the Naval Officer in Charge (NOIC), had left the day after the raid for a new post and been replaced by Commander Eustace J. Guinness of the Royal Navy, who was still playing catch-up. In addition, the officer in charge of security, Port Commandant Lieutenant Colonel Marcus Sieff, had only just returned from attending a conference in Cairo, leaving Major Harry Wilkinson, his deputy adjutant and quartermaster general, as the acting port commandant on the night of December 2. It was obvious that all concerned had a ready excuse as to why they did not have the answers to his questions.

The meeting with the British officials, coming as it did at the end of a long day, provoked in Alexander a mixture of frustration and foreboding. Weary and thus the blunter for it, he again demanded to be informed of the presence of mustard gas in Bari Harbor. This was again "absolutely denied." Alexander nodded, said little, and left unconvinced. He was in no position to argue. All he had to go on was his own competent medical opinion. What he needed was proof that his diagnosis was correct.

Despite the lack of any official directive about poison gas, the medical staff at each of the hospitals he visited had drawn their own conclusions and surmised that the bombing victims might be contamination cases. Each doctor Alexander interviewed confided, "Something funny's happening on my ward." Each nurse said, "You know, something is happening on my ward, too." Each group of patients he saw only confirmed his suspicions and reinforced his "gut feeling" that the culprit must be mustard gas. But this was not the familiar menace he had studied at Edgewood. This was some diabolical new form of the invisible horror, "mustard gas poisoning through a different guise than that recognized from WWI."

———— •◆• ————

CHAPTER THREE

"Angels in Long Underwear"

When he finally got to his room that night, Alexander took time to scribble a quick note to his fiancée before turning in. He had learned that the wire announcing his tragic demise in the plane crash at Bari Airport that afternoon had caused "significant grief" at his headquarters, especially to the lovely young nurse to whom he was engaged. A second cable correcting the error had quickly followed on the heels of the first. He took some comfort in knowing that her period of mourning had ended almost as soon as it began. If anyone could weather such a sudden reversal of fortune twice in one day, however, it was Bernice "Bunny" Wilbur. A tall, slender woman who imbued her khaki uniform with an elegant formality, she had glossy brown hair, deep-set, widely spaced blue eyes, and an attractive smile that, even briefly bestowed, was warm and wide. She was a compelling presence, emanating good humor and intelligence, but with a regal air that could shift from feminine to formidable with lightning speed. Officers quickly learned that the female lieutenant, responsible for 4,500 nurses stationed in the Mediterranean Theater, was a force to be reckoned with.

Since he was the "new boy" at AFHQ, Alexander's colleagues had happily handed him the telephone when she called one morning from the base hospital in Oran with a long list of demands. Standing behind him, flashing knowing grins and chuckling, Gen. Blesse, Col. Standlee, and the others had listened while she berated Alexander for his department's incompetence in failing to obtain enough nurses to staff her field-hospital operating rooms, and she sternly instructed him to "carefully take down" everything she wanted done. He had stuttered an apology, promised to expedite the transfer orders, and hung up to a chorus of laughter from his colleagues, who warned him she was "a strong-willed woman" and to watch his step. Four days later, she called back to say the transfer orders had still not come through, that it was a matter of urgency and she was tired of waiting. The next thing he knew, she had caught a transport plane to Algiers and was in his office, accusing him of being "an obstructionist." After they started courting, Blesse joked that they were the last two people he thought would end up together, given the way they "fought over the phone."

Bunny Wilbur had already made quite a name for herself in the North African Theater of Operations by the time they met. Alexander had seen a dozen or more glowing newspaper stories about her, each accompanied by a photograph in which she appeared beautiful if somewhat intimidating in the Boston mode. She had attended Simmons College and the New England Deaconess Hospital Training School for Nurses and had worked as an operating room supervisor before heading to Europe with sixty-two other nurses as part of the American Red Cross–Harvard Field Hospital Unit in the spring of 1941. They made the dangerous crossing in an assortment of freighters and whalers with a detachment of Canadian troops and came under submarine attack. Two of the boats were torpedoed. Six nurses drowned. Nineteen others got into lifeboats and were afloat on the cold Atlantic for twenty-one days, staying alive by eating barnacles scraped off the bottom of the hull.

Wilbur, whose ship managed to zigzag away from the pursuing

U-boats, arrived in England in the final weeks of the Blitz and was sent directly to Bristol to help deal with a dangerous typhoid epidemic. Within ten days, she and her fellow nurses accomplished their medical mission of tracing approximately 228 cases of fever until they identified the source—their very own "Typhoid Mary" in the form of a cake decorator at a local bakery. The woman responsible was in the habit of putting the icing for her confections in a paper tube and biting off the end before squeezing out the contents, effectively spreading her germs to all her customers. Wilbur's successful investigation was followed by a congratulatory visit from the Queen, tea with Mrs. Churchill, and a commendation. She volunteered to stay in England another eighteen months and spent most of it in Salisbury, battling the infectious diseases that broke out in the wake of the German bombing campaign.

When the US Army took over the Red Cross–Harvard Unit in July of 1942, Wilbur traded her nursing whites for fatigues. She was chosen to serve as chief of nurses for Eisenhower's invasion forces at the same time Alexander joined Patton's wedge of Operation Torch. She made the journey to North Africa as the sole woman aboard a transport ship with 4,447 men. When her landing barge took a direct hit, she waded ashore with the troops. Harassed by flying bullets and pounding waves, they lost most of their supplies. They rolled into Oran in armored tanks but never made it to the French military hospital that was supposed to be their destination. Instead, they had to settle for an abandoned civilian hospital that had been stripped bare by the Nazis. Even the beds had been taken.

Wilbur and the other nurses ripped up their clothes and underwear to make bandages, gave blood for transfusions, and fed the patients from their own C rations. She took to wearing the GIs' coveralls and boots and slept in men's woolen long johns at night to stay warm. Surgery was performed in the most primitive of conditions. For a week, she worked twenty hours at a stretch, while the *whoomp* of explosives and the chattering cough of machine-gun fire made it hard to steady her hands as she held clamps and sponges over suppurating chest wounds. The doctors performed heroic feats, but Perrin Long, full of admiration for Wilbur and her team, later insisted it was their undivided attention "night and day" that determined whether those with broken bodies, and broken spirits, pulled through. "The biggest morale factor in this theater," he told the *New York Times*, "is the nurses."

Wilbur spent months serving close to the front lines, helping to set up and run the tented clearing stations. She was inspecting a new evacuation unit in Tunisia in April 1943 when the call came that Lieutenant General Lesley J. McNair, chief of the Army Ground Forces, had been seriously wounded by a German mortar. After an operation to remove the shell fragments in the back of his head and repair his shattered left shoulder, he was taken to the medical evacuation unit, where Wilbur took over the care of their important patient. The next day, the Associated Press reported that the pretty head nurse "hid his clothes" to keep the die-hard soldier in bed—BOSTON NURSE BOSSES MCNAIR—but she later told reporters there was no truth to the story and that his uniform was cut off prior to surgery. She added, however, that the general was "in an awful hurry to get back to the war." When air transport was arranged at the end of the week, the fifty-four-year-old McNair requested that Wilbur accompany him back to the United States and continue to look after him. She agreed to go on the condition that he would promise her a round-trip ticket. She did not want to get stuck stateside and miss out on the action. While she had the general's ear, she told him about the dismal conditions in North Africa, the shortage of nurses, and the overburdened field hospitals. McNair took up her cause and arranged for her to travel to Washington and tell the Army brass how to better marshal their resources.

Before her brief home leave was over, Wilbur was promoted to lieutenant colonel and appointed director of nurses, serving the North African Theater. The jump up the ranks was so unexpected that there was no time to order the new insignia before her departure. In an impromptu ceremony at the airfield, Colonel Florence Blanchfield, superintendent of the Army Nurse Corps, removed the silver oak leaves from her own shoulders and pinned them on Wilbur's uniform.

The Army trotted their star nurse out to the press as a model of wartime service. Wilbur was more than game, and she turned out to be a gift to the public relations department. She made a series of appearances at blood banks, appealing for donations "so that others might live," and she recorded radio appeals urging more civilian nurses to volunteer for duty. Asked by a reporter what advice she would offer a young woman who wanted to be useful, she replied without missing a beat: "I'd tell her not to expect glamor or sitting by a bed stroking a fevered brow with a smooth white hand. I'd tell her not to expect glory or medals. Her glory will be the gratitude of the boys she takes care of." The publicity tour culminated with a feature story about "Bunny" in the *Saturday Evening Post*. The article, entitled "Angels in Long Underwear," lionized the valiant young Army nurse and her cohorts, "facing the horrors of war with the courage of men."

When she returned to the front, Wilbur was the highest-ranking woman in the Mediterranean Theater. Cocktail parties and dinners were good for morale and lubricated Allied relations, and she did not want for invitations or suitors. A favorite with the generals, she became especially close to Eisenhower and was a frequent guest at his villa in Algiers. Patton admired her moxie, solicited her opinion about ways to improve their efficiency, and always asked if there was anything he could do to make sure they were all measuring up to her high standards. In the primitive, tedious staging areas, she endeared herself to him by insisting on living the same unadorned life as the soldiers, without complaint. During big pushes, she was up at dawn and worked nonstop, oblivious to the peril. She traveled constantly, inspecting battlefield hospitals in Sicily, mainland Italy, Algeria, Morocco, and Tunisia. Along the way, she developed a sharp eye for military mischief. At one isolated replacement depot, she discovered the Air Force pilots had a habit of doing flybys when the nurses were showering in the open tarpaulin stalls, and the new arrivals were too green to know what to do. She gave the squadron leader a piece of her mind and quickly put a stop to it. After noticing the wear and tear that weeks of frontline duty exacted on "her girls," she initiated an R&R program and later took over a hotel on the liberated island of Corsica, where they could go for a restorative break far away from the noise and stress of combat. On the lodge's opening day, the staff paid tribute to her by christening the white, four-story sanctuary "Wilburnice."

It was near the end of that long, hard summer that the whole theater was convulsed in the controversy surrounding Patton's angry outburst while visiting the wounded at the 15th Evacuation Hospital in Sicily on August 3, 1943. Alexander had the story firsthand from a doctor who witnessed the unforgivable attack on one of his patients, a battle casualty. The general had reportedly heard of one soldier's particularly brave action on that day and had wanted to go and commend him in person. He went and knelt by his bed, spoke to the lad, pinned a medal on him, and said, "Let's pray together." When Patton got to his feet to leave, weary after a trying day, he saw another enlisted man coming in and asked what was wrong with him. "General, I guess it's my nerves," he replied miserably. Still in an emotional state after seeing the tent full of bloody and broken bodies, Patton lost his temper and hurled a torrent of abuse against the man.

A moment later, when he encountered a second soldier who admitted being "nervous" rather than physically hurt, Patton completely lost control. He took a swing at the hunched figure of Private Charles H. Kuhl, striking him across the face with his folded gloves. "You coward, you get out of this tent!" he bellowed, dragging him by his collar to the tent entrance and shoving him out. As he continued to rage about not wanting "gutless bastards" in his army, the doctors and nurses intervened, coming between Patton and Kuhl in an attempt to shield their patient from the violent tirade.

A week later, he did it again. Encountering another suspected malingerer on a tour of the 93rd Evacuation Hospital, Patton waved his pearl-handled revolver in the face of the soldier, struck him with the flat of his hand, and threatened to shoot him on the spot. When the quivering private, Paul G. Bennett, started to sob, Patton wheeled on him again, striking him so hard he knocked his helmet to the floor. Once again, the horrified doctors and nurses looked on, unsure whether they should restrain him. "I can't help it," Patton confessed afterward to hospital commander Colonel Donald E. Currier. "It makes my blood boil to think of a yellow bastard being babied."

Word of the "slapping incidents," as they became known, quickly made the rounds of the theater hospitals. An unofficial report of Patton's egregious conduct was sent to AFHQ Chief Surgeon Blesse, who forwarded it to Eisenhower. Blesse and theater medical consultant Perrin Long were asked to ascertain the truth of the allegations and investigate the incidents. Four newspaper correspondents were so disturbed that they went to Eisenhower and said they would publish the story unless Patton was fired. Eisenhower prevailed on the reporters to stay mum and give him time to deal with the situation in his own way, but news of the incidents inevitably reached the home front, sparking a huge uproar in the press. Families of the boys fighting overseas were distressed to think they were being treated in such a brutal fashion. Washington wanted Patton removed from his command.

Eisenhower was faced with a difficult dilemma: He did not want to lose an able leader at such a critical moment in the war, but he also had to assure himself that Patton's temper would be channeled correctly and his abuses curbed. In the end, Ike wrote him a sharp letter of reprimand and demanded he apologize to Privates Bennett and Kuhl. Doctors later testified that Pvt. Kuhl was seriously ill at the time with malaria and running a temperature of 102. Patton also had to appear before the officers and representatives of the enlisted men of each of his divisions to assure them that his impulsive remarks did not detract from his high regard for the average fighting man.

Eisenhower's letter, which he subsequently read aloud to the press, was hand-delivered to Patton by Gen. Blesse:

I must so seriously question your good judgment and self-discipline as to raise serious doubts in my mind as to your future usefulness. . . .

No letter that I have been called upon to write in my military career has caused me the mental anguish of this one, not only because of my long and deep personal friendship for you but because of my admiration for your military qualities, but I assure you conduct such as described in the accompanying report will *not* be tolerated in this theater no matter who the offender may be.

By the time Wilbur encountered him, Patton was sulking and on the defensive, if not exactly contrite. He knew she ran the nursing corps with a firm hand, and he hoped she might see things from his perspective. "Tell me why they are making all this fuss?" he asked. "I didn't do anything serious to the young man. Admittedly, I didn't know he was sick, but I didn't like the way he talked and that's not the way I felt a soldier in my army should talk." Wilbur knew Patton could not abide anything that smacked of "shirking." She also knew that the diagnosis of psychoneurosis, or "battle fatigue," was all too real and not a sign of cowardice or an act put on by weaklings trying to dodge their duty. She preferred the term *exhaustion*, employed by the British Eighth Army, which pretty well summed up how the patient was feeling without the stigma of mental illness.

Patton had not been popular with the Medical Corps even before this latest diatribe. "Old Blood & Guts," as the aggressive general was known, did not always appreciate their risk assessments when planning maneuvers, and at times made it clear that he considered the battlefield physicians more of a hindrance than help. He also felt free to dispense his own advice for managing casualties, as he did in an infamous speech in January 1943: "If you have two wounded soldiers, one with a gunshot wound of the lung, and the other with an arm or a leg blown off, you save the sonofabitch with the lung and let the goddam sonofabitch with an amputated arm or leg go to hell. He is no goddamn use to us anymore." Col. Edward Churchill, chief surgical consultant for AFHQ, once compared Patton's refusal to accept responsibility for the care of the sick and wounded in the Seventh Army to "a maniac driving a machine at high speed without pausing to oil or service it."

Facing him squarely, Wilbur told Patton, "The problem, General, is that you do not understand about sick people." When he blustered that he thought he understood perfectly well, she said, "Let me put it this way: you have an ammunition dump about a mile and a half down the road." When he nodded, she continued in her best ward-matron voice: "I want it moved two miles off to the West." Patton, surprised by her peremptory tone, looked confused and said, "What? Col. Wilbur, you don't know the first thing about where ammunition dumps should be located."

"Of course, I don't," she replied tartly, "in the same way you don't know the first thing about how hospitals should function." Combat breakdowns needed rest and care, and he had better understand that if he wanted to conserve manpower. The general respected her answer and they remained on very good terms.

Alexander smiled at the memory. He thought he could use some of Bunny's negotiating skills in dealing with the obdurate British military bureaucracy. She did not think twice about scolding Patton, and he fancied she would have handled the port commandant better than he did.

All he had managed to establish thus far was just how sensitive an issue poison gas was with the British. As for his questions about the possible presence of a chemical agent in the harbor, he would have to raise them again in the morning. Their answers had not rung true.

As HE LAY IN BED THAT NIGHT, Alexander's thoughts drifted to something his colleague Ed Churchill had told him when he first joined Eisenhower's medical staff in Algiers. "It is impossible to plan for war with intuition as your sole guide," he had advised the young chemical warfare consultant. "It must be planned on the basis of experience." The portly, balding Harvard surgeon had then warmed to one of his favorite topics: how ill-prepared the Army Medical Corps was to deal with combat casualties on a large scale. He was particularly critical of the Army's "frantic but somewhat fruitless effort at secrecy" in the early months of the war. Any written document about the care of British wounded during the Blitz had been carefully guarded by the Office of the Surgeon of the Army, and the "hush-hush" memoranda were only circulated to a select few. After the bombing of London, scarcely any information was available on the medical crisis facing the blacked-out capital, and the little that American doctors heard was distorted by rumor and exaggeration. Finally, John Farquhar Fulton, an acclaimed Yale physiologist and medical historian, made the trip across the Atlantic and brought back invaluable knowledge about treating the so-called blast injuries that British doctors were encountering, and he later published an important article on the subject in the *New England Journal of Medicine*.

According to Ed Churchill, Americans were still amateurs at war. There were "great gaps" in the US Army's appropriations, planning and training for how to deal with the mass casualties incurred in global conflict. Too many Medical Corps officers lacked battlefield experience, and they changed only slowly and reluctantly from the entrenched practices of earlier days. At the end of the North African campaign in May 1943, he helped start a medical circular designed to summarize the experience that forward surgeons had gained in the management of wounds and medical evacuation in the combat zone. Oddly enough, one of the most memorable articles was an analysis of the famous Cocoanut Grove disaster, the deadliest nightclub fire in American history. Although it took place in Boston, the massive fire transformed the treatment of burns on the battlefields of World War II and provided an early template for what became known as "disaster management." Many of the lifesaving measures devised by doctors on the spot were subsequently adopted by the military and quickly became standard practice in frontline hospitals. Alexander remembered the story well, and he ruminated on its eerie parallels to the Bari disaster.

On Saturday night, November 28, 1942, the Cocoanut Grove, the swankiest club in Boston, was hopping. It was a busy Thanksgiving weekend in the college town, and the popular supper club was packed with more than a thousand students, football fans, and servicemen enjoying a bit of leave. Suddenly, at about 10:15 p.m., a small fire broke out in the basement lounge, then quickly worked its way up the decorative palm trees before spreading across the ceiling. The panicked crowd started to flee the premises, but within minutes of the first flames, the entire club was engulfed. The heavy toxic smoke funneled up the stairwell, which acted as a chimney and made visibility impossible. Dozens of patrons were trampled and crushed in the chaos before succumbing to the fumes. So many people pushed into the revolving door at the front of the club that it was soon clogged with bodies. The building, filled to double its legal capacity, was quickly consumed, and many of the exits were blocked or sealed, leaving hundreds trapped in the inferno. In less than fifteen minutes, the conflagration would claim 492 lives and injure another 166. The casualties were mainly due to asphyxiation and extreme body-surface burns sustained in the fire.

More than a hundred partygoers, still in their evening clothes, filled the long brick corridors of Massachusetts General Hospital (MGH). The majority of these were dead on arrival. Many survived for a few minutes but did not live long enough to undergo treatment. The doctors were so overloaded—victims were arriving on the average of one every fifty seconds—it became necessary to dispose of the dead quickly so they could care for the living. Adding to the mayhem, ambulances delivered too many of the casualties to the same backed-up emergency room, but by the time they discovered their error, it was past mattering. There was simply no precedent in civilian life for such a medical crisis.

Fortuitously, the staff at MGH had been holding bombing disaster drills ever since Pearl Harbor and had developed new modes of emergency treatment. They immediately inaugurated a prearranged plan of action. Teams of medical interns manned the door and sorted out the victims, ushering the living patients, still on stretchers, directly to the emergency ward, where they were placed on wooden sawhorses. Nurses administered injections of morphine close to the entrance, started intravenous fluids, and covered burned surfaces with sterile towels. Treatment continued as they were taken from the emergency ward to the isolation room, where doctors employed the novel procedure of simply covering the burns with boric-ointment-infused gauze and pressure bandages, dispensing with the usual steps of debridement and cleansing, which were time-consuming and tended to increase shock. Blood plasma was administered for shock, another new therapy that helped resuscitate severely burned victims. Dr. Churchill, who was chief of surgical services, helped his staff manage the crush of patients over the next three days and was a constant presence in the emergency ward and corridors, monitoring the treatment procedures.

In the aftermath of the horrific fire, investigations were conducted by several agencies to determine why so many had perished—among them, many officers and enlisted men of the Navy, Marine Corps, and Coast Guard. A busboy who did not fully extinguish a match used while trying to change a light bulb in the dimly lit lounge was believed to have sparked the blaze, but witness statements varied, and others attributed it to faulty wiring. In the end, a grand jury indicted ten people, but only one was convicted of a crime and that was the club's owner, Barney Welansky, on one count of manslaughter. The disaster led to sweeping changes in the country's fire safety codes and emergency response tactics, especially when it was revealed that nearby hospitals could have shared the patient burden under a more coordinated evacuation plan.

The Cocoanut Grove fire had an immediate impact on medicine and helped spur a number of innovations in burn treatment, including the first comprehensive descriptions of inhalation injury, improvements in the topical treatment of burns, resuscitation of patients in shock, and infection prevention. At the time, burn victims, especially those who underwent skin grafts, were extremely vulnerable to staphylococcal infections, and many died. Penicillin, which had been discovered in 1928 but was not used to treat humans until 1941, was still an experimental drug, expensive and difficult to procure. With the nation shocked and in mourning, the government ordered that it be made available to the doctors at MGH to treat some of the Cocoanut Grove victims. Under a police escort, the pharmaceutical firm Merck & Co. rushed thirty-two liters of medication containing penicillin from its headquarters in New Jersey to Boston. As a result, the doctors at MGH were able to save thirty-nine patients, who served in a kind of mini-clinical trial, proving the drug's efficacy.

The success of the antibiotic, along with sulfadiazine, in controlling infection in the wounds persuaded the US Surgeon General to set up a pilot study program for penicillin therapy at a Utah military hospital.

After the disastrous Allied defeat in Tunisia in February 1943, hundreds of ailing soldiers were shipped to the Utah hospital and showed immediate improvement after being treated with penicillin. As media reports of the "miracle drug" spread, the Army launched an all-out effort to increase the manufacture of penicillin, convinced it was vital to the prosecution of the war. Within six months, the antibiotic was in use in combat theaters.

Dr. Churchill, who by then had been inducted into the US Army and made chief surgical adviser in the Mediterranean Theater, decided to write about the Cocoanut Grove fire in the spring of 1943, to "rescue something constructive from the catastrophe" and ensure that the advances in burn treatment would be widely disseminated at the front. There were also many lessons to be learned from their handling of mass casualties that might apply to a military operation or accident, where they might have to deal with large numbers of injured soldiers and sailors. Alexander remembered the Harvard professor's instruction: When confronted with disaster, it was "essential to preserve an open mind." What was true in the textbooks, and under one set of conditions, might not hold true for a different situation. Observations would be fragmentary at best. Facts would be thin on the ground. Complete data would be next to impossible to obtain in combat conditions. Yet, as a doctor, he would be asked to make a barrage of decisions in a very short time.

In wartime, he counseled, "when external violence reaches epidemic proportions, one is forced to think in practical and simple terms." The bombing of Bari had been more jarring and violent than anything Alexander had encountered in the past, and he would have to draw on every ounce of his training to deal with the extraordinary challenge ahead.

———— • ◆ • ————

CHAPTER FOUR

"Journey into the Nightmare"

Stewart Alexander was up at first light, intent on beginning his reconnaissance of the harbor with as little official interference as possible. As he entered the dockyards, slowly picking his way through the mounds of rubble, he surveyed the fantastic, twisted, black-and-gray skeletal remains of the Allied convoys. It was hard to believe anyone had emerged alive from that Dantesque netherworld. The whole line of vessels berthed along the length of the outer mole must have been hit and gone up in flames, the force of the consecutive explosions taking the doomed ships down like a row of dominoes. He had been told the American Liberty ships—the wartime workhorses known affectionately as "the ugly ducklings" for their ungainly appearance—had taken the brunt of the attack. The Luftwaffe had delivered a thorough drubbing. All the dockside installations were smashed. Huge loading cranes had been toppled and lay forlornly on their sides. Warehouses, dry docks, and graving docks were in shambles.

To their credit, the British Navy and US Army engineers had already made an impressive start at cleaning up the mess, a sign of how badly they needed the harbor. Out on the mole, men were working like ants, removing jagged chunks of concrete and scrap metal. The port, which had been closed for five days and swept for mines, had partially reopened that morning. There was tremendous pressure to get the convoy traffic moving again and the flow of food and fighting equipment into the hands of the soldiers of the Eighth Army. It was a far cry from business as usual, however, and Alexander imagined the half-submerged wrecks would make navigating hazardous for weeks to come. A number of burned-out vessels had already been towed out to sea and sunk or blown apart with explosives. Any ship able to move under its own steam had been diverted to one of the nearby ports. A coal barge still smoldered on a quay close by, and the fly ash stung his nostrils.

The harbor basin was littered with an astounding amount of rubbish and debris. The oil-slimed water looked sinister, dark, and sluggish. One sailor had recalled that the floating oil had been a foot thick on the surface of the water after the raid. It was a mixture of high-octane gasoline and fuel from two dozen Allied ships and, Alexander suspected, mustard gas or a derivative, possibly dropped by the Germans among the incendiary bombs.

There was no longer any way of telling where the seventeen destroyed Allied ships, and another eight that were badly damaged, had been located in the harbor when the Luftwaffe struck. If it was an aerial gas attack, determining which ships were hit and in what order would help him understand which crews suffered the most direct exposure, as well as those on neighboring ships who might have been affected to a lesser degree. Even men not on the water would have inhaled liberal doses of the noxious vapor as it spread insidiously across the harbor—some of it sinking, some burning, some mixing with the tons of oil floating on the surface, and some evaporating and mingling with the clouds of smoke and flame. If Alexander was right, the effects on the individual men should be in direct relation to the degree of exposure experienced, and the type of exposure—namely, vapor or liquid mustard. The strength of the mustard and the length of exposure would also have had a bearing on the injuries. This would mean another confrontation with the British port commander. He would need a full briefing on the German air raid—the direction from which the enemy planes came and the type and size of the bombs dropped. He was still troubled by the fact that no gas alarm had been triggered during the attack. It was imperative to find out why the nature of the risk was not appreciated at the time so that simple protective measures could have been taken.

The Allies, fearing Hitler might wage gas warfare, had been assiduously shoring up their defenses in preparation for an attack. It was dismaying to think they had somehow been caught so off guard. Throughout the fall of 1943, the threat level had steadily ratcheted up. Alexander had received a series of classified intelligence bulletins warning not only of new warfare gases but also of the increased probability of their being introduced on the battlefield. A most secret War Office memorandum alerted Allied commanders and medical officers to the considerable risk of a novel chemical weapon: "The Germans are now known to possess an odorless gas suitable for surprise attacks by inclusion in H.E. (high explosive) bombardment from the ground or the air." Known as Substance "S," it was thought to belong to the new class of blister gases, nitrogen mustards, which were vesicant agents similar to sulfur mustard in their toxicology. The chief tactical advantage of the new gas was that when used in combination with other bombs and shells, its presence could be concealed until casualties had been produced.

"The principal danger from 'S,'" the memo emphasized, "is considered to be the undetectability of its vapor by smell before damage has been caused to the eyes and lungs." Scientists at Edgewood Arsenal and its British equivalent, Porton Down, were working frantically to develop better methods of detection for the lethal vapor. The existing vapor detector kits could be used to test for the presence of "S" but could not distinguish it from the other blister gases.

The British also passed on worrisome reports about a new liquid mustard mixture code-named "Winterlost." (The German code name for mustard was "lost," from the name of the two chemists, Lommel and Steinkopf, who suggested it could be weaponized.) Designed to be a winter gas, its formulation of 50 percent nitrogen mustard and 50 percent lewisite had a low freezing point and was specifically designed to withstand the subzero temperatures of the Russian front. It reportedly featured the best attributes of both compounds, including the immediate effects and toxicity of lewisite and the greater persistence of mustard.

In a "spray attack," the German planes would drop time-fused bombs that would burst open approximately two hundred feet above ground and release the liquid mustard, which was then transformed into droplets by the slipstream. On their travel to the ground, there would be a loss in volume of each individual droplet due to evaporation. Many factors could influence the quantity of mustard that fell on the troops below. The enemy planes could increase or decrease their elevation, which would affect the size of the droplets, or alter course according to the prevailing wind. Typically, the fine spray of droplets resembled vapor rather than liquid, except when thickened formulations were used, which allowed large droplets to form.

In mid-September, Alexander had received a G-2 memorandum apprising him of a nasty mixture of mustard in synthetic resins that the Germans were experimenting with to control the size of the droplets. Code-named "Zahlost," which, roughly translated, meant "tough mustard," the mixture was reportedly more viscous and would stick to clothing and skin. Concerned that they had no way to defend troops against the new corrosive agent, Alexander had written to Col. Rhoads, chief of the Chemical Warfare Service, requesting more information about the "thickened mustard preparations" as well as improved first-aid procedures. Captured German chemical warfare manuals still recommended removing the thickened mustard by scraping it off with the edge of a knife or some other instrument, which seemed rather primitive, and Alexander had inquired about the availability of solvents.

Contemplating the chemical stew that was now Bari Harbor, Alexander could not be sure what other chemical agents might have been thrown into the mix and might be contributing to the unusual symptoms. The Germans possessed bombs filled with phosphorous oil, which had as its main incendiaries thermite and magnesium; when the particles penetrated the skin, they continued to burn for as long as there was oxygen. It could not be extinguished by dousing with water, and it caused very deep chemical burns and eye injuries. Another possible scenario was that one of the Allied cargo ships had been carrying white phosphorous (WP) for 4.2 shells and smoke pots—used to create a dense chemical smoke screen to mask approaches and unnerve the enemy—and it was released when the vessel was hit and exploded. The Allied forces had begun using white phosphorous for screening in Tunisia, and then "full blast" during the Sicilian campaign.

He had seen a number of victims suffering from the toxic effects of the fragments, which could burn through the skin and needed to be picked out with forceps. In August, when a ship loaded with white phosphorous ammunition exploded in Algiers Harbor, one hundred phosphorous burn casualties were sustained. The individual burns presented no specialized problem, and the handful who died had received extensive thermal injuries but not the phosphorous component. The ammunition ships could likewise have been carrying the new M1A1 flamethrowers that used a gel-like substance called napalm—naphthenic palmitic acid—that generated very high temperatures and produced polystyrene, which was highly toxic. Napalm could well have ignited the intense fires that cremated so many of the ships in the harbor. However, to the best of his knowledge, its action was too violent to correspond to the burns exhibited by the Bari victims.

As part of the scope of his inquiry, Alexander would need a complete list of all the ships in the port that night and their assigned berths, as well as the secret bills of lading. He had to find out exactly what kinds of weapons and explosives the ships had been carrying in their holds before he could definitely rule out phosphorous bombs, let alone a consignment of gas. The more he thought about it, however, the more he found it hard to believe the Allies would have sent a shipment of mustard shells into a busy forward port like Bari, failed to cable in advance the requisite notification of a toxic cargo, and then allowed it to sit around for days as a prime target for an enemy strike. It was not standard practice. Moreover, it did not make any sense.

According to CWS regulations and policy, all ships carrying toxic munitions were given priority and promptly off-loaded. The volatile cargo's "nursemaid squad"—the security detachment, transportation officers, and chemical maintenance company escorting the mustard gas, specially trained in its stowage and handling—would have wanted it discharged without delay. Their task was to check the bomb casings for leaks or split seams and to guard against any signs of wear and tear from corrosion and vibration. Mustard gas bombs were notoriously unstable and needed to be tested for the buildup of pressure inside the casings and vented regularly. The ship's security officers as well as port authorities would have been keenly aware of the danger the gas posed, knowing that an accidental explosion in such a crowded harbor could have dire consequences. The whole scenario was so implausible that he put it to one side and focused his attention on the possibility of a German aerial attack.

Alexander reasoned that a surprise low-altitude spray attack using mustard would have resulted in the general contamination of the Allied ships and their crews in Bari Harbor. If repeated by a number of the German planes, it could result in 100 percent casualties of all those within range. There would have been no escape for the men below, and they would have been drenched in the deadly precipitation and received extensive burns. The mustard would have been scattered over a fairly large area, contaminating all the ships in the inner harbor, including the crippled vessels that remained afloat. It was standard procedure following an air bombardment for the dock superintendent and the port defense officer immediately to undertake a complete inspection of the harbor to ascertain whether any toxic munitions were deployed, and then to cordon off possible areas of contamination with a view to protecting the sailors as well as any ships leaving or entering the harbor.

Yet Alexander had no luck finding any evidence of mustard contamination in his survey of the dock area. No workers were out on the mole laying down lime to prevent further casualties. There were no danger signs posted warning of hazardous materials or fumes, despite the fact that mustard could remain persistent in a standing pool of water for several months. In seawater, the persistence of mustard could effectively be doubled, and it could cause serious injuries to the navy salvage crews. But the only signs on display were those proclaiming No Smoking! in English and Italian.

The Royal Navy personnel he interviewed appeared shocked at the very suggestion that poison gas might have been released in the air raid. "Mustard?" one British officer repeated in surprise, shaking his head. "That's impossible. There's no mustard here." Others, while denying any firsthand knowledge, advised that only the military port authorities could tell him whether there was poison gas in Bari. Alexander thanked them and asked to be informed should any chemical agents be dredged up during the extensive cleanup operation. He also struck out at the Allied War Shipping Administration office at the Stazione Marittima. Under strict orders to maintain secrecy, they refused to divulge any details about the Allied ships' cargo. Information about the transportation of poison gas to the war zone was so classified that Alexander could tell he would never be able to persuade them to make an exception. All his inquiries ran into the same dead end.

The British port authorities were cooperative without being helpful. They politely fielded his questions, but they were no more forthcoming than they had been the previous evening. Under questioning, the stiff-necked officials continued to "state categorically that there was no mustard in the area." If an inspection of the harbor had been carried out after the attack, they clearly had no intention of acknowledging the report's existence, let alone handing it over to an American. So much for Eisenhower's mantra about Allied "unity of purpose."

This time, however, Alexander was not as easily deterred. He decided he could be just as stubborn and bloody-minded as the Brits. Digging in his heels, he once again insisted that in order to make the correct diagnosis and treat the hundreds of contaminated personnel, he needed their fullest possible cooperation. Their answers strained credulity. As he would later note in his report, barely managing to suppress his sarcasm, "It is imperative that guidance and assistance be immediately given the medical officer dealing with the casualties, as the nature of the disaster must be known to proceed intelligently."

Desperate to prod the port authorities into action, he described in detail the ghastly burns he had seen at the 98th General Hospital, and he put it to them that there was no way those injuries could have been incurred other than by chemical exposure. Of the 534 men admitted to the Allied hospitals following the December 2 attack, 281 were found to be suffering from symptoms consistent with some form of mustard poisoning. By that day's count, forty-five had died. More men were being hospitalized with symptoms of contamination every day. Many more fatalities could be expected if they did not receive proper treatment urgently. Every additional hour of delay was causing unnecessary pain and suffering. The vast majority of the victims were British—their own countrymen. If they wanted that on their heads, so be it.

Faced with this sobering assessment, the British authorities began to waver. As Alexander continued to press for answers, they hedged and allowed that if mustard gas was present in the harbor, "it could only have come from the German planes."

Momentarily wrong-footed by this sudden change of tack, Alexander paused to consider the ramifications of the charge that Hitler, in a last desperate gamble, had decided to risk a gas offensive. But coming as it did after a string of firm denials of so much as a whiff of mustard in Bari, it seemed to him to be an altogether too-facile explanation for what had happened, which he now believed was more complicated. It did not take great perspicacity or insight on his part to realize the British, for reasons of their own, were intent on managing his investigation. He had the growing sense that they were endeavoring to cover up mistakes under the guise of military security. While he was in no position to accuse them outright of dissembling or hindering his investigation, he was convinced the withholding of valuable information meant men who might otherwise have been saved were dead and dying still.

Against this certainty, Alexander felt compelled to persevere in his quest to identify the chemical agent and its source, regardless of the official toes he stepped on along the way. In the interest of expediency, and to avoid dissension from becoming a further drag on his inquiry, he agreed that a German gas attack was a possibility. He asked for a diver to be sent down to search the harbor bottom for evidence of German mustard bombs. In order to further substantiate this theory, he also requested the assistance of the port authorities in drawing up a berthing plan that would depict the anchorages of all the ships in Bari Harbor on the night of the raid. He understood it might be an unorthodox request, but it was the only way he could cross-reference the ship positions with the reported casualties and then begin to understand how the mustard gas had been dispersed. It was admittedly a long shot, but worth a try.

What he was thinking, but did not mention, was that if the casualty chart revealed that a predominant number of deaths occurred in and around a single ship, it would support the theory that the source of all the trouble was a toxic cargo of Allied, not German, origin. He would have to cross that bridge when he came to it. He could only hope the berthing chart would help shed light on what happened in the harbor that night. The British officials reluctantly agreed to his proposal and promised to see what they could do.

WITH HIS INVESTIGATION of the harbor temporarily stymied, Alexander returned to the office he had been allocated at the 98th General Hospital. Waiting for him on his desk were the results of the chemical analyses of the harbor waters he had requested the previous day. The tests showed "no trace of mustard." He was disappointed, but not altogether surprised. The fact that the samples, taken so long after the incident, contained no mustard did not necessarily discredit his hypothesis. The mustard could still have been present in the layer of oil on the water's surface for the crucial time period immediately following the attack, when the men had been forced to jump overboard and swim to safety, or tread water while waiting to be rescued. Later, most of the mustard would have been consumed in the raging fire, which reportedly continued to burn on the oily surface of parts of the harbor for another thirty-six hours. Any remaining traces would have eventually dissolved from the oil into the sea, sunk to the bottom, and been broken down by hydrolysis. The tests results, therefore, were inconclusive.

The optimal time for obtaining information in any investigation was in the first twenty-four hours, not several days removed. Most of the evidence was gone or muddled beyond recognition. Alexander was frustrated by his slow progress, but brooding about the precious wasted hours would get him nowhere. With little else to go on, he had no choice but to try to piece together the missing details of the disaster. "To understand the type of trauma involved," he wrote, "it is necessary to discern and delineate the pattern of the casualties as they are occurring. By appraising the nature and volume of the physical and chemical forces applied, the time intervals, and the clinical features and complications as they present themselves, it is possible to sketch the general pattern of the disaster early in the chronology." That was the principal lesson of the Cocoanut Grove fire. Only when the "pattern had been made clear" would he be able to identify who and what was responsible for the mysterious deaths, and then to render the appropriate care for the remaining victims.

He spent the rest of that day, and all of the next, focused on the medical aspects of the investigation. "Reading the reports," he wrote, "is to take a journey into the nightmare of the effects of chemical contamination."

The preliminary postmortem results seemed to confirm his belief that the culprit was a classic blister gas or vesicant, most likely mustard. From his training, Alexander knew that blister gases not only affected the skin, they also had ophthalmological and systemic effects when the vapor or liquid reached the eyes, lungs, or gastrointestinal tract. But systemic effects could manifest by absorption from the skin alone. The human skin is one of the largest organs and is intimately connected with all the other organs, functions, and structures in the human body, and vice versa. The skin and its appendages—hair, nails, sweat, and sebaceous glands—are buffers between the outer world and inner organs, and as a heat-regulating and excretory organ, the skin seeks to protect the body from the onslaughts of the environment. Any toxic agent acting primarily on the epidermis would, therefore, result in delayed clinical signs, cause little or no pain, and present no vascular responses such as redness and swelling (erythema and edema) until later, as was the case with the baffling Bari victims.

The typical epidermal response to irritation was intra- and intercellular edema. If the toxic agent exerted a great effect, the accumulation of fluid between the cells in the intercellular spaces increased and dilated, which could then be detected under microscopic examination. The tissue became waterlogged (spongiotic), and the accumulation of fluid resulted in rupture of the intercellular bridges and fusion of adjacent spaces in the tiny blisters (vesicles), and the fusion of the small vesicles in the formation of large blisters (bullae). If the absorption of the agent allowed it to penetrate the epidermis, causing blistering on its passage, and reached the cutis—consisting mainly of fibrous connective tissue, nerves, blood vessels—it would then result in erythema, edema, nerve injury, induration (hardening), and sensory disturbances.

These were the symptoms and pathology he bore in mind as he studied the case of Seaman Phillip Henry Stone, the young patient who had abruptly died after asking for a drink. His case was of special interest because the doctors had pointed to him as an example of one of the inexplicable "early deaths." The pathologist noted:

> A generalized dusky erythema was seen over anterior chest, abdomen and thighs. The back also displayed this phenomenon but to a lesser degree. A number of large bullae of irregular outline and many smaller vesicles were present on the face, ears, arms, back and external genitalia. The penis was much swollen.... It was observed that the epidermis was easily dislodged on handling the body, the underlying cutis being of livid pink with visible engorgement of the papillae. The lips were dull black in color.

When the chest was opened, the pathologist noted that the esophagus displayed a "curious black longitudinal streaking," probably due to dead cells and tissue (necrosis) and the presence of altered blood. The lungs were very congested and a mottled blackish-red color when sectioned, the bronchi were filled with pus, and the trachea engorged with abnormal accumulation of fluid in the tissue—all signs of chemical irritation. The stomach showed the same black areas, and there were necrotic areas near the opening, most likely caused by swallowing a diluted solution of mustard mixed with oil.

Another case of this early type of death was that of Seaman Stoker McLaughlin, who died two days after the attack of the acute systemic effects of the mustard burns. Casting an eye rapidly down his clinical sheet, Alexander saw that the report also described the "lack of response to the usual methods of resuscitation":

2 Dec 43	Admitted smothered in oil. (1) Swelling of upper lip. (2) Dirty laceration of (Rt.) foot. (3) Shock, Vesication of skin of arms and neck. Conjunctiva injected. 1030 hours B.P. 90/70
	Plasma drip started: 1145 hours I (Unit)
	1330 hours II (Unit)
	1630 hours III (Unit)
	Dangerously Ill List.
3 Dec 43	1800 hours. Under morphia, blisters of neck, arms, chest, back, and both legs aspirated and dusted with sulfanilamide and dressed with dry gauze. Plasma drip continued. B.P. 108/80. Pulse fast 110/mins.
4 Dec 43	Very restless. Sl. cyanosis. Pulse weak. Chest—few moist sounds. 1200 hours cyanosis. Oxygen tried but cannot retain mask. Delirious, very restless. Unrelieved by morphia. 2100 hours, died.

The pathologist reported the striking observation that the surface of the body failed to show the usual appearance of postmortem lividity, the bluish color that sets in as the blood vessels begin to break down after death. The epidermis was deficient and in many parts of the body could be rubbed off except on the face and the ends of the extremities. The skin underneath was pink, and, after the removal of the epidermis, looked like "living tissue." There was practically the identical gross edema and vesiculation of the penis as that of Seaman Stone. When the body was opened, there were similar observations: The tongue was swollen at the base, and both the trachea and the esophagus were markedly congested. On section, the lungs showed an intense hyperemia, a deep-red fleshy color, yet the cut section was relatively dry and only a slight froth could be expressed from the cut bronchiole. Alexander was more convinced than ever that he was correct in his diagnosis of mustard gas exposure, demonstrated by the absence of postmortem lividity, extensive blisters covering the men's bodies, and internal damage to their respiratory tract.

After reading through a thick stack of autopsy reports of the deaths that occurred in the first three days, he concluded that most were due to the effects of total-body-surface burns, and to associated blast injury from the explosion. He summarized the gross findings in the lungs:

It would appear that there were two definite types of pathology. There were the irritative surface damaging effects of inhaled mustard which followed the bronchial tree distribution and were followed by secondary descending pulmonary infection. At the same time, there were present in the lungs the results of direct trauma sustained on the night of the explosions. The frank and clinically recognized blast injuries died shortly after injury or at least within 48 hours. The lung trauma seen in so many of these cases was of a type and degree that would not, in itself, have killed the individual. Were it not for other factors, the individuals would have recovered from the small hemorrhages and larger bruises sustained by their lungs. ... The serious consequences of imposing the mustard vapor injury upon a lung partially damaged or bruised by blast is at once apparent.

Before drawing his conclusions, Alexander removed from the pile of autopsies all the cases showing blast injuries to be the prime factor in the cause of death and placed them in a separate stack he designated as "Blast Deaths." The remaining cases showed blast damage to the lungs that by itself would not have been fatal, but, when combined with doses of mustard vapor, resulted in death. The doctors would have had no way of knowing about the existence of these sublethal blast injuries—such as lung bruises and interstitial hemorrhages—except by X-ray or perhaps by very careful physical examination, and they were only revealed in the pathology reports because the individuals died of other causes.

The striking feature in this group of patients was the severity of the systemic effects and the physiological changes leading to death. The initial changes in blood pressure and pulse might be explained by the total or subtotal body-surface burns. Burns of this extent would produce tremendous changes and death regardless of the causative agent. But the temporary rise in systolic tension above normal levels after the third day, and its later recession, indicated some "grave derangement" of peripheral blood-pressure control. "The systemic effects, and evidence of systemic toxemia, were more marked," Alexander wrote in his summary of the findings, "and more significant than usually expected from mustard." This would need to be explored further before he could form a definite opinion as to why. To learn more about the systemic effects, he needed to see more blood levels and bone-marrow tests. The liver and kidney changes would also be telling, but he would have to await the microscopic studies for that analysis.

Based on the lung and skin phenomena, there was no doubt in his mind that the victims were suffering from mustard exposure. From what he had seen in the preliminary reports, the causes of death could be divided basically into two categories: those associated with severe external chemical burns, and those caused by internal damage due to ingestion or inhalation of mustard. The vapor pressure of liquid mustard was fairly high, and gaseous mustard was given off at normal temperatures, which meant the oil-covered survivors pulled out of the harbor and wrapped in blankets were continuously inhaling mustard. Of this much he was certain.

The following day, Alexander conducted a second rapid study of the harbor. Looking over the notes of his interviews with survivors and their accounts of how they sustained their injuries, he felt increasingly dissatisfied with the British port authorities' latest explanation of events. Using hospital records, he began checking which ships the mustard-contaminated victims had served on. It involved a great deal of laborious research as he discovered the hard way that the Merchant Marine did not keep good records. The merchant ships were not naval vessels, and the crews, mostly composed of civilian volunteers of various nationalities, seemed to disembark or get discharged and paid off with some frequency. It took some doing to figure out who was who and which ship they had been on. The Navy's records were in considerably better order, and he had a much easier time tracing the Armed Guards, usually a contingent of twenty-eight, who served on the boats as gunners and signalmen.

The more he learned, however, the more it made "a German airborne delivery most unlikely." He simply did not see how the Ju-88s could have dropped enough gas to inflict the kinds of injuries he was seeing. He had no choice but to carefully question the British authorities again. "Everyone, including the Post Commander," he later wrote, "denied the presence of American or British mustard gas."

ALEXANDER WAS STILL TRYING TO DECIDE how best to proceed, given the official resistance to his diagnosis, when he received stunning news. A diver searching the harbor floor had found some fractured gas shells. Tests performed on-site revealed traces of mustard. Ordnance officers from the Fifteenth Air Force were immediately called in and identified the casings as being from a 100-pound American M47A2 mustard gas bomb. German mustard gas bombs were always marked with the distinctive Gelb Kreuz, or yellow cross. It was definitely American.

Alexander's first thought was that his instincts had been right—an Allied ship had been carrying a cargo of mustard gas. The shipment had most likely been destined for the chemical stockpile nearby at Foggia, the new home base of the Fifteenth Air Force. In order to improve the US capability to retaliate, the War Department had approved an increase in the amounts of chemical munitions in forward areas and ordered the gas sent to Italy. If the need arose, Doolittle's boys would have dropped the mustard bombs.

As he knew from his training at Edgewood, the M47 was a simple sheet-metal bomb approximately four feet long and eight inches in diameter. It was designed to hold white phosphorous or liquid sulfur mustard. Since it went into use in the late 1930s, there had been many problems associated with the M47A1, including that its very thin casing was prone to leaking and was easily ruptured. The M47A2 model was specifically designed to address these problems, and it was coated inside with a special oil to protect it from the corrosion caused by the mustard agent. But the bombs were still fragile. They would have been blown to pieces in the German bombardment, releasing the lethal mustard into the atmosphere and the oily harbor water.

Alexander found it hard to believe that this was the first time the British officials were learning of the chemical weapons. It remained to be seen whether or not the port commandant or his superiors had known about the presence of the mustard gas from the very beginning, or were unaware of its existence until later, because the ship's crew, along with the custodial officers supervising the movement of the chemical weapons, were all killed in the raid. The circumstances of the tragic accident—because that was what he was now dealing with—would need further investigating. The extent to which the responsible authorities, naval and military, had tried to cover up the escaped gas rather than alert hospital staff to the risk of contamination—thereby exacerbating the injuries and greatly adding to the number of fatalities—would also need to be explored. Alexander would need specific answers to those questions and more.

At that moment, however, his patients took precedence.

Now that his suspicions had been confirmed, Alexander advised the medical staffs in all the Allied hospitals on the proper treatment for mustard exposure. He could now prescribe more specific therapies and thus try to reduce the number of daily deaths. To his dismay, however, some of the British medical staff seemed hesitant to follow his recommendations. They appeared to be waiting for his diagnosis to receive the required official stamp of approval. While he could not fault their conduct or dedication, he worried that their lack of confidence in him might detract from their prompt performance of some of the measures he wanted instituted. He was further hampered by the fact that each Allied hospital in Bari had its own staff and its own way of doing things, so it was difficult to coordinate the medical care and standardize the gas therapy procedures, especially when none seemed very effective.

The task of treating a condition that was foreign to doctors and nurses alike presented innumerable difficulties; in many instances, the best form of treatment was not immediately clear. As no remedy appeared "sufficiently superior to the others to merit specific approval," Alexander realized they had no choice but to go beyond the practiced theories of peacetime and experiment. He kept a running list of the different methods and combinations of treatment:

No dressings—covered with protecting cradle but no local
    therapy used
Starch or talc powder dressing only
Vaseline dressing over Acriflavine (topical antiseptic)
Acriflavine 1–10000 dressing

Sulfanilamide powder dressing
Calamine lotion painting
Dry sterile dressings
Sulfadiazine ointment
Tannic acid locally
Vaseline gauze dressing
Warm saline baths
Vaseline dressing
Ensol dressings
Triple dye

The great majority of patients suffered lesions from both vapor and liquid mustard. As a rule, the more extensive lesions were found on the more seriously ill patients: Fifty-eight patients were recorded as having erythema (redness) involving half or more of their body; eleven had blistering to the same degree. By the end of the first week, the erythema began to subside and the skin peeled off in silvery-gray flakes, revealing new, healthy skin beneath. A few days later, the skin of the blister cases began to slough off, but it left very raw, red areas that were extremely tender and subsequently healed very slowly. Alexander quickly discovered that the conventional teaching of treating blisters contained in the *Manual of Chemical Warfare* was highly impractical, as they were continually ruptured by the patients' movement and torn loose. Seeing this, he ordered the remaining blisters to be punctured and drained, with the outer layer or roof of the blister left intact under a sterile dressing. Dry dusting powders relieved the discomfort in many of the superficial open lesions. Sulfanilamide powder was used to prevent local infection, but when the staff ran short of it, talc proved just as good. About fifty cases were treated with amyl salicylate, but this drug was in very short supply, so it was used sparingly and reserved for fairly circumscribed liquid mustard burns. In any event, it did not appear to heal obstinate lesions any faster.

The simplest treatments proved to be the best. They demanded the least attention from the nurses and caused the patients the least discomfort. After several days of trial and error, the "treatment of choice" for most victims was the slitting of blisters and expressing of the contained fluid, followed by thorough dusting of the entire area with sulfanilamide powder and the application of dry sterile gauze. This method had the added benefit that the dressings were left untouched as long as possible. For a while, this provided adequate protection, but as the lesions dried, the bandages adhered to the wounds and became extremely painful, forcing the staff to try something else.

They tried wrapping the victims in gauze coated with petroleum jelly, one of the innovations in burn treatment that came out of the Cocoanut Grove disaster. It proved to be more satisfactory, but large quantities of Vaseline were necessary to create dressings for the more extensive burn cases, and heavily slathered patients could be difficult to manipulate. When the skin became itchy and irritated, they relied on an application of calamine lotion. In some cases, they used cod liver oil. In one hospital, they sprayed tannic acid solution over the widely burned victims, which hardened the skin and was believed to keep out infectious organisms; in another hospital, triple dye was used on another small group of casualties. On review, Alexander found these cases fared, if anything, "a bit more poorly," and he ordered the treatments discontinued. Unfortunately, a combat hospital was not a laboratory, and Alexander was unable to report on the efficacy of any of these drugs or treatments because they were too rushed to do comparison studies.

Caring for the casualties who were extensively burned presented the biggest challenge. "A casualty with burns approaching full body area in extent required the almost full time attention of one nurse or corpsman," Alexander noted, "and this was quite impossible." The patients required prodigious amounts of nursing in an attempt to maintain even relative cleanliness. The staff found that warm saline baths facilitated the removal of bandages and were especially helpful in relieving the excruciating pain suffered by those with serious burns to the groin and genital region. Cleansing with saline, Acriflavine, or Ensol solution was done between dressings.

Patients with burned and irritated upper respiratory tracts were pre-scribed prophylactic sulfanilamide therapy, but in many cases the treat-ment was not begun soon enough. The hospitals experimented with a variety of local symptomatic aids, but patients continued to deteriorate, and Alexander was forced to acknowledge that the available treatments had met with "a minimum of success." Nose drops, gargles, and mouth-washes offered only a modicum of relief. Inhalation of steam and a compound tincture of benzoin had "relatively little effect" on upper respiratory-tract lesions, tracheitis and bronchitis. When symptoms of lower respiratory-tract infection developed, sulfadiazine therapy was increased, fluids were forced, and oxygen therapy was started, but it was not clear how much this helped. The severity of the burns in many of these cases presented a considerable nursing challenge. Patients cried out in agony as fluids were forced down raw, painful throats, and pro-viding adequate nourishment was a constant problem.

On the whole, the treatment of the respiratory-tract lesions was "most discouraging," Alexander noted wearily. "Another way of stating this observation would be to say that some of the men continued to die very early in the course of their pneumonia."

INSTEAD OF BRINGING MATTERS to a close, Alexander's discovery that the mustard gas had come from the "Allies' own supply" made a dif-ficult job that much more complicated. The diplomatic tensions he had been keenly aware of since his arrival in Bari had burgeoned into a full-blown crisis. The twenty-nine-year-old doctor realized that the poison gas disaster was of "frightful international import"—all the more so because it was, at least in part, a self-inflicted wound. The British authorities' attempts to obfuscate and possibly conceal evidence rankled, but that paled in importance compared to their effort to shift responsibility for the chemical casualties to the Luftwaffe. It was not a harmless fabrication. "If they were going to accuse the Germans of dropping mustard when the Germans had not. . . ." He shuddered to think of the "grave political implications."

In the spring of 1943, President Roosevelt had issued a stern warning that any use of chemical weapons would be followed by the "fullest possible retaliation." That phrase kept returning to nag him now. "The political significance, as well as the military significance, of any error in interpreting the factor of and source of mustard gas in Bari was," he knew, "horrendous." It could potentially lead to widespread chemical warfare if the Allies drew the faulty conclusion that the enemy had deployed chemical weapons. It also placed him, as the sole advocate of the truth, in a terrible position. The situation was indeed alarming.

Adding to his anxiety, the daily death toll from mustard contamination, which had started to decline by the end of the first week, suddenly spiked again on Friday, December 10. By the time he left the hospital that evening, nine men had died in one twenty-four-hour period. This second peak in the death curve—the first came on the third day—demonstrated the secondary effects of pneumonia imposed upon patients already weakened by chemical exposure. The hardest thing for the hospital staff to accept was the fact that the number of deaths was increasing, even though he had diagnosed the toxic agent as mustard gas and arranged for the patients to receive proper treatment. There was no way to predict how many more men would die, or the final scope of the disaster.

Alexander felt he had to inform AFHQ as soon as possible. He wired Gen. Blesse in Algiers, giving him the initial findings of his medical investigation. His memorandum, written nine days after the bombing, was brief and to the point:

T.C.C. 1215 hrs

The burns in the hospitals in this area labeled "dermatitis n.y.d." are due to mustard gas. They are unusual types and varieties because most of them are due to mustard which has been mixed into the surface oil in the harbour.

There are three factors to be considered in apprais-ing the deaths that have occurred in the group:

(1) Blast injury
(2) Immersion and exposure
(3) Mustard poisoning

In the majority of the cases i believe the mustard poisoning is the most important factor.

There are still many cases seriously ill, some of whom i am sure will die.

(sgd.) STEWART F. ALEXANDER

Lt-Colonel, M.C.,

Consultant.

11 DEC 43.

By the end of that day, another nine men had died.

With a growing sense of urgency that he needed to set the record straight and have his diagnosis approved at the highest levels, Alexander sent high-priority cables to both the president and the prime minister, informing them of the nature of the casualties at Bari and the almost certain origin of the mustard gas on an American Liberty ship. Since he had met both leaders at the Casablanca Conference, he felt this was the best course of action, given the extraordinary circumstances. Because the messages were sent through channels, Alexander expected no reply, so he was surprised and relieved when Roosevelt appeared to accept his findings and responded: "Please keep me fully informed."

Churchill, however, was unimpressed with his medical detective work. Alexander was informed that the prime minister had sent a terse reply to the effect that "your man in the field must have made a mistake," and that he did not believe there was mustard gas in Bari. He reportedly asked that the situation be reevaluated.

Alexander was speechless. He felt the color rise in his cheeks and privately cursed the fair skin that made him so transparent. He recovered his composure sufficiently to express his astonishment and loudly protest that he had "proof," but he quickly saw there was no point in arguing with the messenger. He could not fathom the logic of continuing to officially deny what had happened in the face of such overwhelming evidence. It was impossible to tell at such a remove whether Churchill and/or his advisers failed to appreciate the magnitude of the disaster or refused to do so.

Alexander admired Churchill and thought he was a great military and political leader. In spite of his own indignation, Alexander understood that Europe was far more vulnerable to a gas attack than America. Churchill's overriding concern, he knew, was that "we not acknowledge we had poison gas in that theater of operation because if the Germans retaliated they would be dropping poison gas on England." While not questioning the wisdom of this command decision, he felt at the same time that, in the midst of a chemical disaster, Churchill should yield to the "scientist on the ground." Instead, Churchill's ongoing opposition was undermining Alexander's credibility and ability to do his job. The British medical personnel in Bari were not going to follow his lead confidently unless they knew it had been approved in London. The question was, What to do?

Hoping to clear up any misunderstanding, Alexander sent a second telegram, citing his medical findings at much greater length and stating, "beyond any doubt," that these casualties were due to mustard exposure. In due course, Alexander was informed that Churchill still maintained that "the symptoms do not sound like mustard gas," and there must be some mistake, as he had "seen many mustard casualties in World War I and they did not in any way resemble the present casualties or situation." His instructions were the same: "The doctor should reexamine his patients."

Alexander was flummoxed. He was not sure what to make of the "strange exchange of messages"—or precisely how a "lowly, lonely American medical officer" was supposed to respond to a challenge to his expertise in the field from the indomitable British war leader. When he appealed to the liaison officer for advice, the man coolly advised him: One did not argue with the Prime Minister.

———·◆·———

CHAPTER FIVE

"A Special Affinity"

After a sleepless night, Alexander returned early to the 98th General Hospital determined to prove there had been no mistake about his diagnosis of mustard gas poisoning. Churchill was undoubtedly a brilliant man, with an uncanny instinct for the salient fact, and he had put his finger on the most important question about the Bari victims: Why were the toxic effects manifest in this group of mustard casualties so much more profound than any other recorded in military history? Why were these symptoms so unique they went unrecognized—first by the Allied doctors and then by Churchill himself? According to Alexander's calculations, far more patients were dying of mustard-induced symptoms at Bari than on the battlefields of World War I, when the fatality rate had been around two percent among those hospitalized with gas injuries. The death rate in Bari was many times higher—with close to 13 percent of the casualties proving fatal. And before it was all over, it would climb even higher.

The difference, he believed, was that this was an entirely different order of mustard exposure than the asphyxia that brought British soldiers to their knees at Ypres. In the Bari disaster, relatively few men suffered gas inhalation alone, so the massive pulmonary congestion characteristic of victims of the last war was only "minimally present." Moreover, in the past it had always been assumed that there was an insignificant amount of systemic poisoning after simple exposure to mustard splash or vapor. What was unusual about the Bari victims was the amount of mustard absorbed through the skin from the unprecedented, intimate, and lengthy contact as a result of being immersed in the oily harbor water. "In this group of cases," Alexander postulated, "the individuals, to all intents and purposes, were dipped into a solution of mustard-in-oil, and then wrapped in blankets, given warm tea, and allowed a prolonged period for absorption." It was these almost optimum conditions that permitted such "significant exposures" and penetration by the mustard molecules. No doctors or medical researchers had ever before encountered such an extraordinary level of mustard gas toxicity. Thus the systemic effects of the mustard could be seen clearly for the first time.

As he sat there reviewing the British doctors' medical case sheets and pathology reports that morning, seeing again the toxin's devastating impact on the bodies, one recurring observation leapt out at him: the effects on the patients' white blood cells. He flipped rapidly through a thick stack of records, checking the blood counts. There it was again and again—the white blood cell counts fell off sharply. What he was looking at made the hair on the back of his neck stand on end. Alexander had seen these exact results before, but never in human beings.

He slowed down and carefully went back over the results of dozens of blood tests. Then he double-checked the clinical sheets. He started making notes based on the relevant cases: "The effect upon the white blood cells in the circulating blood was most severe," he jotted on a pad. When admitted, many of the Bari victims had a marked hemoconcentration, a reduced blood volume often associated with hemorrhage due to blast injuries. It was reflected in the loss of fluid into the skin and subcutaneous tissue. In the severe cases, hemoglobin determinations of 135 percent to 140 percent were not uncommon and were associated with red blood cell counts in the normal six million range. At the same time, the white blood cell count tended to be in the range of 9,000 to 11,000 per cubic millimeter. In the patients who recovered, the hemoconcentration was corrected by the second or third day. But in some cases, beginning on the third or fourth day, the white blood cell count began to drop:

Observations thereafter traced a steep downward trend. White blood cell counts of 100 cells per cubic millimeter or below were recorded. The lymphocytes [white blood cells found in the lymph organs and of importance to the immune system] were the first to disappear. The granulocytes [the most numerous type of white blood cells, which are important mediators of the inflammatory response] were just as severely affected, but were a day or so behind the lymphocytes in demonstrating their sharp fall. All cases did not demonstrate this fall in white blood cell counts, but all casualties with an extremely low count died.

Alexander was riveted by the case notes. He was convinced that what he was seeing in the Bari victims was the very thing he had witnessed in laboratory experiments with rabbits at Edgewood Arsenal before the research project was shut down as "not beneficial" to the war effort. "It all added up to the same conditions I had seen in my prewar animal work," he later recalled. "Blood cells disappeared, and lymph nodes just melted away." He immediately saw the possible connection to cancer, a disease characterized by abnormal, unrestrained cell growth. Since mustard appeared to suppress white cell division, Alexander reasoned it might also slow the rate of division of cancer cells in relentlessly progressive carcinomas. He remembered thinking, "If mustard could do this, what could it do for a person with leukemia or lymphosarcoma?"

He closed his eyes, recalling the overwhelming sense of frustration he had felt when ordered to abandon his Edgewood research into mustard's medical potential to focus on its combat use. It had been in March of 1942, only a few months after Pearl Harbor, when the country's entry into the conflict had ratcheted up the pressure on the laboratory to prepare for the possibility of gas retaliation. At the time, they knew through intelligence sources that the Germans were stockpiling large quantities of new chemical agents. Edgewood had just received two classified samples of unknown chemical warfare agents that had been smuggled out of Germany at great risk. Dr. Howard Skipper, head of the Medical Research Laboratory's toxicology section, immediately tested the samples and identified the compounds as highly potent blister agents. He went on to break them down and determine their chemical composition. He found that they were amines, a relatively simple compound containing one or more halogen atoms attached to nitrogen, and that each had a beta-chloraethyl radical attached. One had two radicals and the other had three: dichloro-diethyl-amine and trichloro-triethyl-amine. Because their chemical structure

$$
\begin{array}{c}
\text{H} \\
\text{H} \mid \text{H} \\
\backslash \; / \\
\text{H H C H H} \\
\mid \; \mid \; \mid \; \mid \; \mid \\
\text{CI-C-C-N-C-C-CI} \\
\mid \; \mid \quad \mid \; \mid \\
\text{H H} \quad \text{H H}
\end{array}
$$

closely resembled the structure of sulfur mustard gas

$$
\begin{array}{c}
\text{H H} \quad \text{H H} \\
\mid \; \mid \quad \mid \; \mid \\
\text{CI-C-C-S-C-C-CI} \\
\mid \; \mid \quad \mid \; \mid \\
\text{H H} \quad \text{H H}
\end{array}
$$

the Edgewood scientists proposed calling them nitrogen mustards. For security purposes, the German samples were assigned the arbitrary code names 1060 and 1130. They were then turned over to Alexander, head of the Medical Research Laboratory, to study what the new German gas could do to humans.

Alexander and his colleagues immediately initiated detailed experimental protocols to determine the toxic agents' mode of action on all the organs of the body. The first tests were performed on rabbits, which were considered a good experimental proxy for human studies. The rabbits were burned or gassed with lethal applications of compound 1130, permitting study of the toxic agents' action on the animals' skin, eyes, and respiratory tract. The results were very much in line with sulfur mustards and what was expected from this kind of vesicant.

They then set up an experiment to determine the effects of 1130 on the hematological system, the blood and blood-forming organs. A selection of twenty rabbits was made at the time the stock animals were delivered, and after a week of being maintained on a regular diet, only the healthiest and best nourished were used. Blood samples were taken daily until thirty-six hours before the experiment. All the hematological data collected during this control period were compared to data previously established on animals chosen at random from typical stock, and any animals not falling within the normal distribution of total white blood cell count and differential white blood cell count were discarded. In this way, the "normalcy" of the group of test rabbits could be assured. The rabbits were then depilated, their hair removed from around the ears and abdomen, and exposed to lethal doses of 1130. The report described the results:

> The changes in the hematological system were found to be most severe within four days following gassing or burning. During this period the white blood count, absolute numbers of granular and non-granular cells were decreased severely in both the gassed and burned animals. . . .
>
> While the mortality rate for both gassed and burned animals

was about the same, the white cells of the gassed animals were affected more quickly and the white cells of the burned animals were affected more severely.

To the research team's astonishment, a strange thing happened to the white blood cell count of the rabbits—it dropped to zero or points very close to zero. No one at the lab had ever seen such rapid destruction of white blood cells and the accompanying deterioration of lymph nodes and bone marrow. They consulted the literature and found no reports of the same kind of rapid leucopenia, the reduction of white cells in the blood, or, for that matter, anything that had the same effect. At the time, Alexander's first thought was that they must have had a "bad batch of rabbits." But when they repeated the experiment with a new group of rabbits, the results were exactly the same.

The observations were so shocking that he ordered the tests to be repeated with various other laboratory animals to rule out the possibility of poor animal stock or species sensitivity. They tried guinea pigs, rats, mice, and goats. Each time, they achieved the same dramatic effects: Sudden, severe leucopenia, severe lymphopenia, reduction of reticulocytes, lymph node depletion, and marrow depression were constant, repetitive findings. After exposure to the toxic agents, the white blood cell count rapidly disappeared completely, and the lymph nodes were almost completely dissolved and left as "shrunken little shells" of what they had been before. Alexander and his colleagues went back and performed the same tests on the hematologic system using sulfur mustard gas, but they were unable to reproduce the changes in the white blood cell count they had seen with the nitrogen mustards.

Alexander was fascinated by the idea that mustard was a chemical agent that interfered with the body's mechanism for producing blood cells, especially white blood cells. Because of the dramatic and reproducible effects, he could not help but wonder about the possibility of using the compounds directly or in modified forms on human beings with diseases of the blood. He recognized that if nitrogen mustard attacked white blood cells, perhaps it could be used to help control the form of cancer known as leukemia, with its unrestrained white blood cell growth, by using different dosages to destroy some but not all of the excess cells without annihilating the patient. When he proposed an ambitious new set of experiments, he was told first by his chief, and then, on appeal, by the National Research Council, that this was not the remit of the Edgewood laboratory. There was not enough time or money to pursue collateral lines of investigation that did not facilitate the national defense. He was ordered to put the project aside and return to his work on methods of mustard casualty management, treatment, and decontamination. Chasing miracle cures was something that would have to wait until after the war.

Alexander's nitrogen mustard experiments, conducted under the highest military security, were begun on April 13, 1942, and completed two months later. Their original research was published on June 30, 1942, as Medical Division Edgewood Arsenal MD (EA) Memorandum Report 59, *Preliminary Report on Hematological Changes in the Rabbit Following Exposure to Lethal Doses of 1130*. The report was signed by Alexander, who supervised the work, and the five men who participated in the research: T. W. Kethley and C. B. Marquand, the authors, as well as O. E. McElroy, B. P. McNamara, and G. A. Neville. Twenty-one copies of the classified report were printed and distributed to leading scientists and investigators working under the auspices of the National Defense Research Council. It was one of a series of research papers published over the following few months dealing with the lethal effects of compound 1130.

Alexander waited impatiently for a response. He was hoping to win support for his recommendations that further studies should be done to evaluate the application of these compounds in the treatment of leukemia or lymphosarcoma. But he heard nothing—no comment, no advice. Not a word.

ALEXANDER'S PARADOXICAL SUGGESTION that a poison could have curative properties was hardly new. Every age had its alchemists and everyone its cancer elixir. Arsenic was the first medicinal double-edged sword, used for centuries both as a poison and as a treatment for ulcerating lesions. The Ancient Greeks, Egyptians, and Chinese all experimented with potions for tumors, including herbs, plants, and salts of heavy metals—mercury, lead, iron, copper, and gold—resulting in a vast array of remedies, many of them ineffectual at best and deleterious at worst. The most controversial of these so-called cures was probably the one put forth by Anton Storck, a Viennese physician, who claimed in a medical essay in 1762 that his hemlock extract was highly effective against breast and uterine cancers. Despite widespread skepticism, however, various hemlock concoctions remained in use for decades. Faced with so many quacks and false claims, many doctors became resigned to the view of the French surgeon Bernard Peyrilhe, the first to treat breast cancer by radical mastectomy, who wrote in 1776 that the long search for a chemical agent to treat cancer was not only in vain but absurd: Such was the similarity between normal and malignant tissue that any agent damaging to one was bound to damage the other.

By the turn of the nineteenth century, advances in the basic sciences were gaining momentum, and chemists produced a whole range of new substances to investigate. In 1898, a German biochemist named Paul Ehrlich embarked on a quest to isolate a toxin that, when injected, would activate "antitoxins" or antibodies that in turn would immunize the individual against subsequent invasions by the infectious-disease-causing microbe. He began by experimenting with various fabric dyes to stain animal tissue, and, after noting their selectivity—for specific organs, tissues, and cells—started testing the chemicals to determine their therapeutic value. After a bout with tuberculosis, he focused his attention on bacterial toxins and learned how to develop high-grade blood serums extracted from immunized animals, in the process perfecting a serum against the diphtheria toxin from the blood of horses.

Recognizing the limitations of serum therapy for diseases for which no antitoxins could be found, Ehrlich started experimenting with synthesizing new chemicals, or "chemotherapies," that could kill parasites or arrest their growth without damaging the organism. He eventually hit on a ruby-colored chemical dye, trypan red, which proved effective against the parasites that caused trypanosomiasis, the so-called sleeping sickness in horses. He followed up with a much bigger discovery, a molecule with what he called a "special affinity" for the highly infectious organism that caused syphilis. His compound 606, later called Salvarsan, achieved worldwide fame as the "magic bullet" against the dreadful disease that had plagued Europe for hundreds of years. Ehrlich devoted the rest of his life to a systematic search of his vast stores of chemicals for one that would seek out and target cancer, but to his dismay he never found a substance with a special affinity for malignant cells.

Following World War I, scientists held out hopes for poison gases' possible usefulness in medicine, but relatively little had come of it. In the early 1920s, after the Spanish influenza pandemic had killed millions, Lieutenant Colonel Edward B. Vedder, head of the Medical Research Division at Edgewood Arsenal, found that guinea pigs inoculated with a concentration of mustard and tuberculosis bacilli did not develop the flu when other control animals did, and he carried out various experiments to test its health benefits. After an accidental leak at one of the CWS production plants, Vedder then latched onto the idea that chlorine gas might be therapeutic for respiratory diseases, as subsequent tests showed that proportionally fewer of the exposed workers came down with colds than the rest of the staff. Based on this hypothesis, he conducted a series of experiments on patients suffering from everything from bronchitis to whooping cough and pneumonia, exposing them to nonlethal amounts of chlorine gas pumped into a sealed chamber, and published the results in the *Journal of the American Medical Association.*

There was no disputing chlorine as a powerful antiseptic, and the gas cure caught on. The CWS, eager to rehabilitate its postwar image and find new civilian applications for its chemicals, helped popularize the idea with a lavish publicity campaign. In May 1924, an ailing President Calvin Coolidge, who succeeded Warren G. Harding after the latter succumbed to a flulike illness, underwent three doses of the gas in a chlorine chamber and declared the treatment successful. A representative of his administration informed reporters that the president felt much better, and that "all of the depression and lack of energy that accompanies a cold . . . had disappeared." The next year, in its effort to convince Americans that breathing the fumes was beneficial, the CWS staged an event on Capitol Hill in which they blocked off a committee room and gassed 23 Senators, 146 House representatives, and a thousand members of their staff, friends, and families. There was no record of how many had been cured, but apparently they all emerged none the worse for wear.

For a time, this led doctors to begin using the chemical weapon to fight the common cold. This dangerous practice fell out of favor, however, as subsequent research showed the original studies were flawed, and the risk of killing people along with the germs outweighed its benefits. When the University of Minnesota conducted a controlled experiment with patients who had been treated with chlorine gas and those who had not, it showed that both groups recovered at the same speed. Vedder continued to defend the cure, and he endeavored to find ways to portray chemical weapons in a more positive light. In 1925, he published *Medical Aspects of Chemical Warfare*, which contained excellent data on the pathology and physiology of mustard gas, but he was best remembered for arguing for the relative humanity of gas warfare. To that end, he tended to discount any significant long-term effects of mustard gas, arguing that the weapon's iniquities had been greatly exaggerated.

Despite all the dubious science that had gone into proving poison gas's medicinal uses in the past, Alexander was convinced he had stumbled onto something important in his Edgewood experiments with nitrogen mustard. He could not let it go. The possibility that the compound might have the same toxic effect on white blood cells in humans was good reason for doing further testing. How could he allow such a promising study to be shelved alongside hundreds of others in Edgewood's secret archive and collect dust for years to come?

Like any investigator hot on the trail of discovery, he was eager to discuss his research with other doctors and scientists, but he was stymied by the War Department's security directive regarding Edgewood's research. He dared not violate the lab's ironclad restrictions. Desperate to find a way to keep the project alive, he requested permission to consult Dr. Milton Charles Winternitz, the former dean of the Yale School of Medicine, who had full clearance as chairman of the Committee on the Treatment of War Gas Casualties. Winternitz had fathered the Biological Section of the Chemical Warfare Service in World War I, and, finding it reduced to a shadow of its former self by 1940, had helped launch the large and important new medical research laboratory at Edgewood. Having edited and written sections of the definitive text on the pathology of war gases, he was generally regarded as the most prominent man in the field. As soon as permission for the outside consult was granted, Alexander made plans to visit New Haven with an eye to enlisting a powerful ally.

"Winter," as he was known to colleagues and students, had a daunting reputation. Known to be "Napoleonic in outlook and stature," he was a short man with a short temper and a tyrannical teaching method. A legendary firebrand who brooked no opposition, he was reportedly fearless in demanding government funds to study the new chemical agents that had inspired such horror in World War I, ruthlessly quelling all critics, doubters, and prophets of doom. He succeeded in persuading Yale to establish a center to study the biological effects of war gases, as well as an Army laboratory training school. After retiring from the deanship in 1935, he authored a series of important studies on the pathology of shock, and he founded the Atypical Growth Study Unit at the university to explore the pathological process of cancer. He was at the forefront of cancer research and always on the lookout for new ideas and productive approaches.

Alexander arrived for their June meeting armed with a stack of files and charts, but nothing could have prepared him for such a negative reception. He tried to explain about the "bizarre blood findings" in experimental animals, beginning animatedly, "We found that the agent had the most terrible effects on blood and lymph nodes," and describing in detail how the nitrogen mustard selectively destroyed certain cells. Winternitz allowed him to go on at length, but his skepticism showed in the set of his shoulders and the hard, thin line of his mouth. After drilling Alexander with questions, Winternitz told him he did not agree with his findings on the systemic effects. He doubted their validity, adding that such strange effects were not described in either his experimental work or his book. He suggested that errors had been made in observation, or errors in counting the white blood cells. When Alexander attempted to defend the work, Winternitz dismissed the results as probably due to an inferior group of rabbits. He had a sharp tongue and in a disparaging tone made it clear that, in his considered opinion, the Edgewood figures were "unreliable." Although Alexander put up a strenuous argument, Winternitz never budged from his viewpoint that, "if this did happen in animals, it did not happen in human beings because he had seen tens of thousands of cases in World War I and he had never seen this."

Considerably deflated, Alexander realized he was running out of options. Unwilling to give up just yet, he decided to pay an unofficial call on one of his former teachers, Dr. Franklin McCue Hanger, professor of medicine at Columbia University College of Physicians and Surgeons in New York City. Hanger was an outstanding hematologist and a passionate and dedicated researcher. Among his achievements, in 1938 he devised Hanger's Test to measure liver function and cirrhosis. Alexander valued his opinion, but because Hanger was not cleared for classified military information, he could only speak to him about his work in carefully coded terms. The previous night, he had taken a black marker to his papers and redacted any mention of the compounds, their chemical composition, or the location where the research was being done. After reviewing the raw data and some of the graphs, Hanger became extremely excited. "If such a thing really occurred," he declared with an enthusiasm that amazed Alexander, "it is tremendous!"

Hanger told Alexander he would give anything to have samples to study its possible usefulness in treating lympho-hematogenous malignancies in his laboratory. He begged for just "a little bit of the material," or at least information about its composition, so he could carry on further experiments. He was crushed when he learned the classified compounds were out of bounds and, at least for the time being, out of reach of civilian scientists. A few weeks later, Alexander received his travel orders to the front, and that put an end to the matter. But his old mentor's enthusiasm had been reassuring. Alexander had been right to believe in the importance of the systemic effects, and he felt confident that at some time in the future, researchers would follow up on this line of investigation.

Now, sitting in an Allied military hospital six thousand miles away, Alexander held in his hands the incontrovertible evidence: "mustard gas did, in truth, selectively destroy blood cells and blood-forming organs." It had taken a freak accident, and the massive exposures of wartime, to verify in human beings the data demonstrated in laboratory rabbits. Alexander could not save the worst of the Bari mustard gas casualties, but he could make their deaths count for something. It was not much to set against such losses, though it was a silver lining of sorts. There was something larger at work in his self-appointed mission: It had been a one-in-a-million chance that had landed him—one of a handful of doctors in the world who knew of mustard's curative potential—in the middle of a disaster with hundreds of contamination victims. Cruel fortune had handed him a morgue full of case studies. It was a rare opportunity to perform a pioneering investigation into mustard's previously unknown biological effects on the human body. Perhaps some good could come out of this terrible calamity after all. He got up and ran down the hall, yelling for more blood tests.

The medical records of the Bari victims now took on a whole new significance. Alexander went over them with a fine comb, looking for signs of the rapid depletion of white blood cells and severe systemic effects. Several cases stood out at once. He pulled the Clinical Sheet on First Seaman Theodore M. Fronko, age twenty-four. He was a perfect example: admitted on the night of the raid shocked, vomiting, and complaining of burning eyes. He had been rowing a lifeboat and came into contact with the harbor water when helping survivors, and he was covered in thick, black oil. He guessed that he had spent two hours sitting in wet clothes. He developed a sore throat, painful burning eyes, and blisters. Alexander focused on the relevant part of his chart:

6 Dec 43   General condition unchanged. Throat still very painful.
           Thick yellow purulent sputum, blood stained, skin
           irritable. Generalized tiny white vesiculation on body and
           arms. Skin red and hot.
           Otherwise as before.
           R.B.C. [Red Blood Cell count] 4,590,000 per cm. W.B.C.
           [White Blood Cell count] 2,300 per cm. H.C. [Hemoglobin

count] 112%

C.I. [Color Index] 1.2.

7 Dec 43   Throat painful—Sore centre of chest. Cough with yellow
            pus tinged with blood. pulse 120. Chest—Tracheitis—
            lungs normal. Anterior surface of body, chest, abdomen
            still multiple tiny white blisters. Several new blisters Rt.
            arm Lt. thigh. Penis desquamating, soggy.

9 Dec 43   R.B.C. 4,530,000 per cm. W.B.C. 600 per cm. H.C. 109%
            C.I. 1.2.

10 Dec 43   Condition poor. Throat still very sore. Cough and
            bronchitis. B.S. [Breath Sounds] harsh both upper lobes.
            Pulse 120. Soft fair volume. Pyrexia 105. W.B.C. 50 per cm.

11 Dec 43   General condition unchanged. Appeared to be taking
            slightly more notice. Skin desquamating. Erythma fading
            slightly. Sore throat still.
            R.B.C. 3,360,000. W.B.C. 100 per cm. H.C. 97 % C.I. 1.5.

The patient's condition deteriorated, and he was placed on the danger-ously ill list. He was given oxygen, Coramine, and morphine, but he died at 12:45 p.m. on December 12. Alexander underlined the white blood cell counts to emphasize the sharp drop. He pulled out Fronko's postmortem and placed it to one side to be sure he included it in his report.

The Clinical Sheet on Ensign Kopi "Kay" Vesole, age thirty, an American Naval Armed Guard on the US *John Bascom*, followed much the same pattern. The gunnery officer had been wounded in the right shoulder, and had a fracture of the humerus, when his ship was bombed. He was later splashed with oily water when helping rescue injured sailors after abandoning their burning ship, and while rowing a lifeboat to the quay. On the night of December 2, he was admitted in shock and given morphine. His clothes were changed, but he was not washed. By the following day, he had conjunctivitis in both eyes and blisters were beginning to appear on his body. Over the next few days, he received transfusions of plasma, morphia, saline, and atropine drops for his eyes, but he continued to do poorly. Again, Alexander zeroed in on the telling section of his chart:

8 Dec 43   Erythema darker in color, skin being rubbed off back, buttocks, penis, scrotum. Some sepsis in genital region. Dressings soaked and foul smelling. P.M. temp of 103.6. Pulse 120, R 24. Blood count R.B.C. 4 ½ million. W.B.C. 20,000. H.B. 90%

9 Dec 43   Urine acid and NKD. Chest and shoulders peeling. Back and buttocks raw and oozing. Dorsum of feet peeling. Temp high 101-103. Pulse 120-130. Resp 28-34. Very breathless on movement. Chest—no active disease except for poor air entry and quick rate. Sulfadiazine 3 gms followed by 1.5 grs hourly. No food taken. Drinks given ad lib.

10 Dec 43   A.M. Temp down to 99.8 Pulse 120 Resp 24.
            R.B.C. 4 million H.B. 90 %
            White count 550. Slept during night. Some cyanosis. Coramine 2ccs 2 hrly. 1800 hours sodium pentox (A & H) 8% 10 ccs.

11 Dec 43   0030 hours sodium pentox (A & H) 8 % 10 ccs. Poor color. Breathing shallow. Dullness left base. Coughing up sputum. Became irrational during evening, pulled dressings off chest and scraped off skin.
            White cell count—400 per cm.

By the following day, the patient was comatose. He died at 11 a.m. the next morning. Alexander also made a copy of his postmortem.

Gross pathological changes indicative of toxic effect upon the liver, spleen, and lymph nodes were observed. The numerous dark hemorrhages in the chest showed definite signs of blast trauma, but, as he noted in a comment at the bottom, "this case also demonstrates the leucopenia following mustard exposure."

While his investigation into the cause of the mustard gas deaths in Bari was nearing completion, Alexander's medical inquiry into the toxin's effects on the victims was just beginning. He felt a rush of adrenaline as he strode through the labyrinthine hospital complex to the rooms reserved for the pathology exams. Autopsies were also being done at the 70th General and the 3rd New Zealand Hospitals. He would need to speak to all the pathologists and enlist their help in compiling a complete set of gross autopsy studies on all the mustard fatalities. Most of the autopsies thus far had revealed at least some evidence of trauma to the lung, compatible with blast injury. But some of the dead showed no manifestation of blast injury at all. In the deaths that occurred between forty-eight and seventy-two hours, many of the autopsies indicated nothing, while others showed only evidence of blast injury, so that blast could not be considered as the prime factor in the cause of death. "The striking features of this group of patients," Alexander noted, "were the severity of the systemic effects and the physiological changes leading to death."

He made sure that special care was taken in preparing the specimen samples to send to Edgewood for microscopic examination. Each two-ounce sample bottle, labeled with the victim's name, would contain two pieces of an organ, or small blocks of several organs. The tissue would be fixed in Zenker's Solution, washed, and then shipped in 50 percent alcohol. He hoped the specimens would withstand the long journey, and he would write to Edgewood to advise them that the solution should be changed on arrival. The hematological analysis would not be as complete as he would have liked. The heavy burden being carried by the Allied hospitals, and the limited facilities, prevented them from conducting some of the most important tests. There would be no bone marrow studies. No blood chemistry studies. It was maddening, but nothing could be done about it. He would have to badger the lab technicians to do as much as possible in the time remaining. Alexander knew he needed to be scrupulous in gathering all the available data. This time, he wanted to make absolutely sure no one would be able to second-guess his work.

MEANWHILE, THE HOSPITAL STAFF CONTINUED to whisper among themselves about whether mustard gas was the cause of the unusual burns and unexplained deaths. "It was just rumors," recalled Bob Wills, "just talk."

No one knew anything for certain, but by now they were all wearing gloves when handling the bodies. A dental technician by training, Wills had enlisted in the Royal Army Medical Corps and been assigned to the 98th General Hospital in Bari. On the evening of December 2, he had just finished unloading an ambulance train when, without warning, the German bombs lit up the sky and shook the ground under his feet. He remembered running for dear life up a long driveway when the blast wave caught him and sent him sailing through the air, buoyed by a "warm, pleasant sensation." It was the last thing he remembered until he woke up hours later in the back of a truck driven by two American soldiers, who deposited him at the hospital entrance. Unharmed, he was immediately recruited as a stretcher bearer. He then spent the next few days transporting patients to the operating theaters, carrying those too wounded to recover to the "death ward," and taking the deceased down to the temporary morgue, which had been established in the hospital cellar. Somehow—he could no longer recall exactly how—he and six men from his unit ended up being assigned to full-time morgue duty.

The continuous stream of bodies during those first few days was something he would never forget. "There were dead servicemen lying in the corridors because nobody had time to move them," he recalled. There were so many wounded with no hope of recovery that it was hard to know what to do with them all. He remembered seeing a staff nurse bark at a passing soldier, "Cover that man's face up!" When a patient was almost gone, the medics would place a thin piece of gauze over his face so everyone did not have to watch him draw his last shuddering breath. Wills thought it was likely exhaustion, not callousness, that made the soldier step over the body without noticing. They all became somewhat hardened to the situation, with so many lives passing through their hands. But some deaths were so startling they stopped Wills in his tracks, and stayed with him, difficult to shake. There was one particular young cadet who was sitting upright in his bed, larger than life, smiling at everyone. "He looked ever so young and perfectly fit," Wills recalled. "And all he kept saying was, 'Did you hear that bloody bang? Did you hear that bang?' And as he was saying that, he suddenly dropped back dead on his pillow."

They brought the dead down to the cellar and laid them out on boards head-to-toe. There were sixty corpses to start with and more arrived every day. The cellar was long and narrow, some seventy-five yards in length and only eight feet wide, with an earthen floor. It was cold below ground, and pitch black. The men carried Tilley lamps— Army-issue paraffin lamps that produced a flickering light and gave off a low hissing sound—but they did little to alleviate the deep gloom. There were two small rooms where Wills and his group worked to identify the victims and prepare the bodies before they were boxed up and taken to the cemetery south of Bari. They were not "proper coffins"—there was not enough lumber for that—so the local carpenter just made simple rectangular boxes with gaps between the slits, rather like orange crates.

It fell to Wills to gather the victims' personal effects: "We had to take the identity discs off the dead, rings, and watches. We had to go through their pockets, if they had any pockets left, and look for letters and things." Everything they found went into a big envelope labeled with the victim's name. The dead were of twelve different nationalities and races, and it was not always possible to identify them. Some bodies arrived half-naked, with no belongings and what was left of their scorched clothes hanging from them in rags. In some instances, their fingers were too charred for the technician to take prints. When two Soviet Air Force officers stationed at Bari came to arrange the burial of two comrades, they were horrified to see them lying naked and exposed in the wooden boxes. They insisted on a more dignified farewell and returned hours later with two full-dress uniforms, complete with hats for their heads.

Wills witnessed surprising moments of tenderness amid the abject wretchedness of that long week, never more so than when one of the stretchers that was brought down bore the body of a young girl. "We were most surprised to see a girl there," he recalled. "She was a British naval wren [aka WRNS, the Women's Royal Naval Service] who must have been working in the harbor. She didn't seem very old, only in her early twenties." She had not a mark on her, no injuries at all, so they thought she must have been killed by a concussion blast. Wills could not bear to see her dumped unceremoniously in one of the crude pine crates. He nipped upstairs to the closest ward and took a sheet from the supply cabinet. Then he and the other men wrapped her body in the clean linen before placing her gently in a coffin. "Some of the guys could be pretty rough army chaps, but they all treated the dead with the utmost respect and reverence," he observed. "It was touching, really."

The staff never knew how many of the bodies were gas victims, or whether it really was mustard, but they assumed the worst must be true when they were instructed not to mention anything about the raid or its aftermath in their letters home. A complete postal censorship was in effect on all American and British military bases. At one stage, Wills's unit was called to parade and told to keep lips sealed about what they had been doing. Some of his fellow medics wondered what it all meant. "We were sworn to secrecy, that's what it meant," said Wills. "We were told not to repeat anything or talk about what we had seen."

Gwladys Rees and the other nurses were angry at being kept in the dark. "We were at a loss to battle this poison and we couldn't save the majority of the wounded," she noted, struggling to keep her outrage at bay. "Most of those dear boys probably lie buried somewhere in Bari. Some may not even have names." She deplored the decision to draw a veil over the incident, misleading the victims' families about the cause of death and leaving them all in ignorance. "We felt so betrayed," she wrote.

DESPITE THE TIGHT SECURITY imposed on the damaged port, the British could not keep the discovery of mustard gas a secret from the local populace for long. Italian dockworkers whispered about the burned and strangely tanned bodies they had seen being pulled from the murky water. Italian sailors on the *Barletta,* sunk in the air raid, reported that more than fire killed twenty of their shipmates. Italian doctors at the makeshift Balilla Hospital, experienced in mustard gas from the Abyssinian War, suspected the unusual burns might have been caused by the chemical bombs dropped by the Luftwaffe. Italian crews on boats that were ordered clear of the harbor the morning after the raid carried the horrifying news to the neighboring ports of Augusta, Brindisi, and Taranto. The word was that Hitler had finally made good on his threat of retribution against Italy for the "stab-in-the-back" betrayal of the Axis alliance. Convinced the Germans were planning a second retaliatory raid, thousands of refugees refused to return to town and continued to camp out in the countryside. Many feared the Bari raid was the beginning of a new phase of the war—the first salvo in a full-scale chemical war. The British could not control the panic, and the rumors spread.

"There were thousands and thousands of people on the road getting out of town because they didn't know what happened," recalled Sergeant Francis James Vail, a mechanic with the Fifteenth Air Force. "Line for line it was two-wheeled carts, and everybody owned a donkey over there." The long procession of people, animals, and wagons piled high with bags, blankets, and babies clogged the narrow road from Bari to Foggia. He and a friend, a news photographer, were taking pictures of the mass exodus when they were accosted by British MPs and taken into custody. Their cameras and film were confiscated. The provost marshal, presumably attempting to enforce martial law, locked them in a basement overnight with "no explanation." They never saw their cameras again.

When Stewart Alexander tried to learn more about the air raid's impact on the town, he was told by the port authorities that it was a "security issue," and they discouraged him from asking questions. He was led to believe the vast majority of civilian deaths, estimated to be somewhere between two and three hundred—the exact number was unknown, as many bodies were still buried under ruins—were due to the large-caliber German bombs, weighing five hundred to a thousand pounds, that demolished the old part of the city. There were "very few casualties" from mustard vapor, one British officer assured him, adding that the only saving grace was that a "strong offshore wind had blown the stuff out to sea." In addition, since the entire dock area was a military installation and strictly off-limits to the public, the British claimed few Italian civilians had been in the affected area, so the community at large remained unaware of the gas leak and thus unconcerned. Alexander was shrewd enough to discern that the tidy official account presented to him had little bearing on reality. He preferred to rely on his own evidence and interviews with survivors.

American ensign John Whitley, whose minor injuries got him transferred out of the 98th General Hospital to a barren room in the windowless Bari gymnasium on the seafront, saw firsthand how frightened the local inhabitants remained in the wake of the attack. Another air raid at 11 p.m. on the night of December 11 caused people to almost trample one another in their headlong rush to find safety within the sturdy walls of the Castello Normanno-Svevo, the twelfth-century fortress overlooking the harbor. No bombs were dropped on that occasion, but there was a terrific antiaircraft barrage. During that tense period, whenever a German scout plane flew over to observe the condition of the harbor, the sound of the air-raid siren sent people running. Whitley, who was aboard the *Samuel J. Tilden* when it took a direct hit and was lucky to have landed in a lifeboat, understood the daily terror facing ordinary Italians. "Sharing an underground air-raid shelter with the local people crying and praying while standing in water was an experience in itself," he recalled.

The strained relations between the British and the Italians, who resented having their country treated like conquered enemy territory, added to the local conviction that the Allied regime had little regard for their welfare. When doctors at the Balilla Hospital reached out to the British medical officials for confirmation that the cause of so many deaths was poison gas, they received no reply. Wild theories abounded as to why the civilian casualty count was never reported. Under the terms of the occupation, all the Italian newspapers were controlled by the Allied Military Government's Psychological Warfare branch, which saw to it that no mention of the German air raid appeared in print. Even *La Gazzetta del Mezzogiorno*, Bari's main paper and one of the most important in southern Italy, was prevented from running a single story about the attack.

The strict censorship was, at least in part, an attempt to preserve law and order and to facilitate the smooth transportation of supplies and personnel to the front. But the citizens of Bari knew that something was terribly wrong and they were not being told the truth. The tragedy that had befallen them was only discernible in the obituary columns: ten dead in one day, twenty the next. When a dozen names of the deceased were listed as all being from the same street, it indicated where a bomb had fallen on a block of houses. The neat rows of trench graves in the municipal cemetery, however, testified to something else—something silent, invisible, and lethal. It was impossible to calculate how many hundreds of inhabitants had been exposed when the toxic cloud drifted over the town, and had died undiagnosed in the days that followed, their passing left unrecorded. How many lay in their beds choking from unexplained symptoms, and would eventually develop fatal complications, was the subject of fearful speculation.

The discovery of the mustard bomb fragments on the bottom of the harbor gave new fire to reports the Germans had used gas, and the rumors raced up the American chain of command. Communications in the city had not been completely restored, which added to the confusion and the absence of reliable information. The mounting dread of a second German strike forced the chief of naval operations to send a signal reiterating the policy agreed on at the start of the war, that chemical weapons would only be used in retaliation, and emphasizing the need for restraint: "USE OF TOXIC GAS WILL NOT BE INITIATED BY ANY UNITED STATES COMMANDER." Instruction and training in chemical warfare were instituted immediately to ensure that if the enemy's use of gas was verified, Allied retaliation—if and when it was authorized—"would be effective." Gas masks were prepared for imminent use. Orders went out that chemical depots outside the city were to be kept in ready reserve, but offensive materials were not to be issued to combat units. With the soldiers' fears running high, all dumps containing mustard bombs were heavily guarded to prevent the "initiating use of gas under stress."

The rumors also reached the local SS operatives in the port, but the Nazi spies already knew exactly what had taken place. Gruppenführer Karl Friedrich Wolff, the supreme SS and police leader in Italy, had the proof in hand only six hours after the raid. The Germans had sent down their own diver, an Italian frogman still loyal to the Fascists, and he had managed to recover a piece of the bomb casing. Their military headquarters in the north quickly verified that the M47 bomb was a model used by the Americans and typically contained liquid mustard. Wolff relayed the information to Reichsführer Heinrich Himmler, the leader of the SS in Berlin, believing the news that the Allies had unleashed mustard gas was a huge propaganda coup. Wolff's spies were even aware that an American chemical warfare consultant had been called in to investigate and treat the undiagnosed wounds. The German High Command decided to let the catastrophe play out without any additional assistance on their part, though it passed on a warning to their panzer units in Italy: "The Allies could begin the gas war tomorrow." The Hermann Göring Division, responsible for some of the worst civilian massacres in the region, ramped up its chemical defenses accordingly.

On his second or third night in Bari, Alexander heard a report about the incident on a popular Berlin radio broadcast. After a string of Bing Crosby hits, the beguiling host, known as "Axis Sally," interrupted the music program to comment in her come-hither voice, "I see you boys are getting gassed by your own poison gas!" Alexander knew full well that the program, entitled Jerry's Front, was aimed at undermining the morale of the Allied forces and exploited every setback and sunken ship for propaganda purposes. A lot of what passed for news was just plain wrong. But Alexander had a hunch that the Germans might be better informed than he was, and that in this instance he was very much afraid "Axis Sally was right."

CHAPTER SIX

"Recommendation to Secrecy"

When Stewart Alexander next returned to the harbor, he was armed with maps and admiralty charts of the layout of the sprawling port, with its long breakwater constructed in the shape of a crooked finger. Called the Nuovo Molo Foraneo, and rechristened the East Jetty by the Allies, it stretched from the original small marina and dockyard out into the Adriatic Sea to create a sheltered harbor. At the other end, extending from the industrial complex, was the short, straight arm of the Molo San Cataldo, or West Jetty. Two lighthouses—one at the tip of each jetty, separated by a distance of some three hundred yards—marked the harbor's entrance. Submarine netting protected the narrow opening.

It was on the outer eastern mole, lined up side by side in unusually close proximity because of the overcrowding, that four American Liberty ships and a dozen Allied vessels had sat in temporary berths waiting to discharge their cargo. Although the recovered M47 bomb fragments strongly suggested the mustard gas had been in the hold of one of the American ships, the British still adamantly denied that chemical weapons had been brought into the port. Determined to find definite proof that his diagnoses of mustard contamination were correct, and to pinpoint the exact source of the poison, Alexander set about making his own berthing plan of the harbor as it was on the night of the raid and then reconstructing the events that claimed so many lives.

Drawing on interviews with the British port authorities, US military officials, dockworkers, and survivors, he had framed a "mental picture" of what happened. For six days, German Me-210 reconnaissance planes had made regular passes over the harbor, almost as though they were waiting for something. Sailors who had spotted the planes high in the sky recalled feeling a prickling of unease. Then, on December 2, the Luftwaffe pilots saw what they were looking for. That morning, a large convoy of American ships arrived with supplies and ammunition for the stalled Allied campaign. Every dock was occupied. Yet despite this immense haul of valuable cargo, Bari's port defenses were unaccountably weak. The early warning system was primitive and depended on a single unreliable telephone line to sector operations, located fifty miles away. It was out of order on the night of the attack. As darkness fell, the Germans found the strategic port well illuminated and without fighter cover. The Royal Air Force was so convinced the Luftwaffe had been licked in the Mediterranean that officials had instructed some of their wing operations to stand down for the night. Even allowing for the degree of surprise achieved by the carefully planned attack, one British official was forced to acknowledge they had presented the enemy with his target "on a plate."

Squinting into the distance, Alexander could just make out the extreme end of the East Jetty, still under a thin mantle of gray mist, where the first of the Allied ships had been anchored when the bombs began to fall. He had compiled enough information to attempt a rough sketch of what the sardine can of densely packed vessels must have looked like from above to the German pilots. The rudimentary berthing plan, which he had prepared as part of his investigation, showed the relative positions of seventeen merchantmen destroyed in the attack, all of which were in the vicinity of the released mustard gas. But he worried that the sketch was anything but precise. Based in part on British and Italian maps of the wrecks in the ruined harbor, he had been advised that it was difficult for anyone to be sure of the ships' original locations. Many of the mooring lines had disintegrated in the raging fires, and the damaged vessels, battered beyond recognition, had drifted. He just had to hope he had identified them all correctly.

To the best of his knowledge, at 6 p.m. on December 2 the far end of the jetty was occupied by the Dutch SS *Odysseus* and the Norwegian SS *Vest*. (These vessels were penciled in but not assigned a number, as Alexander had no information about the fate of their crews and therefore did not include them in his calculations.) The third from the end was the Italian schooner *Frosinone*. The next three berths were filled by

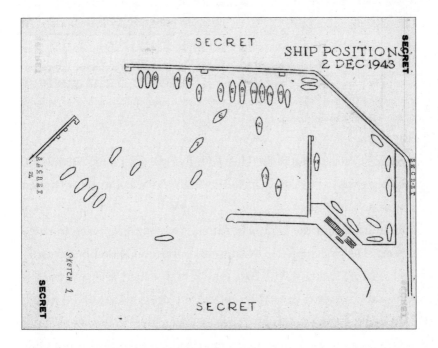

A rudimentary sketch of Bari Harbor prepared for Lt. Col. Alexander as part of his investigation into the cause of the mysterious deaths among the patients in Allied hospitals following the German air raid. (Stewart F. Alexander Papers)

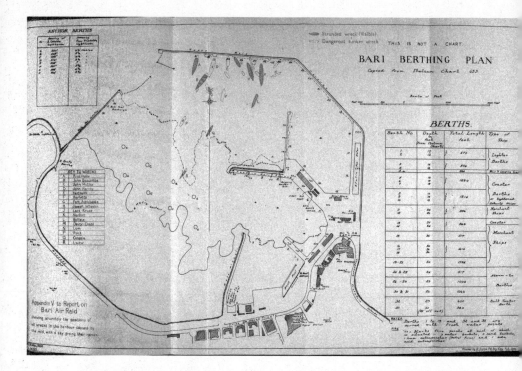

This far more detailed plan of Bari Harbor, showing the approximate positions of the damaged and sunken ships after the December 2 air raid, was prepared as part of the official inquiry into the Bari incident ordered by Gen. Eisenhower. (Courtesy of The National Archives Image Library)

American Liberty ships: the USS *John Bascom*, with a reported 8,300 tons of general army cargo, including high-test gasoline in fifty-gallon drums and acid; the USS *John L. Motley,* which carried 5,231 tons of ammunition; and the USS *John Harvey,* carrying 5,037 tons of cargo described as "war supplies." Next were the British Coastal Forces tankers SS *Testbank*, laden with fifty tons of high-octane fuel, and SS *Fort Athabaska,* carrying general cargo and two captured thousand-pound PC-RS500 German rocket bombs. Next were the USS *Joseph Wheeler*, with a cargo of 8,037 tons of ammunition; and the British (formerly Danish) SS *Lars Kruse,* carrying fourteen hundred tons of aviation fuel.

Then came two Norwegian coal ships, the SS *Norlam* and the SS *Lom,* followed by the small British tanker MV *Devon Coast,* carrying fifty tons of high-octane petrol. The last in line was the French diesel tanker SS *La Drome.* Tied up parallel to the jetty were two British Hunt class destroyers, HMS *Bicester* and HMS *Zetland.* (Alexander also left these last three ships unnumbered.) The USS *Lyman Abbott,* about a ship's length away from the jetty, was at anchor in the inner harbor, along with five other Allied ships destroyed in the attack. Not shown on the sketch was the *Samuel J. Tilden,* anchored two miles outside the harbor's entrance. She took a direct hit, and the sixty-nine-man crew and 209 troops were ordered to abandon ship. Most made it to shore in lifeboats, rafts, and floats, although twenty-seven men were lost.

From careful study of reports of the raid and witness statements, Alexander knew the Ju-88s had come in from the east and "walked" their bombs straight down the line of shipping. At approximately 7:31 p.m., the first bomb tore through the *Joseph Wheeler*'s starboard side and she burst into flames. Immediately another bomb struck the *John L. Motley* and she started to burn. Next, a bomb (or possibly portions of an exploding fuel tanker) fell on the *John Harvey,* igniting a small fire. Anchored much too close to the others was the fourth Liberty ship, the *John Bascom,* which took three hits from aft to forward, ripping through the bridge and deck and destroying all but one of its lifeboats. Then the *Motley*'s cargo of ammunition blew, and the force of the explosion caved in the whole port side of the *Bascom,* which began to sink immediately.

The *John Bascom*'s captain, Otto Heitmann, ordered the most seriously injured to be put in the one remaining lifeboat. Fifty-two wounded, far more than the boat's capacity, were loaded and lowered into the water. Boxed in between two blazing ships, and in imminent danger of a collision setting off the highly combustible cargo, Heitmann instructed the remaining crew to jump overboard and hold onto the seine floats attached to the lifeboat. Many of his crew, along with sailors from some of the other ships, made it to the East Jetty, where they scaled the five-and-a-half-foot wall, hauled up their comrades, and headed to the lighthouse for shelter. Among those trapped on the breakwater, nearly a mile out to sea, was the young American serviceman with the bad eyes, Warren Brandenstein, who prayed a passing boat would spot them through the dense, black smoke rolling over the harbor. Looking back at the mass of flames behind him, he said his only thought was, "This must be what Hell is like."

Alexander had heard of the heroic actions of Ensign "Kay" Vesole, the gunnery officer of the *Bascom,* whose medical chart he had earmarked as showing all the signs of serious mustard exposure. In the midst of the assault, Vesole had gone from gun to gun, directing action, and, despite a broken arm and a vicious shrapnel gash across his chest, had led a rescue party below decks to carry out wounded personnel, personally searched the entire ship for dazed and concussed men, and calmly supervised the loading of the casualties onto the only lifeboat, along with syrettes of morphine and other medical supplies. He had insisted on rowing the lifeboat with his one good arm, and, ignoring the danger from a nearby ammunition ship, managed to pull three or four helpless men from the water and drag them to the bomb shelter at the end of the jetty. Just as he started to return for more wounded, the ammunition ship blew and flung him thirty feet onto the quay, which accounted for all the debris the doctors found buried in his back. As the flames began to sweep over the jetty, and weak from loss of blood, Vesole had the presence of mind to dispatch men with flashlights to the extreme end of the seawall to signal for help before he collapsed from loss of blood.

The first Liberty ship to explode and sink was the *John Motley.* Sixty-four of her crew were reported missing or dead. The only survivors were four naval armed guards and seven merchant seamen—all of whom had been ashore.* On fire and adrift, the *John Harvey* had moved inexorably across the harbor toward the USS *Pumper*, a US Navy tanker with a half-million-gallon capacity. It was estimated that the flames reached the *Harvey*'s cargo hold by about 8:20 p.m., and the ship blew up. The massive explosion shot a fountain of flames, sparks, and smoke six to eight thousand feet into the air. Witnesses said the effect was that of a "huge Roman candle"—brilliant, multicolored, and shedding burning debris all over the harbor. The force of the explosion, combined with the almost simultaneous eruption of an ammunition ship, destroyed several nearby vessels, including the *Testbank*, which went down with most of her crew.

Then the *Joseph Wheeler* exploded, taking almost her full complement of twenty-nine merchant crew and fifteen armed guards. The commanding officer and twelve surviving members of the Armed Guard unit had been ashore. The oil fire quickly spread to the *Fort Athabaska*, and the extreme heat detonated the two German rockets, decimating the ship. Near the end of the line, the *Devon Coast* took a direct hit and sank, followed in quick succession by the *Lom* and the *Norlam*. After dragging the burning *La Drome* to safety, the two British destroyers, *Bicester* and *Zetland*, were diverted to Taranto.

The *Lyman Abbott* escaped with only moderate damage. Two men died, but nearly all the armed guards suffered burns and injuries caused by flying debris and shrapnel. The ship, blown onto its port side and lying in the harbor, must have been very close to the vessel leaking mustard from its ruptured hold. According to Alexander's notes, the fumes were strong enough that, "at some point in the evening, someone aboard the *Lyman Abbott* called 'Gas!' Many of the crew put on their gas masks for about half an hour. None had recognized gas themselves.

---

* The ships' crew and casualty numbers vary widely depending on the source, so the author has relied on Robert M. Browning Jr.'s *U.S. Merchant Vessel War Casualties of World War II*, Captain Arthur R. Moore's *A Careless Word . . . A Needless Sinking*, and George Southern's *Poisonous Inferno*.

Masks were removed of their own volition." It was the only report of gas on the night of the raid, but then the *Lyman Abbott* was eventually righted and most of its crew lived to tell the tale.

At 11 p.m., a small Norwegian coastal steamer spotted the flashlight signal of the men stranded on the East Jetty and sent a launch. In two separate and perilous trips, some sixty men were picked up and ferried to the steamer, before the Norwegian captain informed Heitmann it was too dangerous to remain any longer, as the ship was being carried into the minefields nearby. Fortunately, the *Pumper's* whaleboat was able to pick up a few of the remaining men; the stragglers, Heitmann and Vesole among them, were rescued by a British minesweeper just as the flames closed in around them. Vesole was taken to the 98th General Hospital, where he died days later of his injuries and extensive mustard burns.* Conscious only part of the time, he had worried about his men to the end. The British doctors, realizing the effect his death might have on the morale of his wounded American crewmates, did not tell them. In all, the *John Bascom* lost two officers, two crew, and ten armed guards.

Sensing that he had finally pieced together what had happened, and he now had his quarry in his sights, Alexander returned to his office. He began by logging the whereabouts of each victim of a "mysterious death," labeled as "Dermatitis N.Y.D. [Not Yet Diagnosed]" by the Allied hospitals at the time of the attack. He had already traced which ships the deceased had served on, and he compiled the number of casualties primarily attributable to mustard contamination for each vessel. By correlating the ships' locations with the mustard death tallies, he was able to discern a pattern. Using the sketch of Bari Harbor, he could see the fatalities fanned out in a cone-like trajectory emanating from a single ship, which must have been the one carrying the mustard gas.

---

* In March of 1944, Ensign Kopi "Kay" Vesole was awarded the Navy Cross for meritorious conduct and self-sacrificing actions responsible for saving countless lives. The article about the hometown hero in the Davenport, Iowa, *Daily Times* did not mention mustard gas.

The casualty distribution chart told a grim tale. The focal point of the disaster was the American Liberty ship *John Harvey*, moored between berths 29 and 30. This ship, he had been informed, "no longer existed." It had disappeared without a trace. The captain, Elwin F. Knowles, seventy-eight members of the crew, and nine passengers perished. There were reportedly eight survivors, a Merchant Marine cadet and seven seamen, who happened to be ashore that evening and who had no idea what was in the ship's hold.

Alexander labeled the *John Harvey*—"the mustard ship"—as #1. Designating each of the adjacent ships by number revealed that those closest to the epicenter of the chemical explosion, the *John Harvey*, had been showered with burning oil and liquid mustard, and thus their personnel had suffered the greatest degree of exposure and greatest number of mustard-induced fatalities. According to his information, there were eighteen such deaths on Ship #2, the *John L. Motley*; eleven on #4, the *John Bascom*; nine on #3, the *Testbank*:

Ship #1	no survivors
Ship #2	18 deaths
Ship #3	9 deaths
Ship #4	11 deaths
Ship #5	3 deaths
Ship #6	10 deaths
Ship #7	2 deaths
Ship #8	0 deaths
Ship #9	0 deaths
Ship #10	11 deaths
Ship #11	2 deaths
Ship #12	4 deaths
Ship #13	1 death
Ship #14	1 death

Unknown and Miscellaneous Ships—11 deaths

He then categorized the mustard deaths. Pneumonia or suppurative pneumonia was the dominant feature in thirty-five cases. (These were the later deaths.) In forty-eight cases, neither blast injury nor pulmonary infection could be allowed as *the* cause of death but could be explained as due to:

(1) total or subtotal body surface burns per se regardless of the specific etiology, mustard

(2) systemic effects of the mustard burns upon the peripheral vascular bed

(3) toxic systems of the mustard upon remote organ systems

(4) the sublethal effects of a blast injury added to one or more of the above

(5) undetected bacterial infection in a body severely weakened by 3 and 4 above

The death figures in the chart represented only the mustard fatalities documented by Allied military hospitals to date, and they were not a reflection of either the total number of deaths caused by mustard contamination or the total number of deaths as a result of the Bari raid. As Alexander knew all too well, both totals were being revised upward on a daily basis. The vast majority of the victims died in the inferno ignited by the ammunition ship and the *John Harvey*, and their bodies would never be recovered. Moreover, many injured personnel had been taken onto undamaged ships in the harbor for emergency treatment, and later, when those ships were diverted to other ports, the wounded had been sent to military hospitals nearby.

Alexander did not know whether the doctors in the neighboring "heel" ports had been informed that the men had been subjected to mustard gas or, in the case of fatalities, whether the cause of death was correctly recorded. Given the British preoccupation with security, he very much doubted it. Other survivors who had appeared in good condition had already been transferred to hospitals elsewhere in Italy and in North Africa, the United States, and Britain, in order to free up much-needed beds. In addition, some of the casualties had "aspirated or swallowed variable amounts of the mustard in oil solution." He had no way of finding out whether these men subsequently developed symptoms and received proper treatment. All their charts were labeled "Dermatitis N.Y.D." He fretted that some of these cases had been lost to the vast military medical bureaucracy and would not be tracked down before being discharged, and they would be sent home without ever knowing what was ailing them. Then there were the injured Italian sailors, most of whom had been taken to their own local hospital near the waterfront and not to one of the British military hospitals. Except for ten serious cases who had been transferred to the 98th General Hospital, Alexander had no information about their condition or the number of mustard-related casualties.

Aware that time was running out, he immediately ordered that all auxiliary hospitals in the Mediterranean Theater that had received Bari victims be alerted that the patients were at risk from mustard gas contamination. Even as he gave the orders, however, he knew that it was too late. Much too late. Most of the serious exposure cases would be beyond help.

ANGRY AT HAVING BEEN INTENTIONALLY MISLED, Alexander returned to Navy House intent on getting answers. The British authorities had tried to prevent him from knowing about the mustard gas right up to the point where he "held it up to their nose." Fed up with being lied to, he confronted the acting port commandant with his evidence from the harbor. It was only then, "under pressure" from him, that Maj. Harry Wilkinson admitted that the *John Harvey* had been carrying 540 tons of hundred-pound American mustard gas bombs, in addition to white phosphorous and a tremendous quantity of high explosives.* He had known about the classified cargo all along. A beleaguered Wilkinson "acknowledged the mustard gas was listed on the shipping invoice." But he hastened to add that secrecy about the presence of poison gas in the war zone was so strict that he had been instructed not to reveal the contents of the *Harvey*'s hold to anyone. Under explicit orders "to deny the presence of mustard gas," he had consequently told Alexander he had no knowledge of the chemical weapons when questioned, and he had continued to maintain the fiction in the days that followed.

It did not take long for the War Department to confirm Alexander's findings. The *John Harvey* had embarked from Baltimore with a cargo of war supplies and sailed across the Atlantic to Algeria without incidence, arriving in Oran on November 1, 1943. On November 10, AFHQ issued instructions for the American Liberty ship to be loaded with "5500 tons bombs and ammunition and 720 tons of supplies, destination Bari." Air Force Ordnance Depot No. 2 sent a breakdown of the tonnage allotment to the freight department at Oran, where the *Harvey* took on her cargo of "24,430 Bombs Chemical, HS, 100-lb, M47A2." (HS, "Hot Stuff," is the US military hazard code for mustard.) First Lieutenant Howard D. Beckstrom of the 701st Maintenance Company was assigned to supervise the delivery of the chemical weapons. The ship was also assigned a cargo security officer, Second Lieutenant Thomas H. Richardson of the US Transportation Corps. After departing Oran on November 20, the *John Harvey* sailed in convoy KMS 32, put in briefly at Augusta, and then continued on to Bari in a nine-ship convoy AH10, arriving on November 28.

The official paper trail indicated that more people knew about the presence of mustard gas in Bari Harbor than Alexander had thought

---

* It was later established that the *John Harvey* was carrying one hundred tons of mustard gas.

possible—and some of them were American. A shipping wire and copies of the manifest sent via air courier were forwarded by the US Transport Officer, Adriatic Base, to Bari, in accordance with the usual practice, and were received and signed for by Major A. J. Balfour, the dock superintendent, on November 25. Further, a breakdown of the bombs and ammunition loaded on the *John Harvey* was sent to an ordnance officer in Bari on November 28. Wilkinson, the acting port commandant, received his copies of the breakdown on November 30. Even if the British insisted on maintaining their ignorance, an American port officer boarded the *John Harvey* on her arrival in Bari and was told by the ship's security officer that she carried a "cargo of mustard gas."

Despite the crush of cargo ships, the *John Harvey* was ordered that same day to Berth 29 on the East Jetty and told to await her turn in the unloading docks. When Captain Knowles voiced his concern about anchoring on the already tightly packed East Jetty, he was advised the ship could not remain outside the harbor because of German "U and E boat activities." For the next five days, Knowles, a veteran skipper who was not technically supposed to know about the gas shipment but was doubtless aware of it, made repeated trips to the War Shipping Administration office to petition for an earlier slot in the discharge schedule. The *Harvey's* security officer, Lt. Richardson, also tried to do something about the ship's "low priority." He made no headway, possibly because he felt he could not disclose the real reason behind his request. The acting port commandant, the docks superintendent, and the sea transport officer discussed the *Harvey's* predicament, but as there was nothing to be done about the freight backlog, they agreed she was "in as safe a place as could be found."

Wilkinson was at the wheel of his jeep in the center of Bari when the bombing commenced. The raid was over by 7:50 p.m., and by the time he reached his office in the dockyard, the harbor was in ruins and the entire outer mole was a mass of flames. Seeing the black smoke billowing from the petrol bay on the West Jetty, his attention was focused on the tanker in the midst of discharging high-octane fuel. At the earliest opportunity, near about 8 p.m., he met with the naval officer in charge, Capt. Campbell—Commander Guinness was present and took over as NOIC the following day—and informed him that a number of the burning ships were "dangerous and one was carrying mustard." He also informed Major Joshua F. Bolland, the Port Authority defense officer, of the possible risk from gas. They discussed whether or not to "scuttle" the *Harvey* to prevent the burning hulk, with its toxic cargo, from drifting closer to shore. The order was issued, and a naval officer took the instructions to the *Bicester*, but she was damaged and unable to take any action.

The port commandant, Lt. Col. Marcus Sieff, had just returned from Cairo and was having a drink at the brigadier's headquarters when a bomb fell through the roof at the far end of the building. Shaken but unhurt, Sieff rushed to the NOIC's building; most of the front had been blown in, and he urged Campbell to "order every possible ship to sail out of what was now becoming a holocaust." Sieff then ordered that all the ships' manifests be brought to him immediately. To his "horror," he saw that the *Harvey* was carrying mustard shells and immediately told the NOIC, "If you can't get that ship out, sink it, because if we don't and the wind changes, God knows what will happen to this town tonight." The NOIC said he would have the ship sunk at once.

Four messages sent to the *Harvey*'s master by four different means— two by land, and two by water—ordered him to scuttle the ship if there was any danger of her catching fire. At least one of these reportedly was delivered: A British lieutenant was able to proceed by motorcycle to a point on the mole that was within hailing distance of the Liberty ship. He passed the message to an officer who was on the poop deck, after confirming with the latter that his ship was the veritable *John Harvey*.

Shortly thereafter, two enormous explosions rocked the harbor.

Wilkinson recalled that the shock wave swept over the port: "It picked me up like a feather, hurling me across the full length of the office to finish up on the floor on the other side of the building, which itself seemed to be in an imminent state of collapsing." Wilkinson eventually made his way through the maelstrom of smoke and fire to the discharging dock and ascertained to his relief that the tanker was intact. He had only just turned back to his jeep when "a brilliant white light lit up the night sky, followed by a massive explosion. At anchor a half-unloaded ship, carrying a cargo of petrol cans, blew up."

He was not sure what had happened to the *John Harvey*.* In the blinding smoke, there was some confusion about the charred wrecks, but Wilkinson opined that there could be very little doubt the Liberty ship "sank of her own accord almost immediately after she exploded." The crew, and all ten members of the Army chemical warfare detachment supervising the movement of the toxic load, were killed before they could raise the gas alarm. He considered it likely that the detonation of the ammunition on board took her down and hurled some of her load of mustard bombs into the sky, where they shattered in midair. Some thirty broken casings were thrown onto the outer mole. What onlookers described as "a tidal wave" following one of the explosions drenched everyone in the vicinity. Liquid mustard fell like rain back into the harbor and onto neighboring ships.

George Southern, a twenty-one-year-old gunner on the *Zetland*, was standing on the forecastle facing the *John Harvey* and "just had time to see the massive upheaval" before it engulfed him in a rush of searing hot air. He and the rest of the bridge staff were sent reeling onto the open deck of the destroyer. When he came to, he discovered he was

---

* It remains unclear whether the *John Harvey* was scuttled, was consumed by fire, or received "a direct hit from exploding ammunition," as Lt. Col. Marcus Sieff reported, then split in two and sank.

soaked—not in rain as he first thought, "but with a thick, greasy liquid which was as black as pitch and gave off a foul stench."

Between midnight and dawn, explosions of varying intensities continued intermittently. Fortunately, the huge fires burned up most of the escaped mustard gas, and the strong southerly breeze prevented the worst of the fumes from wafting over the town. As nothing could be done about the film of liquid mustard already formed on the harbor water—most of which the British officials believed would quickly hydrolyze or settle on the bottom and break down into harmless compounds—they apparently were most concerned about the ongoing risk posed by toxic vapor. They were not worried about vapors rising from the water, which they also deemed harmless, but the presence of high concentrations coming from the mustard puddles out on the mole, as well as splashes on nearby boats. An early morning reconnaissance of the harbor confirmed the presence of "some gas in the dock area."

The first "definite" report of contamination came several hours later, at around 10:30 a.m., when the port defense officer, accompanied by the base medical officer, Surgeon Lieutenant John Cosh, boarded the *Vienna,* a Coastal Forces depot ship, which had served as a casualty clearing station during the raid. There they discovered that sick-bay personnel were suffering from eye symptoms and the doctor had a blister on one foot. By 11 a.m. on December 3, several members of the British command in Bari knew they had mustard gas casualties, but all were under the impression that by then the hospitals had received a "general warning."

At 2:15 p.m. that same day, a meeting was hastily convened at the harbormaster's office to consider the extent of the contamination and what should be done. A small group of officials—three British military officers and three US Air Force officers from Gen. Doolittle's Adriatic base—made a series of critical decisions. Lieutenant Colonel Oliver N. D. Sismey, general staff officer for the British headquarters in Bari, informed the gathering that the *John Harvey* had been carrying 540 tons of American mustard gas bombs. Then Lieutenant Colonel Joseph R. Hradel, an American chemical warfare specialist detailed to the Fifteenth Air Force, explained that the bombs were not fused, so the danger would only exist if the casings split and the gas dissipated. Since the worst was over, and the remaining cracked and broken bombs had sunk with the *Harvey*, he considered the only real risk posed by the munitions going forward was possibly to salvage operations.

In the meantime, as an extra precaution, they decided the dock police were to be informed and two sentries posted, one British and one American, to monitor the direction of the wind in case it changed from the south to the more usual north. In the event the wind began blowing toward the shore, the sentries and dock police had orders to cordon off the endangered area and display signs warning of hazardous fumes. Maj. Joshua Bolland, working in conjunction with Major Howard W. Fieber, a Chemical Warfare Service specialist with the Twelfth United States Air Force, would immediately undertake a complete inspection of the docks and test for contamination, and they were to alert Navy House and the No. 6 Base Sub Area of any signs of gas. They also dispatched decontamination squads from the Twelfth Air Force, which was nearby and had the necessary equipment, including gas masks, antigas clothing, and a large supply of powdered bleach.

At the conclusion of the meeting, the British and American officers were "unanimous in their opinion that the concentration was unlikely to be dangerous outside the dock area and that precautions were only necessary within the dock area." It was agreed that, "in order to maintain secrecy, no general warning was to be given now."

The "recommendation to secrecy" was made because they believed at the time that the crisis had passed and the problem was in hand. Many of the ships were still burning, but the fires were under control. Survivors were being brought ashore by all possible means. Measures had been taken to empty the harbor and reroute vessels. The officers were under the impression that hospital staff had been alerted to the danger of gas, but in retrospect it appeared the warnings were impeded by missed calls and confusion about the classified nature of the information. In such a fluid situation, it was inevitable that vital services such as communication would leave much to be desired. However, military security remained at all times paramount in the officers' minds.

Alexander winced inwardly at the full import of these last disclosures. Of all the various officials who knew about the toxic gas, none had felt capable of releasing the classified information to medical personnel. Their reluctance probably stemmed in part from a fear of being held responsible for violating security regulations. The bottom line was that "no direct information concerning the possibilities of mustard exposure was communicated to the hospitals that evening." Then, from the moment of the 2:15 p.m. meeting, all inquiries about mustard gas in Bari Harbor hit a blank wall. No wonder the doctors and nurses had been unable to get any straight answers about what was wrong with their patients. He saw now that he was not only up against the British authorities but also the intransigence of American officials. Someone way above his pay grade at AFHQ must have anticipated there might be "a mustard problem," and had sent him to deal with it, all the while withholding the true facts of the case. He should have realized that it was in the interests of both military bureaucracies to have the Bari disaster hushed up. "The cover-up and stone-walling," he later surmised, had come about after the incident and for the usual reasons. "It was the same factor of not wanting to admit errors in judgment had been made."

It was a conspiracy of silence—a concerted Allied effort to cover up the presence of poison gas in the harbor on that ill-fated day. There was, after all, plenty of blame to go around. The mistakes leading up to the disaster had been cumulative—beginning with the shared decision to leave the lethal cargo in a harbor choked with ammunition ships—and amplified by the failure on all their parts to make sure the threat of gas was fully realized once the raid began. But it was the decision to maintain the highest discretion about the poison gas after the attack that compounded the tragedy and had incalculable consequences. That had been the costliest mistake, the fatal error.

Alexander could only shake his head in disgust. In their haste to conceal any traces of the incriminating chemical agent, the port authorities had also been sloppy. Owing to the large fires still burning in the harbor on the morning of December 3, the inspection carried out by Bolland and Fieber failed to detect numerous heavy patches of mustard deposited on the outer mole by the M47 bombs, some of which were still intact and others were split and leaking. The toxic site, spread over an area roughly 200 by 10 square yards, was not found until December 6, when a second inspection of the dockyard was carried out by a team of chemical warfare technicians from AFHQ and the Eighth Army. A second round of decontamination was immediately ordered before any dockworkers were injured. One ton of dry bleach was scattered on the mole, and the next day it was hosed down to wash the paste into the sea. Not coincidentally, the largest mustard patch was directly in front of Berth 29, where the *John Harvey* had been moored and was now sunk in forty feet of water.

The new information substantially corroborated Alexander's assessment of the cause of death as mustard gas and the source of the contamination as the American Liberty ship. From what he had been told, Alexander estimated that the broken bomb casings discovered on the outer mole would account for the release of "at least 2,000–3,000 pounds of mustard." Although there were injuries due to mustard vapor, ironically they were "not of major degree or significance." The six Allied officials at that crucial December 3 meeting had been worried about the wrong thing, and they missed the real killer in their midst—the lethal mixture of liquid mustard and fuel oil. They could not have known what they were dealing with, because this form of chemical exposure had never before occurred. It went unrecognized by the doctors in the Allied hospitals because these chemical injuries were unlike any they had ever seen. As a direct result of the deference to military security, the contamination went undetected and untreated for too long. Men died because medical personnel and those rendering first aid at the scene did not have adequate information. Alexander knew his assignment was only to investigate the medical aspects of the disaster, and not to bring those responsible to book, but he could not help feeling that a larger inquiry into what went wrong was warranted.

He was now ready to begin writing his preliminary report into the unexplained deaths at Bari Harbor. All he could do was shine a light on events without fear or favor. The facts would speak for themselves. "It was the mixture or solution of mustard in oil that produced most of the severe casualties and deaths," he asserted in the opening section of his report. "Some casualties were due to vapor alone, but the great majority, and the important ones, were those who were covered in oil."

He then outlined the regrettable sequence of events:

The burns sustained by the victims depended upon the amount of mustard in oil contaminating their skin and the length of time the oil remained in contact with the skin. As there was no thought of a toxic agent in the oil, no attempt was made to wash or decontaminate the men. Many men in wet, oil-contaminated clothes were wrapped in blankets, given warm tea and allowed to lie in the oil on their skin all night. The opportunity for burns and absorption must have been tremendous.

He refrained from adding that the "recommendation to secrecy" had resulted in a protracted period of exposure, which in the end was what killed them.

. . .

ALEXANDER HAD BEEN IN BARI almost a week, and there was still no official acknowledgment of his diagnosis of mustard gas poisoning. If Churchill was allowed to bury the truth, Alexander believed it would be a grave injustice not only to the Bari victims but also to all those who might one day benefit from the valuable lessons that could be learned from the tragedy. His greatest fear was that the whitewash in progress would end up expunging any mention of mustard gas from the record, and, along with it, all of the important medical findings on the systemic effects on the body, particularly the depletion of white blood cells.

Being "young and foolhardy," he decided he would not be party to an official lie, no matter the cost to his career. To his mind, the Hippocratic Oath he took as a doctor superseded any vow of loyalty he made when he joined the Army. He would not sacrifice his "professional integrity" to placate a prime minister loath to admit that a poorly defended British port had been subjected to the worst poison gas disaster of the war. After hearing Axis Sally's broadcast, Alexander was no longer persuaded that secrecy was mandated by the exigencies of war. The Nazi propagandist had made it embarrassingly clear that the Germans knew all about the gruesome accident, and she had gleefully announced it to the world. The secret was out. The attempts to suppress the story were largely to save face. Perhaps, if he felt more charitable about their motivations, he could believe the British authorities were concerned about keeping up morale on the front and at home. No father or mother wanted to hear that a beloved son had died a horrifying and unnecessary death. A line came back to him from his days as a researcher at Edgewood: At the end of World War I, the head of Britain's Chemical Warfare Department had observed, "Gas has very few friends, people are only too ready to forget it."

Alexander did not want the Bari victims to be deliberately forgotten, as the survivor George Southern put it, "as if they were something to be ashamed of." Their nations owed them a debt, and if Alexander was right, medical science would as well. He had the full support of his superiors back in Algiers, including Gen. Blesse, his commanding officer and AFHQ chief surgeon, as well as Standlee and Perrin Long. And he knew Bunny would back him all the way. She would never countenance anything that interfered with her ability to perform her duty. Nothing could prevent her from speaking her mind if she believed it was in the best interests of her patients. He might be standing on principle, but standing tall in her eyes was every bit as important to him.

He had spent days studying the victims, checking their charts, poring over their test results and autopsy reports, and searching, endlessly searching, for any answer that might somehow stem the tide of death— all the while knowing time was against him. It had been an extremely difficult, draining, heartbreaking job. The decision at the highest levels to conceal the presence of mustard gas had "complicated the clinical and pathological picture"; added to the delay in his reaching a true diagnosis; and, he had little doubt, contributed to the number of casualties. He was appalled at the instinct to close ranks and keep silent—even at the expense of men's lives. He would not be a pawn for the British authorities and their attempt to rewrite history in a more benign light.

Alexander sent a terse message to Churchill, informing him he had "reexamined all the data" and was standing by his diagnosis of mustard gas poisoning. This spurred a rapid reply: The diagnosis of mustard was not correct and should be discarded. Alexander refused to back down. Furious, he sent his fourth and final message. Courtesy and respect had been deeply ingrained in him since his days at the military academy, but he was capable of abandoning decorum for something more abrasive: "If the Prime Minister does not wish to accept my diagnosis," he fired back, "he is free to make his own."

Churchill's response came in the form of an edict: There was to be no mention of mustard gas in Bari. On the afternoon of December 13, Col. Bayley, the British commander of the Medical Department, District Two, received urgent orders regarding the recording of all mustard gas casualties incurred during the December 2 air raid. He transmitted an abbreviated form of the orders to FLAMBO, an echelon unit of AFHQ:

```
To: Surgeon WFTD Med Flambo
From: Med Distwo
Most secret
In view of deaths suggest mustard burns be recorded
as burns enemy action instead of dermatitis (nyd).
Signal agreement or alternative.
```

The cover-up was entering a new phase. The doctors in the Allied military hospitals were ordered to alter the medical charts of the Bari victims. All references to mustard gas were to be removed, and the temporary diagnosis of "Dermatitis N.Y.D." replaced with the standard war-service diagnosis, "burns due to enemy action." They were further directed that all references to the American chemical warfare consultant be stricken from the medical records. Alexander's British colleagues reluctantly expunged his name and his findings as to the real cause of death. They told him they were not happy about it, but they had no choice. When Alexander balked at falsifying the medical records, he was informed the ruling had been approved by AFHQ and he was expected to comply. Feeling defeated, he acquiesced with bad grace.

Jessie Park Smith, a nursing sister, was tending Bari casualties at the 98th General Hospital when the staff received the long-awaited confirmation that they were dealing with mustard contamination, along with special instructions as to how to classify the injuries. "It was a high secret," she recalled. "One of the Allied ships in the harbor was loaded with mustard gas bombs ready for retaliation if Hitler used this form of warfare. We had to use the term 'Burns Enemy Action' on patients' medical cards."

After the censorship order was imposed, Bayley pleaded with Alexander to stop pushing for official acceptance of his mustard gas diagnosis. He was already persona non grata with the British command at Navy House. No good would come from continuing to challenge the prime minister's verdict. Visibly flustered, Bayley warned the persistent young American doctor that if he carried on, it might even lead to his being "court martialed." Although they had clashed over his handling of the investigation, Alexander liked the brigadier and could see the man was genuinely frightened for his "safety and wellbeing." He sensed his days in Bari were numbered.

CHAPTER SEVEN

"Magnum Opus"

During the early months of the Italian campaign, the war correspondent Ernie Pyle observed that it was axiomatic that "the closer you get to the front, the less you know about what is going on." There were countless times when Alexander wished he could fly back to Algiers just so he could find out what was really going on in Bari. The British authorities' attempts to keep a lid on the disaster continued to hamper his investigation and make even routine inquiries difficult. Several days after his conversation with the port commandant in Bari, he discovered a whole new group of mustard gas victims the British had neglected to report to him. Even though they were right there on his doorstep, lying in another British military hospital only two hours away, he knew nothing about how they were faring.

He had learned that the British destroyer *Bicester* had come through the air raid unharmed, and, as soon as the barrage was over, returned to the devastated harbor and took part in rescue operations throughout the night. After picking up about thirty oil-slicked survivors—many of them Americans from the sunken Liberty ships—the *Bicester* was ordered to clear the harbor and directed to the nearby "heel" port of Taranto. Six hours out to sea, the entire ship's crew began suffering from eye symptoms—the gritty, burning sensation followed by pain. Soon their eyes were so red and inflamed they could hardly see. The commanding officer suspected some kind of chemical irritant was the cause of the trouble and ordered all hands to rinse their eyes with an eyewash, but, over the course of the voyage, the conjunctivitis grew progressively more severe. Eighteen hours later, the symptoms were so acute that the crew, almost completely blind, had great difficulty in mooring her. A large proportion of the ship's company had to be admitted to the British 70th General Hospital in Taranto and treated for injuries caused by exposure to mustard gas vapor. An ophthalmic specialist was sent for, and about forty men were treated for eye lesions.

The first chance he had, Alexander arranged for a driver to take him to Taranto so he could interview the crew and survivors aboard the *Bicester.** Leaving Bari for the first time, he was struck by the beauty of the surrounding countryside and stopped several times to take photographs. Gazing down on the rolling fields, olive groves, and serene inlets, he found it hard to believe anything bad had ever happened here. When he got to the 70th General Hospital, on a hill overlooking the harbor, he spoke to the medical staff about their so-called NYD cases. Then he went in search of the patients. The sailors told him that none of the port authorities had warned them about the risk of poison gas in the harbor, which had been brought on board the ship by the dripping victims, who left a toxic trail wherever they sat, lay, or traipsed on deck. When the ship departed Bari on the morning of December 3, it was necessarily battened down, and sufficient vapor had been disseminated by then to affect the eyes and respiratory tracts of all those tending the casualties, along with much of the crew. Several men recalled hearing someone on deck mention "the odor of garlic" in the course of the eve-

---

* In his preliminary report, Alexander incorrectly identified the ship as the *Bistera,* a misspelling of *Bicester* that created more confusion and led many subsequent authors and historians to believe it was yet another contaminated vessel.

ning, but it was laughed off as part of the local charm. At the time, no one made any connection to mustard gas.

One of the survivors, Alfred H. Bergman, a US merchant marine who served on the *John Bascom,* had been in the hospital in Taranto for ten days with second- and third-degree burns to his right hand and wrist that he told the doctors were "due to leaking mustard gas." His wounds were not visible, as they were coated with a heavy white ointment, but his medical records revealed that portions of the burned area had become septic. The lesions had been cleaned and redressed and were now healing satisfactorily, but he would need at least three to four weeks of hospitalization, and skin grafts might be necessary. Bergman was being transferred to a Red Cross dispensary in Naples, and then to the large American 7th Station Hospital in Oran for further treatment. The cases of eye inflammation suffered by the *Bicester*'s crew had remained severe for three or four days and then rapidly subsided. By the end of the first week, most were no longer experiencing any difficulties. The immersion cases, however, were wrapped in blankets for the duration of the journey. Once again, the extended period of exposure facilitated the absorption of the mustard through the skin and had fatal consequences.

Of the 102 admissions in Taranto, sixteen had died. This was by far the largest group of American casualties. Alexander considered the British authorities' omission in reporting these cases to him a very serious matter, the more so because it precluded him from ensuring that they received prompt and appropriate treatment for their injuries. AFHQ needed to be informed at once, and he planned to send a wire as soon as he got back to Bari.

It did not escape his notice that the crew of the British vessel *Vienna,* which was ordered to leave Bari Harbor just two hours later, was given a gas warning. The ship made it through the raid and successive explosions without sustaining any major damage, and even though pummeled with shrapnel and flaming debris, the only injury recorded was to the resident cat, which suffered a small chest wound. For most of the night of December 2–3, the *Vienna* served as a casualty clearing station and had been crowded with victims receiving first aid and waiting to be taken by ambulance to the 98th General Hospital. Toward morning, the officers and crew reported suffering from sore eyes, and several men were vomiting. The ship's medical officer could not explain the symptoms. Just prior to being ordered to Brindisi, however, the NOIC at Bari informed the ship's commanding officer of the mustard gas in the harbor and advised him to take the "necessary precautions."

After a quick inspection, the ship's medical officer was almost certain the vessel had not sustained direct contamination from the liquid mustard bombs, and the affected men were the survivors who were pulled from the oily water. A decontamination squad was sent in to spread bleach in the sick bay and other affected areas of the boat, and all the victims' uniforms and blankets were promptly removed and tossed overboard. It was later noted that had they been better versed in antigas measures, they would have taken the added precaution of having all the victims hosed down before they were allowed in the unventilated quarters belowdecks. Once they put out to sea, it emerged that the sick-bay personnel who had been tending the victims were suffering from mustard exposure and were unable to perform their duties. On arrival in Brindisi, two officers (including the medical officer), the leading sick-berth attendant, and six Navy ratings (enlisted men) were sent to the nearby 84th General Hospital. Most cases were only mildly affected by the fumes, and there were no fatalities.

Several other British ships that picked up victims that night suffered from the effects of mustard exposure, including the *Bicester*'s sister ship, *Zetland*, the HMS *Vulcan*, as well as a number of MTBs (motor torpedo boats). By far the worst case was the *Vulcan*, which, because of a mistake in reading the signal "owing to temporary blindness," thought her destination was Taranto, but then she received a second signal telling her to correct course and proceed to Brindisi. Before leaving Bari, the ship discharged all the injured sailors, not realizing, as one crew member bitterly observed, that they were "the lucky ones." Soon many of the crew were complaining of burning eyes. The lower deck was cleared and every man was given an eye bath of boric lotion. As gas was not suspected, no countermeasures were taken.

When the *Vulcan* finally limped into Brindisi on December 4, a tug pulled up alongside and towed her to the bay where she was instructed to drop anchor a safe distance from the other ships. According to Able Seaman Bertram Stevens, the port's decontamination squad was waiting for them; within five minutes, a motorboat arrived, packed with medical personnel in overalls and gas masks. By that time, he and most of his shipmates had been without fresh water for thirty-six hours, could no longer see, and many, including Stevens himself, were "covered in blisters." Once they docked, the sailors were told to strip, and their clothes were taken away and destroyed. They were sluiced down on the dock naked as the day they were born, before lining up for a medical inspection. The entire ship's company was admitted to the 84th General Hospital in Brindisi.

Bert Stevens woke up several days later to find himself in a tented field hospital, his eyes bandaged and his hands swathed in masses of gauze. The doctor who unbandaged his eyes told him his vision would gradually improve, and he dismissed the soreness in his throat as caused by dust and smoke. Blisters "the size of an old penny" had begun to appear on his private parts, and the doctor apologized for cutting off clumps of hair so he could treat the sores. A week later, Stevens was discharged from the hospital in Brindisi and given draft papers back to Britain, still no wiser about what had caused his unusual symptoms.

Casualties admitted to the 84th General Hospital consisted of roughly sixty from *Vienna*, forty from *Vulcan*, as well as numerous

MTB personnel. According to Alexander's notes, of the forty-eight "eye-only" casualties, most were resolved by the end of the first week:

```
21 required 4 days hospitalization
 8 required 5 days hospitalization
 9 required 6 days hospitalization
 5 required 7 days hospitalization
 4 required 8 days hospitalization
 1 required extended hospitalization
```

Interestingly, the medical officer on the *Bicester* related that he had not yet been able to file the Hurt Certificates—a document signed by a doctor signifying the bearer sustained wounds in the course of duty—for the mustard gas injuries sustained by the ship's forty-two survivors and members of the crew. He apologized for the confusion, admitting that many of the patients had already been evacuated to other hospitals, and the demand for the paperwork for benefit claims was "universal." It was an upsetting situation, he explained, as the reason behind the mounting clamor for medical forms was that the majority of the men were not convinced they would fully recover their vision, and "their fear was not easily assuaged." He wanted it understood that the delay was not his fault. He had been unable to issue the forms because he was still awaiting "instructions as to the exact wording of the certificates." Apparently the American and British military authorities had not yet agreed on the lexicon of euphemisms to describe the mustard gas casualties.

Advised he should leave Bari before he was thrown out, Alexander began making preparations for his departure. First, he secretly amassed crucial scientific data on all those exposed to mustard gas. Second, he made copies of the medical case records of the mustard casualties in their unadulterated form, complete with the doctors' memoranda on the unusual burns and systemic effects that had been attached to their files prior to Churchill's purge of his diagnosis. Finally, he collected the results of fifty-three autopsies of mustard fatalities. Erring on the side of caution, he ordered duplicate copies of every autopsy report as well as two sets of pathological specimens from forty "representative cases," made up of men from "at least twelve nationalities and races." Once he was back in Algiers, he would review all the data he had collected and finish writing up his notes.

Alexander had taken the investigation as far as he could in his ten days in Bari, but he was still dogged by the feeling he was leaving behind a lot of unfinished business. Vital information was missing. There were still many unanswered questions, and he had grave reservations about removing the mustard diagnosis from the victims' medical charts, especially in terms of omitting information relevant to the long-term health consequences of exposure. He had requested copies of all his bizarre communications with the prime minister, but the British authorities refused to release them. He could not help but look reproachfully at their handling of the crisis, and the costly delays. In the proper time and place, he would address the matter of their muddled response and make his recommendation, "a plea for more adequate planning for possible future episodes of disaster medicine or hostile use of chemical agents."

As he packed his holdall, he also had to admit he was leaving with "a bit of a heavy heart." He wished he could have done more. He castigated himself for not insisting on interviewing the Italian doctors with the aid of an interpreter, and not doing his own reporting on civilian casualties and the effect of mustard fumes on the town, realizing that information would be an important part of any definitive account of the disaster. "But I did have my hands full," he later recalled. "I had no staff, and Bari was completely under British military control where my relationships were somewhat tenuous at the time."

After his plane took off from Bari Airport, it flew over the harbor. He looked down on the masts of sunken ships poking up above the

SECRET   S E C R E T

APPENDIX # 2

SUBJECT: Intermediate Report on N.Y.D. Dermatitis Cases.

                                        Hq, Hs 2 District, CMF.
                                        Tel No. 13611.
                                        9582 H.
                                                15 Dec 43.

D.D.M.S.
AFHQ, Adv. Adm. Echelon.

        Lt. Col. Alexander, U.S.M.C., Medical Advisor in C.W., arrived by air
from ALGIERS on 7 Dec 43 and comenced his investigation.

        A short report submitted by him is attached. It has been discovered
that certain cases were rescued by ships leaving the port of BARI on the night
of 2/3 Dec 43 and were taken to BRINDISI and TARANTO, these going to the
former port were only mildly affected, and there have been no deaths, but
those accepted at 70 General Hospital, TARANTO, were more serious and of the
102 admissions, 16 have died to date.

        A request has been submitted in cipher to AFHQ to diagnose these cases
as burns due to enemy action. If this is authorized evacuation of certain
long term cases can be carried out and liberate much needed beds.

                            (Sgd)
                                    COLONEL
                                    D.D.M.S.

T.C.C. 1215 hrs

Copy to: SURGEON, D.M.S., AFHQ,
          G.O.C., 2 District,
          War Diary (2).
          File

D.D.M.S.
2 District.

        The burns in the hospitals in this area now labeled "Dermatitis N.Y.D."
are due to Mustard Gas. They are of unusual types and varieties because most of
them are due to mustard which has been mixed into the surface oil in the harbour.

        There are three factors to be considered in appraising the deaths that
have occurred in this group:

                        S E C R E T

                        - 30 -   **SECRET**

(Stewart F. Alexander Papers)

water at awkward angles. He thought about the mustard bombs lying in the belly of the *John Harvey* somewhere in the murky depths. There was no telling how long they might remain there.

Just in case he encountered any unexpected plane trouble on the way home, he presented Col. Bayley with a summary of his latest findings on Wednesday, December 15, the day before he was due to leave. Bayley then forwarded Alexander's "short report" to AFHQ, along with a cable explaining in carefully couched language that it had been prompted by the recent discovery of "certain cases" that had been rescued by ship the night of the air raid and taken to hospitals in Brindisi and Taranto. In keeping with the officially mandated censorship policy, Bayley added a pointed reminder to his American colleagues: "A request has been submitted in cipher to AFHQ to diagnose these cases as burns due to enemy action."

Blatantly defying Churchill's edict to omit the term *mustard gas* in all communications, Alexander laid out what he had learned in his ten days in Bari in his parting memorandum, making no bones about the cause and effect:

```
Subject: "observations of casualties burned in Bari
harbour on 2 Dec 43."
To: D.D.M.S. (Deputy Director Medical Services,
Col. J. H. Bayley)
HQ, No. 2 district



1.   During the period of December 7 through Decem-
ber 16 i had the opportunity to see and study many of
the casualties which followed the air-raid on Decem-
ber 2. These included cases in the 98 general hos-
pital, 3 n.z. general hospital, 14 combined general
hospital, 70 general hospital and 84 general hospi-
```

tal. The latter two hospitals being in taranto and brindisi respectively.

2.   The skin burns were definitely due to mustard. Some were mustard vapour burns, but most of the burns were due to mustard mixed or dissolved in crude oil.

3.   All cases had eye symptoms of one degree or another, except two cases from S.S. Lyman Abbott, who had worn gas masks. The eye symptoms were due to mustard.

4.   There were mustard lesions of the respiratory tract in most of the cases that died, though this was in many cases complicated by an associated blast lesion of the lungs.

5.   The systemic effects of mustard poisoning were the most remarkable feature in this group of cases, and were much more marked than in any previous group of mustard burns. They were much more severe than any described in the last war.

6.   A final appraisal of the cause of death or of the most significant factor in the cause of death, must await microscopic study of the pathological changes. blast injury probably played some part in some of the deaths. I feel that most of the deaths are primarily attributable to mustard.

7.   Arrangements have been made with 98 general hospital to prepare pathological specimens for shipment to porton and edgewood by 19 december. if these are forwarded by air courier to the D.M.S., AFHQ, I will arrange for their future shipment. Plans were laid on for clinical and gross pathological records to accompany these specimens.

```
8.   A full report will be rendered to the D.M.S. and
a copy forwarded to your office for your information.
9.   The cooperation of your staff and of your hospi-
tals has been superior.


                 SGD. STEWART F. ALEXANDER
                     Lt-Colonel. Med Corps.
                   Consultant C.W. Medicine.
```

After reading a copy of this latest memorandum, one of Alexander's colleagues at AFHQ added a sardonic note below item number 9. Commenting on the "superior cooperation" of the British Medical Corps, he scribbled, "Superior to what?"

ALEXANDER WAS IN A HURRY to get back to Allied headquarters. He was looking forward to seeing Bunny again. She had agreed to catch a plane to Algiers and spend Christmas with him. Not only was he in a rush to return to friendly territory, he also figured his bosses would be prodding him to file his preliminary report ASAP. Even though he was completely whipped, he knew he was in for a working holiday. Fortunately, Bunny was as busy as he was and did not resent the fact that he would have to dive straight into his report and would have little time to spend with her.

On Christmas Eve, they sat together and listened to President Roosevelt's broadcast from Hyde Park on the portable radio that Bunny had received as a gift from Gen. McNair. FDR announced plans to launch "a gigantic attack upon Germany" and his selection of Gen. Eisenhower to be supreme commander of the Allied Expeditionary Force. Eisenhower had informed his staff of the impending changes a week earlier, but the public statement made it real and irrevocable. He would be relinquishing his command of the Mediterranean Theater on January 1 and moving his headquarters back to London. By the nature of war, Alexander knew it was almost impossible not to form a strong attachment to a military commander, especially one who had also become a friend, and both he and Bunny felt the emotional letdown. They would be very sad to see Ike go.

On December 27, Alexander submitted his preliminary report of the "Toxic Gas Burns Sustained in the Bari Harbor Catastrophe." All told, more than a thousand Allied servicemen were killed or went missing following the German air raid. (This included approximately fifty sailors of the US Naval Armed Guards and at least seventy-five American merchant mariners.) Of the more than 800 casualties who were hospitalized, 628 were estimated to be suffering primarily from mustard gas exposure. Sixty-nine deaths, wholly or partly attributed to mustard, occurred within two weeks of the incident. But it was probable that there were many others whose records could not be traced. In the introduction to the comprehensive, minutely observed twelve-page account of the chemical disaster, Alexander wrote, "The facts are related as of December 17, at which time many of the detailed data, and especially the histo-pathology, are not available. Many of the observations in this report are based upon statements made by casualties, or by medical officers and nurses who attended the cases, and only later study of the case records and data analysis will permit accurate appraisal and evaluation."

He then went through his investigation step by step, methodically laying out the events of the December 2 air raid and the days that followed, beginning with the first-aid treatment and the nature of the injuries and continuing to the symptoms, eye injuries, clinical observations, and pathology reports that led to his diagnosis of the casualties as "due to mustard vapor and to a mustard-in-oil solution's being in contact with the skin for a protracted period of time." The systemic effects and evidence of systemic toxemia were manifested strikingly by a depression of white blood cells. Gross pathological changes indicative of toxic effects were noted in the liver, spleen, and lymph nodes. His conclusion was unequivocal: "The point should be clearly made that these exposures were due to mustard and not to other agents. It was not a new agent, but a new, and rather unique, method of applying an old agent."

From a chemical warfare perspective, the Bari incident was instructive in terms of defensive measures and treatment for chemical accidents, but it did not represent an immediate military threat. Such a large number of casualties were "not likely to be reproduced to this degree in any tactical employment of mustard," Alexander wrote, "since such an opportunity for prolonged exposure will not be the common situation." From the point of view of "disaster management," it was almost an object lesson in what not to do. Although he had to be careful not to overstep his mandate, he implied that the authorities had been remiss, pointing out both the lack of warning that there was gas in the harbor and the failure to decontaminate the victims before rushing them to the hospital.

In the last line of the report, he returned again to the "severe systemic effects," in particular the destruction of white blood cells, in human beings—the singular medical insight that had been purchased at such a steep price. In his modest conclusion, he noted only that the effects were of "far greater significance than has been associated with mustard burns in the past." It was still too early to make any great claims for his observation, but the tantalizing suggestion was there: The toxic effects of mustard gas might hold promise for the treatment of certain types of cancer.

COL. EDWARD CHURCHILL, chief surgical consultant for AFHQ, reviewed Alexander's report, confirmed the release of toxic gas, and concurred with his findings of mustard contamination exacerbated by prolonged, full-body exposure. He also agreed that serious errors had been made. "The lack of warning that mustard gas was loose and the failure of decontamination precautions before rushing the injured to hospitals," he wrote, "violated one of the principles of disaster management." He then pointed to one of the fundamental lessons learned from the experience of the Cocoanut Grove fire: For the treatment of mass casualties to be effective, "the pattern and nature of the trauma must be ascertained by observers who are not responsible for rescue work and first aid efforts."

Eisenhower, assured by Gen. Blesse and his senior medical staff that Alexander's diagnosis of mustard gas contamination was correct, approved the preliminary report. If he was aware of the dispute with Churchill, it did not stop him from rendering the Bari report into the official record, though it was immediately classified. Col. Standlee, Blesse's deputy, sent five copies of the report to Colonel Shadle, adding in a cover letter that Alexander "calls particular attention to the systemic effects manifested in this group of casualties." Shadle in turn forwarded the report to the Office of the Chief of the Chemical Warfare Service in Washington and to the War Office, with his own note inviting them to mark the systemic effects of mustard.

Alexander had been granted permission to send copies of his report to appropriate chemical warfare experts who could benefit from his experience, as well as to Edgewood Arsenal and Porton Down, along with pathological specimens of forty representative cases. One of his first letters was to Col. William Fleming, who had recruited him into the Chemical Warfare Service and was now chief chemical officer for the European Theater. Apologizing for not filling him in sooner—"I have really been busy for the past several weeks"—Alexander explained what had been monopolizing his time, and he enclosed a copy of his preliminary report. "I am a bit ashamed to say that more effort was extended in trying to save lives than was directed towards scientific investigations," though he believed he had still managed to "collect quite a bit of data." He continued:

> The most amazing part of the picture presented, and I am sure you can read between the lines, was the severity of the systemic features, and the magnitude they assumed. I am sure you will remember how I considered the systemic effects of mustard [at

Edgewood].... This group of cases, and it is important to point out that they were quite different from the usual cases in the last war, certainly presented dramatic effects. I am a little hesitant about stating how striking they are in an official report until I have my pathological data and clinical case records available for study, but there is little question in my own mind.

Alexander promised to write again at greater length when he had "a little more time and a bit more distant perspective upon the whole group," adding, "I would not like to make a hasty or ill-advised statement at this time."

The following day, he wrote to Colonel John R. Wood, director of the Medical Research Laboratory at Edgewood:

27 December 1943

Dear Colonel Wood,

I am enclosing a preliminary report of a group of mustard casualties I recently had the opportunity to see. The report is somewhat sketchy in places but I believe it will give you a general picture of the problem as I saw it.

The point I am most anxious that you and Dr. Winternitz's group consider is the picture I have tentatively described as systemic effects. The blood changes and liver changes I think are very definite. The blood changes might be explained, as I have alluded in the report, by the subtotal body area burns even though of relatively mild degree. Many of the cases had some degree of lung trauma from the blast, but they did not die respiratory deaths. We may grant that blast effects accounted for some of the later deaths, but it still leaves many cases that died with neither of these factors being significant. As you will gather, it was a most interesting group of cases, and left plenty of room for mental gymnastics....

I should like you to:

1. Acquaint Dr. Winternitz with the features of this group of cases.

2. Send me your microscopic findings.

3. Send me your comments on the medical aspects of the episode.

With kindest personal regards,

> Stewart F. Alexander
>
> Lt. Colonel, M.C.

The British officials in Bari and Porton Down never acknowledged his report. Sometime later, however, Alexander received a personal letter from Col. Bayley, who made cryptic reference to his "magnum opus." Gen. Blesse and other senior members of AFHQ's medical section lauded the exceptional job he had done collecting and evaluating the data under difficult conditions, but, because of the secrecy surrounding the disaster, recognition of his work was necessarily unofficial and restrained. He was told a commendation was withheld for fear of "offending the Prime Minister." Nevertheless, admiration for Alexander's Bari report poured in from leaders of the Chemical Warfare Service. Col. Rhoads, chief of the Medical Division, hailed Alexander's meticulous investigation:

15 January 1944

Dear Colonel Alexander:

I would like to let you know of the high praise that has been given your report of the Bari Disaster. It provides us with such complete information as to represent almost a landmark in the history of mustard poisoning.

We plan to use this report as a model in the plants where industrial accidents may occur. I am sure it will be most useful.

Sincerely yours,

> Cornelius P. Rhoads

Alexander also heard from Captain George M. Lyon, a Johns Hopkins physician responsible for preparing chemical defenses for the Naval Command in London. Alexander had written to Lyon, advising that the disaster scenario presented by the Bari incident should be a wake-up call for the Navy, and was "worth bearing in mind" because of the possibility of a recurrence in future shipping accidents. Thanking him for sending a copy of his preliminary report, Lyon observed that Alexander had certainly made his mark: "Col. Shadle was most generous in his praise of you and what you are doing. I know of nobody who could have done a better job in that famous incident you stated so masterfully. I think your contribution in that will be one of immense value."

Col. Fleming sent a hasty note to say he concurred with Alexander's conclusions about the mustard-in-oil and was "quite bursting with pride with the excellence of the report." He indicated that the Bari report was quickly becoming required reading among the Allied commanders planning the next phase of the war, and calculating the odds the Germans might use gas against the Allied armies when they assaulted the beaches of France. "Such solutions, by the way, have been lately mentioned to us as a deliberate use of the agent in landing operations," Fleming added in an oblique reference to the D-day preparations, codenamed Operation Overlord, then being developed in detail. "The present episode certainly suggests the effectiveness of such."

The following week, Fleming wrote to Alexander again, enclosing copies of the new Chemical Warfare Service memorandum and medical bulletins that were being circulated to all Allied port commanders, based on the information gleaned from his Bari report. The new medical directives stressed that all personnel involved in any chemical warfare accident involving fuel oil remove all clothes and traces of the oil from their bodies "at the earliest possible moment." A warm shower and thorough soaping were recommended, but because the vesicant could be difficult to remove, all port surgeons were ordered "to secure and hold 100 gallons of liquid petroleum for this purpose." Above all, Alexander's report had served to increase awareness of the risks involved in the transport of lethal gases. "Chemical intelligence" was now regarded as of the utmost importance. Transport authorities, security forces, as well as surgeons, were to be provided with full and up-to-the-minute information about the presence and kind of chemical weapons in port or expected. "Your report scooped the situation here and has aroused most intense interest both military and medical," Fleming told his protégé. "All of which increased my pride in you. Further reports will be welcome."

As to the friction with his British counterparts in Bari, Fleming assured him it was par for the course: "Relations with the CWS here, are, on the whole, happy, both of us having the silly idea that it is the same war for both of us. This does not mean of course I do not fight with them—that is my way of doing business. But both sides appear to enjoy the scrap."

Even before Alexander's preliminary report reached Allied officials, the bickering between the Americans and the British over how to handle the Bari incident occupied the highest levels of government. In a meeting of the British War Cabinet on December 17, 1943, Sir Andrew Browne Cunningham, commander in chief of the Mediterranean Fleet and newly promoted to first sea lord, registered his displeasure that details about the Luftwaffe attack had appeared in American newspapers, and that a press statement by Henry Stimson confirmed the damage that had been sustained as a result of the air raid. Fearful that the American secretary of war's loose lips might cause the whole sordid affair to erupt into view, Cunningham requested that a telegram be sent forthwith to the American chiefs of staff, who "should be left in no doubt as to the misgivings with which disclosures of this nature were viewed by the British Chiefs of Staff."

During the last two weeks of December, a blizzard of cables flew back and forth among London, Washington, and AFHQ Algiers concerning their divergent strategies for handling the potentially damaging fallout from the chemical warfare incident and any adverse publicity that might result from the gas casualties. All the different branches of the British services involved in the Bari disaster weighed in with their individual concerns and self-serving desires for continued secrecy. "The Royal Navy took up with the Admiralty the policy in respect of how to report the gas casualties resulting from the Bari air raid," Lowell Rooks, Eisenhower's assistant chief of staff, advised G-1, AFHQ, on December 22. "The Admiralty have replied that entries in the medical records would be covered so as to keep secret the real cause of those casualties which resulted from burns due to gas."

By contrast, Rooks asserted that he, Commodore Royer Dick, and Deputy Chief of Staff General J. F. M. Whiteley were all agreed that as the United States made "no secret of the fact that we have adequate stocks of chemical warfare materials immediately available," and if necessary could retaliate in kind, the policy should be to "report these casualties truthfully and openly." If the matter is brought up publicly, he added, "We should state the plain facts of the case." He suggested the matter should be put to the Combined Chiefs of Staff to get an approved policy.

In a draft telegram dated Monday, December 27, Rooks stated Eisenhower's preference for full disclosure: They proposed reporting "the straight facts," indicating the lessons learned and recording the incidence of gas casualties in normal casualty reports "without concealment." That suggestion was quickly shot down, the December 27 memorandum was rescinded, and a very different set of guidelines had been cobbled together by the end of the week. Eisenhower cabled the British War Office the new nomenclature for reporting chemical casualties: all skin affections-burns would be listed as due to "enemy action"; lung and other complications as due to "bronchitis, etc., enemy action"; and all deaths simply attributed to "shock, hemorrhage etc. enemy action." It was considered that "these terms will adequately support future claims by those injured for disability pensions."

In the event questions arose about the US holdings of gas, or enemy propaganda attempted to exploit the accident, Eisenhower proposed to restate that "Allied policy is not (repeat not) to use gas unless and until the enemy does so first but that we are fully prepared to retaliate and do not deny the accident, which was a calculated risk." After another flurry of cables, and the addition of the Air Ministry's suggestion that "injuries to eyes" should also be classified as due to "enemy action," the new terminology for the Bari gas casualties was approved by the chiefs of staff and the British War Office.

The Allies continued to worry that news of the toxic release was on the verge of "breaking" at any minute. Thus far, the papers had only reported on the air raid, but how long would it be before the news-hounds started poking around the rumors of poison gas. Air Vice Marshal Richard Peck, assistant chief of the Air Staff, fretted that "a large party of war correspondents"—one group of Australians and another of Americans, including *Time-Life*'s Will Lang and George Rodger—were present in Bari on the night of the raid, and there might be "repercussions." A discreet check into their whereabouts determined that the pool reporters had all departed early the following morning and appeared to have had little opportunity to learn more about the incident. It was advised that the journalists should be left well enough alone. "I agree that it is best to let sleeping dogs lie," Peck cabled in reply. As an added precaution, a prepared statement was drafted by the Political Warfare Executive in London and "kept on ice" in case it should become necessary to counter any negative publicity or enemy propaganda on short notice.

By then, however, Eisenhower had concluded there was little hope of containing news of both the air raid and the chemical accident, and he scrapped plans for a confidential inter-service briefing of commanders and surgeons. He had been given to understand that the fact that a ship carrying gas bombs had been hit in the attack was already well known in Bari, and he "strongly recommended" the British take no further action other than the postal censorship that had already been imposed: "It is believed that the knowledge is now so dispersed among divergent groups including civilian population in the Bari area that no, repeat no, effective briefing can be accomplished."

In the course of the negotiations, there had been sufficient finger-pointing by the British with respect to the presence of the American mustard bombs in the harbor to persuade Eisenhower to order a complete review of the disaster. (The first sea lord pleaded complete ignorance as to the gas consignment, and the Air Ministry was demanding a full report as to why it was there in the first place!) Among his own advisers, Air Chief Marshal Arthur Tedder, commander of the Mediterranean Allied Air Forces, was also pushing for an official review, upset that his staff was coming in for an "unjust distribution of blame" for the obvious shortcomings in the port's protection. "Even had the defenses not had the defects noted, the effect of the raid would in all probability have been precisely the same in the circumstances," Tedder protested in a December 23 memorandum, noting that it was one well-placed bomb that struck an ammunition ship, which in turn ignited the other ships, including the *John Harvey* and its toxic payload. "It would be quite erroneous to allow the extent of the damage to bias views on the effectiveness or otherwise of the air and A.A. [antiaircraft] defenses."

Eisenhower, already aware of the many missteps and miscommunications outlined in Alexander's report, did not need convincing. There were compelling questions about the accident that needed answers. He announced that he would be appointing a Board of Inquiry to investigate and report on the circumstances resulting in the chemical casualties in the Bari air raid.

In a cable from Cairo on December 29, Churchill, who had been uncharacteristically silent on the matter during a fortnight's illness, signaled that he was paying close attention: "The Prime Minister has already been informed of this by Gen. [Harold] Alexander who shared his astonishment that a ship with such a cargo should have been sent to Bari. The Prime Minister awaits the results of the enquiry with the greatest interest."

The next day, newspapers across the globe printed a "thank you letter" from Churchill, expressing gratitude for the many kind messages he had received during his illness, which had been the subject of rumor and cautious press reports. For his protection, the prime minister's movements were necessarily furtive and clandestine, so the Nazis would not have the benefit of knowing he was in North Africa. He reassured the world that he was on the mend but would be taking a holiday in an "unknown destination," as he needed "a few weeks in the sunshine" to restore his physical strength.

Worn out and admittedly "at the end of his tether" after weeks of travel and high-level war meetings, Churchill was not in the best of shape, physically or mentally, by the end of 1943. He had been on the go continuously since leaving England for Egypt on November 12 to confer with Roosevelt ahead of the Cairo Conference, which was crammed into November 22–26, and was followed two days later by the Tehran Conference, where they held their historic first talks with Soviet Premier Joseph Stalin, the most important and far-reaching Allied strategy sessions of the war. It was at Tehran that the "Big Three" finalized plans for Operation Overlord and shaped the postwar future of Europe. On December 2, Churchill had immediately returned to Cairo for another round of discussions with the president, this time to review the important question of Turkey's participation in the war.

After the back-to-back meetings ended on December 11, Churchill had intended to go to Bari. He had planned to tour the Italian front with General Sir Harold Alexander, but he caught a bad cold on the flight to Tunis. Sitting on one of his suitcases on a desolate airfield where they had been waylaid temporarily, he felt "so tired out" he changed his mind about going to Italy. The weather there was reportedly "absolutely vile and all advances were fitful." Instead, he asked Eisenhower whether he could stay and rest for a few days at his beautiful seaside villa in Carthage, which by coincidence was known locally as the "White House." Churchill dined that night with Eisenhower but awoke the following morning with a fever. For the next six days, he was seriously ill with pneumonia and an irregular heartbeat. His personal physician, Lord Moran, aka Dr. Charles M. Wilson, was so worried he confided to Harold Macmillan, the British resident minister at AFHQ, that he thought the sixty-nine-year-old bulldog politician was going to die.

Churchill sent a telegram to President Roosevelt on December 15: "Am stranded amid the ruins of Carthage, where you stayed, with fever which has ripened into pneumonia. All your people are doing everything necessary, but I do not pretend I am enjoying myself. I hope soon to send you some suggestions for the new commands. . . ." FDR responded two days later: "I am distressed about the pneumonia and both Harry [Hopkins] and I plead with you to throw it off rapidly. . . . The Bible says you must do as just what Moran orders, but at this moment I cannot put my finger on the verse and chapter. . . ."

By Saturday, December 18, Churchill's temperature was back to normal and he began to rally. On Christmas Day, he was well enough to preside over a festive holiday gathering, welcoming his guests while attired in a blue silk dressing gown decorated with dragons and wearing bedroom slippers that bore his initials in gold. Eisenhower arrived for a morning meeting to find Churchill propped up in bed, flanked by the new British commander-in-chief of the Mediterranean, General Sir Henry Maitland Wilson. Frustrated by the impasse in Italy, Churchill harped on his obsession with assailing Germany through the "soft underbelly" of Europe and stressed the importance of keeping up the tempo of their attack in the Mediterranean. At Cairo, he had proclaimed, "Whoever holds Rome holds the title deeds of Italy."

The real matter under discussion was his plan to put an invasion force ashore at Anzio, thirty miles south of the capital city, which he believed would break the deadlock at Cassino and open the road to Rome. With most of the top theater brass in attendance—including Air Chief Marshal Arthur Tedder and Generals Alexander and Wilson— the pajama-clad PM held forth on the merits of the amphibious flanking operation, code-named Operation Shingle, which had been on the drawing board for two months. The Americans were opposed to any new operations in the Mediterranean unless in a supporting role for the Normandy invasion. Eisenhower still regarded the maneuver as a "risky affair." Not only did it mean shifting precious resources and landing craft from Operation Overlord to the Italian attack, but he doubted that even then they would have sufficient troops to compel a German retreat. Churchill was nevertheless committed to the operation, and he argued strenuously that Rome must be taken quickly or the whole Italian campaign would be counted as a failure and the Allied cause would suffer. He and his staff prophesied prompt success. Eisenhower repeated his reservations but agreed to support the plan as long as he could have the landing craft back the moment the two Allied divisions were established on the beach.

Later on Christmas Day, after the meetings, Churchill cabled Roosevelt, begging him to save Shingle, the amphibious attack on Anzio, even though it meant pushing back the Normandy landings, tentatively scheduled for May, by a month. What, he asked the president, "could be more dangerous than to let the Italian battle stagnate and fester on for another three months? We cannot afford to go on and leave a vast half-finished job behind us."

By December 26, Lord Moran declared Churchill had made good progress and was healthy enough to leave Carthage, but only if he agreed to a three-week rest cure in Marrakesh. Despite his illness, Churchill reportedly continued to work "at an alarming pace" from his bed, ignoring the protests of his doctors. He also resisted the advice of cabinet colleagues to delegate some of his manifold duties to other ministers. The Mediterranean strategy occupied the long hours spent on his back. Macmillan, who had returned to Algiers, had his own way of gauging that the patient was improving: "I judge he is recovering, because telegrams are beginning to arrive—some rather disturbing!" he noted in his diary. Cranky in convalescence, Churchill was more querulous and demanding than usual and was soon phoning Macmillan at AFHQ almost hourly.

In one of the most poignant and personal communiqués ever issued from 10 Downing Street, the prime minister concluded his message to his countrymen and Allies by insisting that despite being laid up in Africa, he was never idle: "I have not at any time had to relinquish my part in the direction of affairs and there has been not the slightest delay in giving the decisions which were required from me." At this point, it seemed to Stewart Alexander that the prime minister "doth protest too much." Looking back on their disconcerting exchange about the medical crisis in Bari, he could attest to Churchill's exertions, if not his coherence, during the feverish period in question.

CHAPTER EIGHT

"Forgotten Front"

For Gen. Eisenhower, the Bari disaster was the worst setback on his watch. It was the last "serious blow" that forces under his command suffered from the Germans in the Mediterranean. In ordering the strike on the Allied ships, Field Marshal Albert Kesselring, commander in chief of the German troops in Italy, had hit them where it hurt most, halting the vital flow of men and supplies. The air raid put the strategic port out of commission for a week, and at half strength for more than a month, and the heavy losses slowed the buildup of the Fifteenth Air Force at Foggia and the advance of the Eighth Army. The campaign on land had flagged—bogged down by the incessant rain, muddy roads, and forbidding mountain ridges. The delay in reinforcement could have consequences for the "end-run" to Rome, the amphibious attack on Anzio scheduled for January 22, and even for the assault on the coast of France now fixed for June 1944. By not being able to assist the forward movement of the Army to the extent planned, it had become impossible to take Rome before the transfer of Eisenhower's theater command. He felt this last failure keenly, but it was not in the cards. Shingle was no longer his problem. He had to focus all his attention on planning Overlord.

Before leaving on New Year's Day for a short home visit before assuming his command in London, Eisenhower appointed the members of the Board of Inquiry to look into the "disturbing incident" that occurred in Bari. The board would consist of twelve officers—six American and six British. Four members of the board, including Stewart Alexander, were experts who had been summoned to Bari shortly after the raid for the express purpose of investigating various aspects of the chemical accident, and their personal knowledge and experience would be given additional weight. Eisenhower left instructions that the board, in addition to reporting all pertinent facts, should comment upon and submit recommendations as to the actions required to avoid a recurrence of similar accidents. He also requested "specific answers" to the following questions:

a. Why was a consignment of gas at Bari?
b. By whom and on what authority was it loaded?
c. The extent to which the responsible authorities, military and naval, were aware of the presence of the cargo?
d. Effects on individual men in relation to the degree of contamination experienced?
e. Decontamination methods employed and their effectiveness?

The Board of Officers convened in Algiers the first week of January 1944 and began accumulating contemporaneous reports and interviewing medical personnel and commanding officers, including masters of the ships *Bicester*, *Zetland*, and *Vulcan* and captains of the Coastal Forces and Royal Navy. In some instances, where further information was required, they made their own inquiries or obtained statements from the individuals concerned. Another small board of a half-dozen officers was convened in Bari to answer questions—delivered by airmail from Algiers—that required on-the-spot investigation. Of special interest: Who exactly in Bari received the ten copies of the *John Harvey*'s manifest that apparently had been forwarded from Oran, and who—if anyone—in authority did they inform in view of the nature of the cargo?

In all, twenty-two witnesses testified to what took place in Bari on December 2–3, 1943. For the most part, the assembling of the timeline of who knew what, and when, about the mustard gas in the harbor, proceeded along the same lines as the investigation Alexander had conducted himself. In the manner of most in-house reviews, it uncovered little in the way of anything new. Some of the discrepancies that had troubled Alexander had been glossed over, and some of the gaps were filled. By now, of course, all the various military and naval authorities had had ample time to get their stories straight. The inquiry identified the same list of Allied officials as having prior knowledge of the consignment of mustard bombs, and they all stated for the record that they did not inform anyone else of the gas shipment, as "it was not normal practice to do so," and that in an operational port like Bari, the toxic cargo was not seen as "an abnormal risk." It proved impossible to trace any of the missing manifests, or to establish that any responsible authorities were informed prior to the raid. Only vague explanations were offered as to why no gas alarm was sounded during the attack and no hard warning ever reached the appropriate quarters.

A first draft of the "Report on the Circumstances in Which Gas Casualties Were Incurred at Bari on 2/3 December 1943" was completed on February 6 and circulated among those concerned for comment. The British, who had compiled their own official account, had many suggested alterations and additions. A final draft of the report, comprising eleven sections and nine appendices, was completed by March 14. A multitude of sins was covered by the proviso, stated at the top: "Some of the details of events are, and will probably remain, obscure." In his summary of their findings, the president of the board,

Brigadier Raleigh Chichester-Constable, wrote, "We considered that no useful purpose would be served by delaying the report in order to chase down witnesses, now widely scattered, in the hope of clearing up these uncertainties."

The Board of Officers Report found that on the night of the raid, several messages warning of possible gas casualties went astray in the pandemonium that followed. As a direct result, the casualty clearing stations on ships, first-aid posts, and hospitals were ignorant of the danger, and their initial treatments exacerbated the mustard's toxic effects. They ascertained that, on the night of December 2, a Lieutenant Harry Richardson Gray of the 30 Commando Unit took a group of casualties to the 98th General Hospital and told the medical officer that he had heard a rumor that one of the ships in the harbor was carrying gas bombs. However, Surgeon Lt. John Cosh, who discussed the matter with Gray the following day, "had the impression that the warning he gave was a general one, and he did not suspect the casualties delivered by him to be [contaminated], nor did he at the time realize the possibility of contamination through the medium of oil fuel."

Gray stated that, on his return to Navy House at midnight, he went to the operations room to see whether he could obtain more information on the gas situation. Upon learning the rumors were true, he asked the duty operations officer, a Lieutenant Shearer, to telephone the hospital to that effect. Shearer did as instructed, spoke to a medical officer and informed him of the gas risk, and received his assurance that the warning would be passed on to all the hospitals concerned. According to the official account, the fate of this message was not known. Lt. Gray left for England shortly after the raid and was unavailable to provide evidence on this point.

Most unfortunate was the conclusion that the 98th General Hospital's telephone call to Navy House on the morning of 3 December failed to obtain official confirmation of mustard gas in the harbor, though "whether the alleged informant was ignorant of the facts or was impressed with a supposed desirability of secrecy is not clear." The board's investigation brought out that the "reticence of authorities" generally to disclose the presence of mustard impeded proper gas precautions from being taken and the proper treatment of victims, and that this "unnecessary reticence" could have been dispelled by clear direction from the Combined Chiefs of Staff. Rather than attempt to pass censure on specific officers, the report sought to be instructive in its portrait of the complete chaos on the ground, the absence of any coherent command structure, and the extent to which the majority of men involved were acting on their own initiative. Addressing the lack of any official gas warning, the board concluded:

> The outstanding fact which emerges from our inquiry is that a number of persons suffered from mustard burns which might have been allayed and possibly prevented if the true nature of their injuries had been appreciated from the beginning. . . .
>
> It is probable that had the appropriate medical authorities received definite information that a ship carrying mustard gas had exploded in the harbor they would have been able to reach a true diagnosis a good deal earlier. As it was, they were confronted with patients exhibiting the ordinary symptoms of shock, exposure, burns etc., who therefore received initial treatment actually favorable to the absorption of mustard. The particular clinical picture was unusual. The burns were not typical of mustard because they had been brought on by long exposure to a solution of mustard in oil, aggravated by resuscitation treatment involving in some cases a long period in blankets.

The board recommended that the existing procedures for gas shipments be supplemented and that, going forward, toxic ammunition should always require "special notification": Cables should be sent from the port of dispatch to port and ordnance authorities at the port of discharge with details of cargo and dates of arrival, as well as all ports of call, and in every case acknowledgment would be required. Furthermore, stowage of "mixed cargo"—toxic munitions and explosives on the same ship—should be avoided whenever possible, and these shipments should not be sent into large, busy ports in forward areas. More training in chemical warfare was also recommended, with new instructions to include warnings about the danger posed by poison gas dissolved in oil, with particular reference to all persons working on ships, in harbors, and in armored fighting vehicles (AFVs). There was an implicit reproof in the wording of the board's conclusion:

> If there is reason to believe that gas has escaped from a ship, through an air raid or otherwise, the Port Authorities should immediately warn the area HQ and the Commanding Officers and Masters of ships, giving the fullest information available. It must be the responsibility of the naval and military commanders concerned to pass on the warning for the information of hospitals, first aid posts etc., and definite arrangements for a speedy dissemination of this information should be made beforehand.

Perhaps the most surprising disclosure was that on the night of Friday, December 3, at the request of General Clarence L. Adcock, Col. Shadle, chief chemical officer at AHHQ, and Major K. J. B. Earle, a British technical officer, were ordered to fly from Algiers to Bari the first thing the next morning to inspect the damaged harbor. Due to extremely bad weather, they were grounded at Naples for a night and reached Bari at 9 a.m. on Sunday, December 5. They reported to the new NOIC, Comm. Guinness, who was "very much concerned" about the toxic munitions aboard one of the cargo ships and whether the harbor was contaminated. According to Shadle's account: "In checking the manifests of the ship, *John Harvey,* we learned that she carried approximately 200,000 100-lb. H [mustard] bombs and 700 cases white phosphorous smoke bombs, 100-lb." They immediately undertook a complete reconnaissance of the harbor with a representative from the port manager's office, at which time the positions of various ships that had sunk or were damaged were pointed out. During this inspection, and later inspections, they located a contaminated area on the outer mole as well as ruptured mustard-bomb casings. Shadle stated that it was "most evident that more of these bombs were exploded in mid-air and which was the cause of many of the survivors being contaminated." Immediate action was taken to place the area off-limits to personnel and to decontaminate the area.

On completion of their inspection, and extensive diving operations, Shadle and his technical officers apprised the NOIC that it was likely that "at least some of the casualties" were caused by contact with the film of mustard-in-oil solution floating on the water's surface. The danger from this had passed, and the only remaining hazard lay in direct contact with pools of mustard trapped in low points underwater during salvage operations. They also advised him that the amount of white phosphorous in the water was not hazardous—eleven and a half gallons taken internally would be required for fatal results—and would slowly oxidize, producing harmless phosphoric acid and "red" phosphorous, which was not toxic and would not ignite spontaneously in air. The only risk might lie in phosphorous-saturated wood from the wrecks that, on drying out, could ignite spontaneously. The technical team's inspections were completed on December 6, the day before Stewart Alexander arrived in Bari. However, the crucial information about the mustard and the white phosphorous listed on the manifests and found in the harbor was never shared with Alexander or hospital personnel. One hand of the Chemical Warfare

Service did not let the other know what it had discovered. Secrecy once again trumped common sense and concern for the welfare of the victims.

When it came to military security, and the rules and regulations governing shipments of poison gas, the board attempted to clarify its position: "There appears to be nothing secret about the Allies' policy with regard to chemical warfare; it has been proclaimed that we intend to retaliate if the enemy begins." Therefore, it was to be expected that there would be shipments of poison gas, along with other kinds of bombs and ammunition. The board considered that the "recommendation to secrecy," taken both at the 2:15 p.m. meeting and later by Shadle's reconnaissance party, "was made (it is understood) because it was believed that by then anyone who had to take action or could be affected by the information had already been warned; and it was undesirable, as a routine matter of secrecy, to spread the news any further to individuals not directly affected."

Here was the one lesson from the Bari tragedy that stood out clearly in the fog of wartime confusion and miscommunication. The board stressed that "the relationship between secrecy and safety" be impressed on all those who might possibly have to deliver a decision in such matters in the future:

Normally, the principle of secrecy and safety work together; but if they come into conflict, the former should give way where toxic ammunition is concerned to the needs of the latter. Obviously, the enemy should be kept in ignorance as far as possible of the presence of toxic ammunition in any particular place, but warning must be given when any danger arises, whether the ammunition concerned is our own or the enemy's.

The specific answers required by Eisenhower were furnished at the end:

a. This consignment of gas was at Bari because it was required by the Air Force at Foggia to comply with [Allied] policy [to accumulate mustard reserves on the Italian mainland].

b. The cargo was loaded at Oran on the authority of NAASC [Northwest African Air Service Command], pursuant to the policy of AFHQ.

c. The following responsible authorities in Bari were aware before the raid of the presence of this cargo in that port:

Port Commandant
Dock Superintendent
Port Officer (U.S.)
Transportation Officer (U.S.) Adriatic Base Station

There is some doubt whether the Sea Transport Officer was informed.

d. The effects on individual men were in direct relation to the degree of contamination experienced. The degree of contamination was regulated by several factors; namely, the absolute amount of mustard in contact with the skin, the type of exposure (either vapor or mustard in solution), the strength of the mustard in oil producing contamination, and the length of exposure either to vapor or the mustard in oil solution. The subject is dealt with in detail in Appendix G [Alexander's medical report].

e. The decontamination methods employed and their effectiveness are dealt with in [the body of the report and Appendix I].

The Board of Officers Report was careful to spread the responsibility equally between the two Allied forces. Certain weaknesses in the port's defenses and security organization had been exposed—the NOIC blamed the port commandant for allowing too many ships in the harbor, and Lt. Col. Sieff testified that on two previous occasions he had expressly asked Capt. Campbell to disperse them—and actions were being taken to remedy the situation. But it was understood that setting up and coordinating an adequate air defense system in a newly captured port was always difficult. The problems presented by the enemy's use of *Düppel*, or "Window," foil strips to interfere with radar, could not be immediately solved, as there were no effective countermeasures, but it could be reduced by familiarizing ground and air radar operators with the new tactic and improving the flexibility of their defensive organization. The abnormal congestion in the harbor had made a bad situation worse, but it was agreed that none of the ships could have been dispensed with, and the problem lay in the shortage of warship accommodations on the east coast of Italy. (In the meantime, Manfredonia was being developed as an advance naval port to ease the burden on Bari.)

The Italians also came in for their share of criticism: According to testimony by several Royal Navy captains, the local tugs fled the port rather than participate in rescue operations; and the turmoil in the dockyards was compounded by the fact that the laborers—the majority of whom were Italian, both civilian and military—had no experience with bombing raids, and it took the best part of three hours to coax them out of the shelters and get them working again after the "all clear" was sounded. The accident had served to highlight a general ignorance of antigas precautions, and, as a result, a number of ships were knocked out of action for days, owing to the avoidable contamination of both the vessels and their crews. "It was an unlucky raid," Gen. John Whiteley, Eisenhower's assistant chief of staff, observed to a War Office colleague in London. "There's no one person who can be hanged for the affair."

Perhaps the most chilling testimony was given by Commander Guinness, who had not yet taken over as NOIC but was present during the raid, and thus was a dispassionate and informed witness to the events of the night of the attack. In light of the raging fires, continuous explosions, and the very real possibility of the wind shifting from the south to the more usual north toward land, he maintained that a far greater catastrophe could have taken place had the *John Harvey* not sunk when it did, taking the majority of its toxic load with it. "Had the ship concerned exploded," Guinness stated, "the whole town and dock area and all ships in the vicinity would have been contaminated." Instead of the harbor being unusable for a few days, the whole town and surrounding area would have been uninhabitable for weeks. The commander's view was that the port of Bari had had a very narrow escape.

Eisenhower acted on the board's recommendations but kept the findings secret and saw to it that the report was sequestered. The last thing he wanted was for information about the many errors and undiagnosed injuries to reach the press and then cause a hue and cry at home about the gas casualties. Not even Alexander was permitted to see a copy of the completed report.

The Allied authorities feared the poison gas accident would further erode public support for the war, especially since the Anzio gamble had not paid off. Beginning with the Battle of the Rapido, aka "Bloody River," the carnage during the crossing of the waterway was so great that survivors of the decimated 36th Infantry Division demanded a congressional investigation into the botched operation. For the Americans, February 1944 was the deadliest month in the Mediterranean to date, with nineteen hundred bodies and counting. According to Captain Harry Butcher, Eisenhower's naval aide, with Anzio bogged down in yet another stalemate, the ongoing bitter fighting in Italy, and the recent revelation that twenty-three American transport aircraft lost in the Sicilian operation had been downed by their own naval gunfire, AFHQ's relations with the press were at an all-time low. "It added to the apprehension of the professional public relations people who think that because of this [the Sicilian friendly fire accident], the Bari disclosure, and the Patton incident, the public has lost confidence in the armed forces' willingness to release bad news about its operations."

The cascade of depressing news from the front drove home the Allies' painfully slow progress. Stateside editors wanted upbeat pieces featuring battlefield heroics of American combat soldiers—"gung-ho" marines and glamorous flyboys—not a ceaseless stream of stories about suffering and senseless death. The strict censorship, the dearth of information, and the fact that even most of the Bari survivors themselves never knew what really happened to them, meant that the cover-up, such that it was, succeeded in enshrouding the truth about the chemical-weapons tragedy. None of the Allied news releases about the air raid ever referred to mustard gas. With action in the Mediterranean developing so fast, and more pressing problems dominating headlines, the Bari incident soon faded from memory. The release of poison gas remained hidden under a veil of secrecy—obscured by mystery, deception, and official lies.

DESPITE HOW CLOSE THEY HAD COME to disaster, Allied shipments of chemical weapons to the front continued unabated. As plans for the June 1944 invasion of France took shape, Eisenhower and other military planners at Supreme Headquarters Allied Expeditionary Forces (SHAEF) became increasingly concerned that Hitler might employ poison gas on the Normandy beachhead to cause panic and disrupt the landings. "While planning the Normandy invasion, we had weighed the possibility of an enemy gas attack and for the first time speculated on the probability of his resorting to it," General Omar Bradley wrote in his memoir. "I reasoned that Hitler, in his determination to resist to the end, might risk gas in a gamble." Roosevelt and Churchill ordered the stockpiling of a sixty-day supply of chemical munitions at secret depots in England. By mid-May, less than a month before D-day, the theater command considered the threat of German gas warfare serious enough to order combat-ready toxic bombs sent to operating air stations "so a retaliatory strike could be launched in a maximum of twenty-four hours."

There were also growing fears that the Germans might try using "biological warfare," which the US Army broadly defined as the use of bacterial or toxic agents to produce disease or death in population groups and render large areas unsafe. The Nazis had shown an interest in biological warfare, and there were rumors they had conducted experiments for its use in offensive action. From the intelligence available, it appeared there were "two principal types of biological attacks": a mass tactical or external attack, such as the Japanese used in China; and sabotage or an internal attack from behind the lines, paralleling incidents in World War I, when the Germans tried to spread infectious diseases such as glanders and anthrax amid the horses on the Western Front. Over the winter, Alexander received a number of G-2 bulletins warning them to guard against the grave new danger. "Due to his steady deterioration, the enemy may in desperation resort to biological warfare," one Most Secret memorandum admonished. "It is therefore imperative that all intelligence officers, medical officers, and others concerned be keenly alert to possible methods of attack, and be alert to recognize any presumptive evidence of its contemplated employment or attempted use."

On January 7, 1944, Alexander wrote a memo to John P. Marquand in the War Research Service, advising him that they had received a scrap of intelligence warning of German activity, which had immediately been relayed to Washington and London. While it was not of the "highest evaluation"—the information came via Spain but was believed to have originated in France—he regarded it as a "definite report":

```
The germans are at present actively engaged in prepar-
ing for bacteriological warfare, probably as a result
```

of the bombings of germany, there is one very important factory at LUDWIGSHAVEN, and forty others in germany at Large.

The chemical war had taken an ominous new turn. In an attempt
to "neutralize any such an action," Alexander was put to work investigating whether the Axis armies were preparing to use biologicals. For
clues to the enemy's intentions, every effort had to be made to capture
medical documents and supplies, especially German and Italian biological products, vaccines, and blood serums. Samples of captured matériel
were to be forwarded without delay to G-2, AFHQ. They were advised
to keep a lookout for the appearance of German chemical troops who
had been specially trained and prepared for biological warfare.

Alexander was ordered to take blood samples from German POWs,
captured at Anzio and elsewhere, to check for any unusual types of
inoculations and to search their packs, pay stubs, and papers for any
indication of recent immunizations. He also collected blood samples
from Allied soldiers whose divisions had recently been stationed in
occupied parts of France and Italy and forwarded them to the Army
Medical Center in Washington for analysis. Any unexplained illnesses
or outbreaks of disease of unknown etiology were to be reported at
once. Any sign of enemy chemical units, field laboratories, decontamination apparatus, or new or reissued protective gear should be regarded
as suspicious. "This is to let you know we are keeping our ears and
eyes open," Alexander assured Marquand. "Unfortunately, captures [of
biologicals] have been very slim and not remarkable, and one cannot
investigate what one doesn't capture!"

At the same time the D-day planners were building up their chemical reserves, they also had to accumulate sufficient gas-warfare protective equipment for the entire Allied Expeditionary Force. The invasion
plan called for every soldier to wear protective outer garments for the

landing and carry a gas mask, cellophane protective covers, eye shields, eye ointment, one can of shoe impregnate, and one package of protective ointment. Most soldiers were also equipped with sleeve detectors—an armband made of poison-gas-detector paper procured from the British, and information cards detailing the signs and symptoms of gas poisoning. As added insurance, Chemical Warfare Service decontamination units would land right behind the infantry on the invasion beaches, prepared to clean the coastline for the troops in the event the Germans deployed chemical weapons to counterattack.

The most important single piece of equipment, the gas mask, had been improved since the start of the war. As the new models began arriving, chemical officers examined the fit and made adjustments on every individual, from privates to the supreme commander. Once again, the new masks did not work on men who wore glasses. Some things never changed. Alexander promptly contacted the chief surgeon of the North African Theater of Operations: "It is recommended that steps be taken to procure gas mask spectacles for all men in this theatre requiring same," he wrote in reference to his own invention, now in early production. "In the event of hostile chemical attack, the lack of gas mask spectacles for those men with significant refractive correction will seriously impair their efficiency and perhaps jeopardize their safety."

In a folder of CWS memoranda, Alexander had saved a Bill Mauldin cartoon that captured the grim reality of modern industrial warfare and the constant race for technical supremacy. It showed one haggard GI telling another, "I see Comp'ny E got the th' new style gas masks, Joe." Behind them is a torched battlefield strewn with abandoned and obsolete gas kits.*

---

* It was not until after the war that Alexander learned German scientists had invented two new rapid-action, extraordinarily powerful nerve agents, tabun and sarin, for which they were totally unprepared.

EXCITING NEWS FROM EDGEWOOD arrived in April. Alexander's Bari report was generating great interest. The response from the scientists and laboratory researchers was "tremendous." Col. Rhoads, chief of the Medical Division of the CWS, wrote to Alexander from his Washington office, requesting additional slides of pathological specimens taken from the Bari casualties so that they might be coordinated with the individual cases. "Your cooperation in furnishing the previous report and slides is greatly appreciated," added Rhoads. "It is felt that the report and slides make a distinct contribution to the medical aspects of the agents concerned."

Alexander felt the same electric thrill he had experienced two years earlier when he had first stumbled on the bizarre blood effects at Edgewood. This was the first sign that researchers at the CWS grasped the significance of the systemic effects in human beings and were pursuing the potential medical applications of mustard compounds. It was exhilarating to be part of a larger effort to see whether the Bari data indicated they were onto a possible treatment for cancer. He quickly dispatched a set of forty case records for the Bari victims from whom the original slides had been taken.

On April 17, 1944, he sent Rhoads a lengthy memorandum providing the necessary background information and context for the misleading diagnoses listed in the medical case sheets and path reports: "It is most necessary to point out that none of the medical case sheets make any mention of a vesicant agent because of the security regulations that were immediately applied at the time," he wrote. "The use of the term 'N.Y.D. Dermatitis' was a command decision." He went on to explain that the immense pressure under which the hospitals were working prevented the accomplishment of many of the laboratory tests that he had requested, and this accounted for the sometimes "scanty" observations in the case notes. For the same reason, he would be unable to provide additional slides, as the only existing sets of tissue blocks had been sent to Edgewood and Porton Down, and nothing was retained at the busy forward hospitals.

Alexander noted that, with the luxury of time, and after close study of the clinical material, he had modified some of the impressions and opinions in his preliminary report. In the intervening months, the death toll had risen. Of the 617 documented mustard casualties, eighty-three, or 13.6 percent, were fatal. The results of the treatment of sulfur mustard casualties proved discouraging. He was preparing a more detailed final report and was awaiting the results of the microscopic studies at Edgewood. The changes in the liver, kidneys, and hematopoietic system had yet to be explained. "The systemic effects continue to be the most interesting aspect of the picture and provocative of thought," he wrote. "Any advice, help, or suggestions would be most welcome so the best possible use may be made of the information gained in this episode."

On May 18, two Edgewood researchers, Arnold R. Rich and Arthur M. Ginzler, completed their study of the "Pathological Changes in the Tissue of the Victims of the Bari Incident." Although hampered by the "inadequacy of the material available for study"—due to postmortem changes and poor fixation of the specimen samples, as well as the lack of bone-marrow and small-intestine samples—they were intrigued by the systemic action of the absorbed mustard. "In general, the course of events in these casualties, as described in Alexander's report, bears out to a considerable degree the present conception of the action of mustard," they wrote in their discussion of the cases, citing the extensive microscopic lesions to the lungs, kidneys, and skin. "The outstanding question raised in this report is whether, because of the apparent differences listed between the type of shock occurring in the Bari cases and ordinary traumatic shock, the former might have been due to a systemic action of mustard absorbed through the skin from the mustard-in-oil solution in which these victims were so long immersed. The suggestion is made by Alexander of a direct toxic action on the peripheral blood vascular bed."

While it remained questionable whether the shock syndrome was necessarily a manifestation of the toxic effects of mustard, Rich and

Ginzler concluded that the profound leucopenia (reduction of the number of white blood cells) in some cases clearly demonstrated that "systemic mustard intoxication did occur." Since a full explanation could not be given from the material provided, they recommended that "a study be made of the effects of very extensive skin burns due to mustard or mustard-in-oil in animals, directed particularly to the possible production of a clinical picture similar to that seen in the Bari victims."

Alexander smiled to himself as he read the last sentence. A study would be made! The toxic legacy of the Bari disaster would continue to be explored. It was a small triumph, perhaps, but he savored it nonetheless. Checking the classified circulation list at the end, he could see that the Edgewood tissue study, along with his Bari report, was being sent to more than a dozen National Defense Research Council scientists and laboratories for further evaluation. Most gratifying was the name of the American poison gas expert who had rejected his earlier work—Dr. Milton Winternitz.

TAKING ADVANTAGE OF THE RELATIVE LULL in action that spring, prior to the big buildup ahead, Alexander thought he had better marry Bunny before she was promoted again and outranked him. She would be accompanying a group of nurses being sent to France with the invasion force, so they would soon be parted. Time was precious. They were married on Wednesday, April 29, 1944, and made history as the first time two colonels in the United States Army had ever married. The popular radio commentator Walter Winchell announced the unprecedented "silver leaf merger" on his Sunday night broadcast. The colorful civil ceremony took place in Algiers City Hall with a French magistrate officiating, complete with French and American civil and religious rites, followed by a military ceremony at the hospital guesthouse overseen by an army chaplain. Gen. Blesse, the couple's commanding officer, gave the bride away. Eisenhower offered them his villa for their

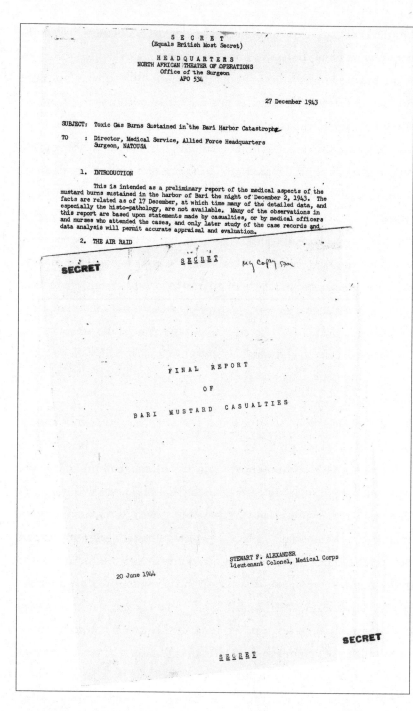

SECRET
(Equals British Most Secret)

HEADQUARTERS
NORTH AFRICAN THEATER OF OPERATIONS
Office of the Surgeon
APO 534

27 December 1943

SUBJECT: Toxic Gas Burns Sustained in the Bari Harbor Catastrophe

TO   :   Director, Medical Service, Allied Force Headquarters
         Surgeon, NATOUSA

1. INTRODUCTION

        This is intended as a preliminary report of the medical aspects of the
mustard burns sustained in the harbor of Bari the night of December 2, 1943. The
facts are related as of 17 December, at which time many of the detailed data, and
especially the histo-pathology, are not available. Many of the observations in
this report are based upon statements made by casualties, or by medical officers
and nurses who attended the cases, and only later study of the case records and
data analysis will permit accurate appraisal and evaluation.

2. THE AIR RAID

SECRET   SECRET   my copy 57a

FINAL   REPORT

OF

BARI   MUSTARD   CASUALTIES

STEWART F. ALEXANDER
Lieutenant Colonel, Medical Corps

20 June 1944

SECRET

SECRET

(Stewart F. Alexander Papers)

honeymoon, but they were too busy to take him up on it, so they made do with a week's holiday in Oran.

At Alexander's bachelor party the previous night, his best man, Perry Long, proposed a tongue-in-cheek toast to the intrepid investigator of the Bari disaster. "This officer," he declared, "systematically located and charted a city-wide network of bars, brasseries, wine shops, back rooms and blind tigers. Single-handed and alone, and with utter disregard of the consequences to his stomach, ulcers and liver, he sampled the wares of said dispensaries." Raising a glass, and speaking above the raucous cheers, he continued: "No sot in this theater has shown such indefatigable enthusiasm, even when he was obviously overburdened with the weight of his evening's tour of duty. During one critical period, with the assistance of only three other officers, he successfully destroyed the liquid contents of seventy large bottles. Incapacitated but undaunted, he bravely urged his companions on to greater efforts, and waving an empty cognac bottle, was carried from the scene of action on a stretcher." Needless to say, they all got roaring drunk.

WHILE WORKING ON THE CHEMICAL DEFENSES for Overlord, Alexander continued to spend every free hour laboring over his analysis of the Bari casualties. He incorporated the results of the microscopic studies from Edgewood, revising his opinion about the impact on the liver and placing even greater emphasis on the depression of the hematopoietic and lymphatic systems. He submitted his "Final Report of the Bari Mustard Casualties" on June 20, 1944. But by then it was old news. Two weeks earlier, on June 6, the Allies had landed a massive invasion force on the Normandy beachhead, and the troops in Italy, who had been through so much, were relegated to the "forgotten front."

———— •◆• ————

CHAPTER NINE

"A Riddle Wrapped in a Mystery"

The poison gas disaster in Bari may have been an accident, but Col. Rhoads knew that the startling discovery of mustard's therapeutic potential was not. Stewart Alexander's detailed, systematic study of the horrific casualties was nothing short of a "classic medical paper," and it clearly pointed the way to a chemical that could possibly be used as a weapon in the fight against cancer. Although the Allied authorities tried to have the records of the embarrassing episode sealed, Alexander had succeeded in extracting invaluable data from the morass of human suffering and official secrecy and disseminated his findings. The inquisitive young physician had been the right man, in the right place, at the right moment in history, and Rhoads intended to ensure that Alexander's efforts did not go to waste.

As chief of the CWS Medical Division, responsible for coordinating all research related to war gases and their effects on soldiers, Rhoads was perfectly situated, and powerful enough, to make certain the Bari report was not relegated to oblivion but instead was transmitted to a top research laboratory operating "under military security." He wanted the mustard gas in Bari Harbor studied in a controlled setting to test Alexander's observation of its capacity to decimate white blood cells and to determine whether the harmful substance—in tiny, carefully calibrated doses—could be used to heal.

One of the country's foremost cancer doctors, Cornelius P. Rhoads—everyone called him "Dusty"—had long been on the hunt for a cure. As a pathologist, scientist, and renowned clinical investigator, he had dedicated most of his career to the slow, frustrating search for a medicine that could vanquish cancer, even as the origin and nature of the fatal malady remained elusive. He often joked grimly that Churchill's observation that Russia was "a riddle wrapped in a mystery inside an enigma" was better applied to cancer than the impenetrable Soviet state. Researchers could not even agree whether cancer was a single entity or many different afflictions lumped under one title. The idea persisted that the disease might be beyond their ken, that it was "scientifically inaccessible." But Rhoads refused to subscribe to this defeatist philosophy. Cancer, for him, was the ultimate foe, and it would continue to ravage the young and old until it was conquered. Propelled by a sense of urgency, the forty-five-year-old Rhoads left no one in doubt that he regarded the war as an inconvenience. He was in a hurry for the fighting to be over so he could get back to his real work—beating a disease that annually took a heavy toll on human life, causing one out of every seven deaths in the United States alone.

Long before the Bari disaster, a close brush with death had made Rhoads a believer in chemical cures and shaped his career. Born in Springfield, Massachusetts, the son of an ophthalmologist, he graduated from Bowdoin College and Harvard Medical School in 1924 and then trained under the eminent neurosurgeon Dr. Harvey Cushing. While a surgical intern, he spent one summer at the Grenfell Mission Hospital in Labrador, studying tuberculosis. TB is highly contagious, and by the time the young medical student returned to Boston, he was coughing up blood. He spent a year recuperating at the Trudeau Sanatorium, in Saranac Lake, New York, where he met Strachimer Petroff, a member of the revered "Trudeau Group," whose groundbreaking work on tuberculosis had achieved worldwide fame. Inspired by Petroff, Rhoads began conducting his own experiments and developed a lasting interest in and devotion to laboratory medicine. After his own illness, his interests turned from surgery to pathology, the science of the causes and effects of diseases. In 1928, he joined Manhattan's Rockefeller Institute for Medical Research, where he worked under the distinguished pathologist Dr. Simon Flexner. After only two years, Rhoads became head of his own special service at Rockefeller for hematological disorders, eventually concentrating on leukemia, the most common cancer arising from the blood cells. By the time he returned from a research stint in the tropics in 1932, during which he and a team of doctors made significant advances in controlling the once-fatal disease known as pernicious anemia, he was more determined than ever to find a cure for cancer.

Ironically, Rhoads himself became the passive object of research when he fell victim to a fulminating streptococcal infection in 1936. At the time, common bacterial infections loomed large as killers, and even minor cuts and scrapes could prove fatal. The doctors at Rockefeller treated him with an experimental antibacterial drug already in use in Europe but still regarded with suspicion in the United States, and Rhoads became one of the first Americans saved by the original miracle drug, sulfanilamide. He would later tell people he was lucky to have lost only one finger instead of his life. The experience instilled in him an abiding faith in the possibility of medical advances in the future, along with a predisposition to dismiss the "melancholy statements" made by skeptics regarding other disorders for which progress might be just around the corner.

Despite a reputation for arrogance and overzealousness that did not always make him popular with his colleagues, Rhoads continued to make a name for himself as a gifted clinical instigator, and in 1940 he was appointed professor of pathology at Cornell University Medical College. Brilliant, charismatic, and fiercely driven, he also became the director of New York's Memorial Hospital for the Treatment of Cancer and Allied Diseases, the oldest and finest cancer hospital, now ensconced in a large facility on 68th Street and York Avenue on land donated by John D. Rockefeller Jr. Vowing to use Rockefeller's gift to redouble their commitment to laboratory research, he announced plans to develop new experimental methods and scientific tools to conquer the disease.

Rhoads knew they faced serious hurdles. Little progress had been made in the treatment of cancer since Hippocrates first gave the disease its name and issued his famous prescription, "What drugs will not cure, the knife will." For centuries, surgery was the only remedy. Using a simple but brutal procedure, doctors cut out the malignant lumps and masses and hoped they would not return. Marie and Pierre Curie's discovery of radium in 1902 led to the first treatment that brought relief to some patients. But while the invisible rays shrank tumors and pulverized lymphomas, they worked with an indiscriminate shotgun effect, targeting healthy as well as diseased tissue. It soon became apparent that radiation also caused some tumors to grow rapidly, eventually killing Marie Curie and many of the early pioneers of the procedure. While it marked the dawn of radiation oncology, the treatment had its limits, was corrosive in excess, and turned out to be largely ineffective against progressive metastasized cancer. More than forty years had passed, and radiotherapy and surgery were still the only two means of combating cancer.

For Rhoads, who had scarcely embarked on his plans for Memorial when the war came, the convergence of the Bari report and his intense search for a cure crystallized into a single mission—to exploit the military research into poison gas to find a chemical that could selectively injure or kill cancer cells in the way sulfa drugs worked on streptococci.

While science had established the cellular origin of cancer rather than bacterial infection, Rhoads still believed the bacteria-eradication model was a winning strategy: that cancer cells, like bacteria, were foreign invaders that had to be eradicated at any cost. By mentally substituting the rampaging cancer cells for the invasive bacteria, "cancer might be regarded as not so inaccessible, but rather as vulnerable to attack by accepted techniques."

If Stewart Alexander was right, mustard gas might represent a treatment breakthrough. The autopsies of the Bari victims revealed that mustard's toxic effects specifically targeted white blood cells, which almost vanished, while lymph tissue "melted away." Rhoads seized on this as convincing evidence that mustard was a "most promising substance," and certainly an impetus to further research. He was enthralled by Alexander's suggestion that the suppressive effect of the poison might be harnessed to target rapidly growing cells that run wild in the body and then invade healthy tissue. "Since mustard gas was found to destroy normal blood-forming cells," Rhoads wrote, "it was theorized that it might destroy cancer."

A monumental question remained, however: Could mustard's toxic effects be harnessed to target *abnormal* or malignant white cells, while at the same time not doing too much damage to the rest of the patient?

Similar observations of mustard's effects had been reported at the end of World War I, but the bitter public backlash against chemical weapons put a damper on poison-gas research. In 1919, two American pathologists at the University of Pennsylvania, Edward and Helen Krumbhaar, analyzed the physical effects of the German mustard gas Yellow Cross, used at Ypres, and found that it produced noteworthy changes in the blood and bone marrow of the victims. The blood of the gassed soldiers revealed below-normal white blood cell counts. They also observed signs of "disturbed bone-marrow function," leaving it depleted and the production of blood cells sharply diminished. The

Krumbhaars concluded the changes were due to severe mustard poisoning, but they missed its larger significance, instead pointing out that the reduced number of white blood cells left the patients vulnerable to secondary infections. Typically, patients then contracted pneumonia, which they did not survive. All too aware that of the 1.2 million World War I soldiers exposed to mustard gas, 91,198 had died, their observation of the gas's "direct toxic action" did not seem to represent any more than an academic contribution to the problem. Their paper was filed away and forgotten and did not even rate a mention in Winternitz's definitive text on the pathology of war gases.

During the interwar period, a few lines of investigation indicating the toxin might be used as a treatment began to emerge, but they too received scant attention. In 1931, a pair of young researchers at Memorial Hospital, Frank Adair and Halsey Bagg, showed that mustard gas, in addition to causing nasty blisters, could be used as a topical agent to treat superficial skin cancers. After curing animals of induced skin cancer, they tried their dilute solution of mustard gas on thirteen human patients and reported that there was no evidence of the disease after four months of treatment. Inspired by their immediate experimental success, they wrote: "We fully recognize that this agent has been applied in our case too recently for us to report cancer cures. But as it takes so many years to report cures, we are hoping that such a preliminary report may suggest possibilities to other investigators."

The next development came from a British pathologist named Isaac Berenblum, who carried out a series of studies on mustard gas's action on tumors and suggested that it was conceivable that it could be used to inhibit the growth of malignancies. Mustard's possible "anti-carcinogenic action" should have attracted interest, but Berenblum himself did not rate his findings as being in any way conclusive, and he advised that a much larger series of tests needed to be done before the pathological changes could be explained.

Ten years and another world war later, Alexander's report on the Bari casualties had put mustard's anticancer activity back under a microscope and grabbed the medical community's attention. Rhoads recognized this was the kind of opportunity that only came along once in a lifetime—the serendipitous discovery of a miracle drug that might be the equivalent of a "penicillin for cancer." The idea was not as far-fetched as it sounded. The history of medicine was full of examples of major innovations inspired by horrendous battlefield casualties. A French barber named Ambroise Paré perfected the ligature when confronted with hundreds of butchered limbs during the 1537 Siege of Turin. Anesthesia had been around for years, but it took the terrible injuries of the American Civil War in the nineteenth century before it was put to regular use, and technique rather than speed became the hallmark of surgical excellence. The Bari disaster provided Rhoads with a huge set of data from a most unfortunate group of human subjects, a war dividend no doctor in the field of neoplastic disease could ever have dreamed of. Galvanized by the wealth of new information, he recognized that it might enable him finally to solve the cancer puzzle.

To Alexander, the dynamic, forward-looking Rhoads, with his boundless energy and optimism, was a "tower of strength in reopening and pursuing the medical application of mustard gas." His tenacity and personal magnetism were irresistible. He had an intuitive instinct for people who could help him get the job done, and he in turn had a catalytic effect on others. Although some of his peers thought it was folly for Memorial's director to throw himself into what looked like a repetition of Paul Ehrlich's futile search for a medicine to cure cancer, nothing would deter him. In his headlong pursuit, Rhoads made enemies and gave sustenance to his critics, but Alexander never doubted that he was on the side of the angels. "Dusty, as I knew him, was a most remarkable man," he recalled. "In him were combined tremendous scientific and investigative talents with great administrative and leadership ability. He, from the first, saw the enormous potential in the use of this compound and its possible modifications."

UNBEKNOWNST TO ALEXANDER, Rhoads had every reason to be excited by the Bari report. By dint of his position, the CWS chief was privy to a top-secret Yale study that underscored the importance of the Bari findings in providing overwhelming evidence that mustard gas was a cell poison that had a powerful effect on human beings. As a member of the Committee on the Treatment of Gas Casualties since 1941, Rhoads knew that shortly after Pearl Harbor, the Office of Scientific Research and Development (OSRD) had awarded some two dozen contracts to laboratories around the country to evaluate chemical warfare agents and attempt to develop antidotes. He also knew that Winternitz, who was chairman of the committee and keen to remain on the cutting edge of cancer research, had arranged for Yale to receive the contract to investigate the new group of offensive agents, the nitrogen mustards. The new compounds were a close cousin of sulfur mustard, the nitrogen analogs methyl *bis* and *tris* beta-chloroethyl amines, which belong to the family of alkylating agents.

In early 1942, Winternitz assigned two pharmacologists, Louis S. Goodman and Alfred Gilman Sr., to conduct a nitrogen mustard study on animals. This was carried out concurrently with Alexander's experiments at Edgewood Arsenal. The Yale study was similarly guarded about the classified compounds, referring to them in their records only as "substance X."

Ignoring the gibes of their colleagues that "the enemy did not intend to attack with hypodermic needles," Goodman and Gilman carried out a series of tests on the lethal effects of the virulent poison, and the efficacy of various antidotes, using "a battery of syringes and a horde of rabbits." Like Alexander, they immediately noticed the agents' severe toxicity and observed that the tissues that renewed themselves most rapidly were the ones most susceptible to destruction, primarily lymphoid tissue and bone marrow. They, too, appreciated the connection to cancer and nitrogen mustard's therapeutic potential. Unlike Alexander, however, the Yale scientists were permitted to quickly change the focus of their investigation, and they began exploring how the chemical warfare agent might be used to treat malignant lymphoid tumors.

No doubt Winternitz was bound by strict military confidentiality, and not a desire to monopolize the data, when he declined to apprise Alexander of their parallel investigation into the nitrogen mustards when the young CWS physician visited him for advice in the spring of 1942. And then, without telling him, he went through channels to obtain a copy of Alexander's classified Edgewood study—EA MD Report 59—which Winternitz promptly supplied to his Yale team. But his cruel and utterly disingenuous dismissal of Alexander's work on mustard-induced leucopenia in rabbits does not reflect well on him and is not in keeping with the true spirit of scientific inquiry. Writing about their clinical saga two decades later, however, Gilman separated himself from such compulsive secrecy and was at pains to share the credit for their rapid progress. Numerous military research centers, including Edgewood's Medical Research Laboratory, were working on the compounds at the same time, and "close contact" was maintained through circulated reports and frequent consultations. "The point to be emphasized," he wrote, "is the collaborative nature of the basic investigations on the nitrogen mustards which led to the clinical trial."

For their part, Goodman and Gilman were fascinated by the "unique properties" of the compounds, and they found their type of action on cells was unlike that of any known chemical. In some respects, it resembled radiation and might possibly have the same palliative effect without scorching the patient's insides. By comparison, sulfur mustard, because of its extreme chemical reactivity, did not lend itself to medical use. They were struck by the special "sensitivity" of the normal lymphoid tissue to the cytotoxic or cell-killing action of the nitrogen mustards, and they wondered how the agents would affect fundamental cell processes, particularly fast-spreading cancer cells where the mechanism of controlled growth had gone awry. "The problem was fundamental and simple," Gilman later explained. "Could one destroy a tumor with this group of cytotoxic agents without destroying the host?"

Anxious to apply their theory, and not wanting to wait to round up a whole group of experimental animals with natural or induced cancer, they turned to a Yale colleague, Dr. Thomas Dougherty, in the Department of Anatomy, for help. Dougherty, whose research on mice included transplanting lymphomas, supplied them with a "lone mouse" with a fairly advanced tumor. After just two administrations of the compound, the mouse's tumor began to soften and regress, soon shrinking to the point it could no longer be felt. "Amazement," declared Gilman, choosing the one word that summed up the team's reaction upon observing the remedial action of the mustard. "This was quite a surprising event," wrote Dougherty of the initial results and the thrilling couple of weeks that followed.

The mouse remained in remission for more than a month. Then a very slight growth began to appear at the tumor site. A second treatment of nitrogen mustard produced a regression again, but not as complete as before. When the tumor finally began to grow again, a third round, administered some three months later, had no impact. The doctors' hopes were dashed when, after eighty-four days, the mouse died. On the bright side, however, it lived nine weeks longer than untreated mice with the same tumor, the latter lasting only twenty-one days. Dougherty described the difference as a very impressive "prolongation of survival time." Nothing had ever achieved results like this.

Next came many animal experiments in which they used different kinds of lymphomas and varied the dose of nitrogen mustard and the number of administrations in order to try to find a proper treatment method. As it turned out, they achieved by far their best result with the first mouse. Along the way, they surmised that there might not be one therapy that worked for all tumors, but they concluded that if one agent was found to have an effect on a tumor, it should be tried on them all. The conventional research approach until then had been to think in terms of a general treatment for all types of cancer, or at least a certain species of cancer. Dougherty believed that it was only because they had begun to accept the probability that there was not going be any one compound that would inhibit the growth of all cancer cells, that they "therefore came up with a compound which had an effect on at least some cancers."

Although Gilman later acknowledged that the idea of injecting a cancer patient with a poison—let alone one ominously marked "compound X"—would have been viewed by most physicians at the time as "the act of a charlatan," he felt they could not ignore the implications of their still-secret data. Their research into nitrogen mustard occurred in a singular moment in medical history, when clinicians were given license by the OSRD to try almost anything. "Without consulting anyone, without FDA requirements, and no peer review, we just decided we were going to give this drug to a patient," he recalled in 1983. "If the current restraints had been in effect then, I don't think these drugs would have been used."

In early December of 1942, Goodman, Gilman, and Dougherty approached Gustaf Lindskog, a thoracic surgeon, with a proposal: If he agreed their experiments on mice were "sufficiently encouraging," would he consider a therapeutic trial of nitrogen mustard in a human being? After reviewing their research, Lindskog decided it had merit and took the initiative, only days later finding them a suitable tumor patient. "Any drug that gave any promise of controlling malignancy seemed to me worth trying," he recalled. "The patient readily agreed to accept the chance of help."

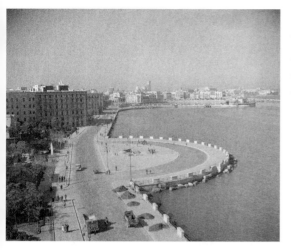

The magnificent waterfront at Bari, a strategic Allied port on the Adriatic coast of Italy, had escaped the war almost unscathed.

Sailors unloading the tons of vital cargo needed to supply the Allied armies in the bloody Italian campaign and the long march to Rome.

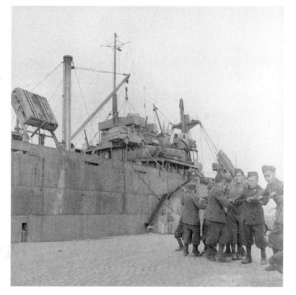

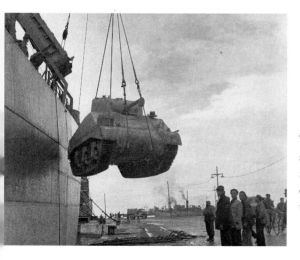

The usual blackout precautions were suspended in order to facilitate soldiers in the round-the-clock discharging of urgently needed staff cars, tanks, trucks, fuel, and ammunition.

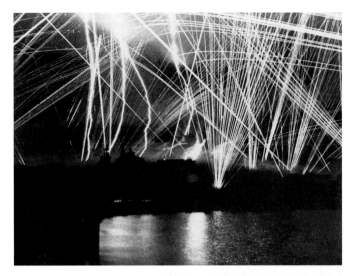

The Nazi air raid on December 2, 1943, took the Allies by surprise, and chandelier flares and antiaircraft fire lit up the night sky over Bari as the bombs rained down on the vulnerable harbor.

The Luftwaffe "walked" their bombs down the line of American Liberty ships moored almost hull-to-hull in the over-crowded harbor.

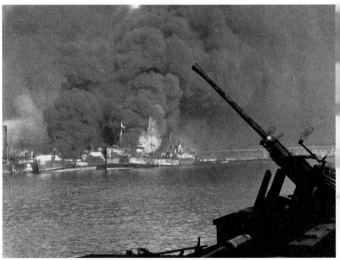

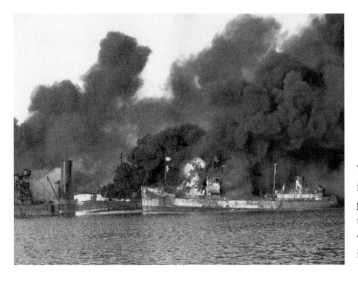

Thousands of tons of fuel from the damaged freighters gushed into the harbor, and the flames swept across the water like a prairie fire, leaping from ship to ship.

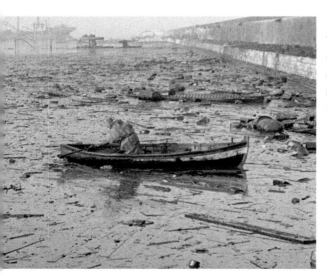

The next morning, rescue boats of all sizes searched the oily, debris-filled harbor waters for survivors but mostly brought up remains of the dead.

A British port official surveys the smoldering ruins, a tragic scene made all the more poignant by the NO SMOKING sign posted in English and Italian.

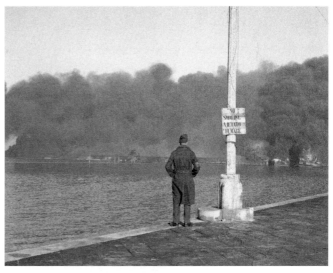

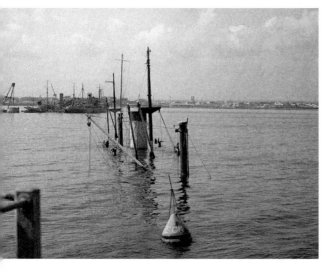

The devastating attack on December 2, 1943, dubbed the "little Pearl Harbor," was the worst Allied naval disaster of the war, with the loss of 17 ships and over 1,000 casualties. Pictured here is the mast of one of the sunken vessels.

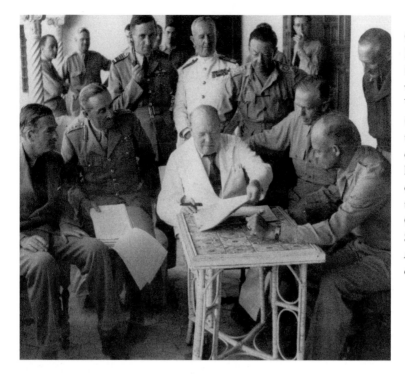

Gen. Dwight D. Eisenhower (front right) met with Prime Minister Winston Churchill (center) and his top advisers to discuss their plans to knock the Italians out of the war at the Allied Planning Conference at the St. George Hotel, AFHQ in Algiers, on June 4, 1943.

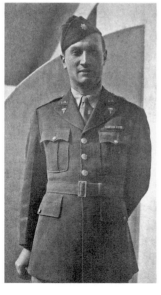

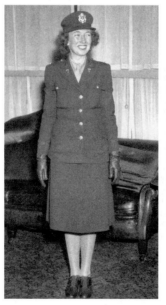

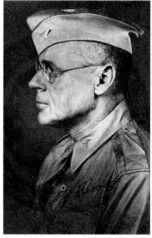

Lt. Col. Stewart F. Alexander was assigned to General Eisenhower's staff at AFHQ after the general requested the services of a chemical warfare consultant in response to the growing threat that Germany might resort to poison gas.

Lt. Col. Bernice "Bunny" Wilbur, responsible for 4,500 nurses stationed in the Mediterranean, was already a force to be reckoned with when she crossed swords with Alexander, and won his heart, at AFHQ.

Despite Churchill's objections, Alexander wrote two classified reports on the Bari mustard-gas casualties and sent them to Col. Cornelius P. "Dusty" Rhoads, chief of the Medical Division of the Chemical Warfare Service, calling special attention to the depleted white blood cell counts and systemic effects.

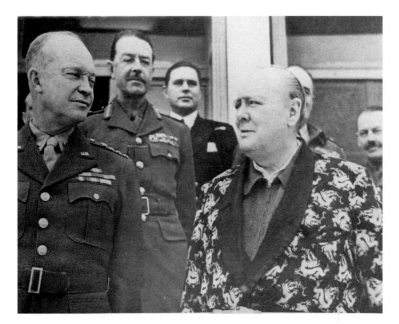

Eisenhower invited Churchill, clad in a dressing gown, to recuperate at his villa in Carthage, Tunisia, during the last two weeks of December 1943. Gen. Harold Alexander, in the rear, arrived for a Christmas Day strategy meeting.

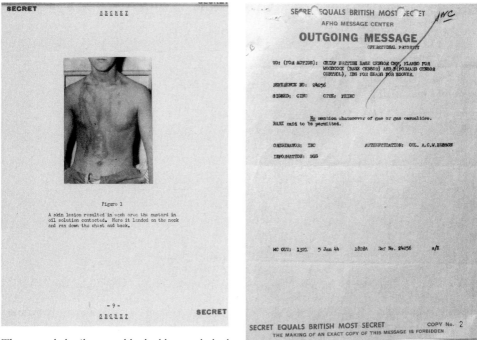

The wounded sailor stated he had been splashed following an explosion in Bari Harbor. This photograph, taken eight days later, shows the skin lesions caused by contact with what Alexander believed was a toxic solution of mustard in oil.

One of dozens of telegrams that flew back and forth between British and American military officials, imposing a policy of secrecy on the Bari mustard-gas incident and casualties.

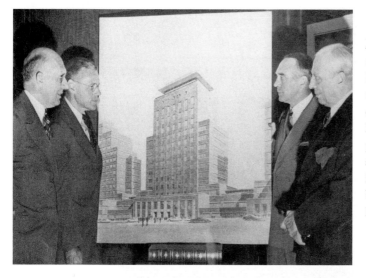

Alfred P. Sloan Jr. (front right) and Charles F. Kettering (front left), the chairman and wizard chief engineer of General Motors, announce their plans to create the most advanced cancer center in the world, to be led by Cornelius "Dusty" Rhoads (rear left).

Rhoads (center) recruited researchers from the US Army's Chemical Warfare Service to form the core staff of Sloan Kettering, including C. Chester Stock and David Karnofsky (right), Joseph Burchenal (left), and Fred Philips (far left).

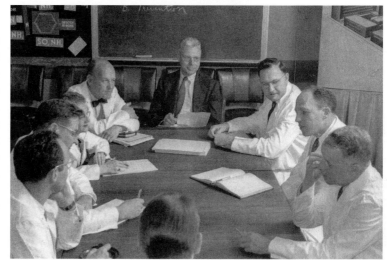

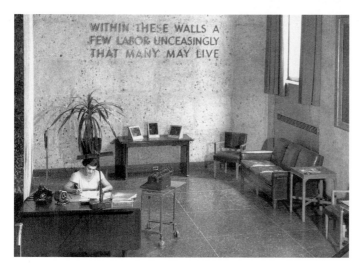

The lobby of the newly opened Sloan Kettering Institute in 1948, which the *New York Times* hailed as the "most concentrated assault on cancer so far in history."

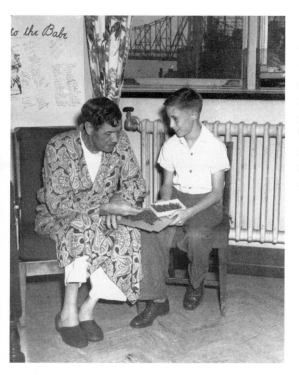

This is one of the last known photographs of Babe Ruth, wrapped in a bathrobe at Memorial Hospital, receiving a donation from a young fan for the Babe Ruth Foundation. The slugger, who died a week later, made medical history as one of the first patients to receive experimental chemotherapy.

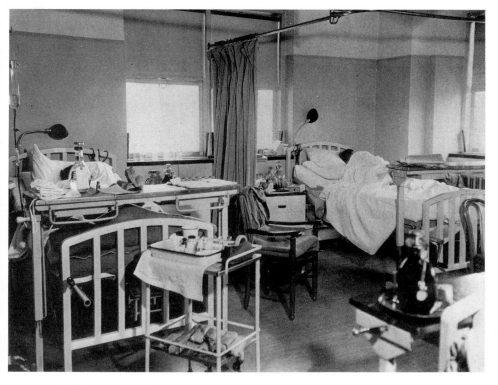

Children on the leukemia ward receiving treatment at Memorial Hospital. At the time, acute lymphoblastic leukemia was the most common childhood cancer and was invariably fatal, causing death within a few weeks or months.

After the war, Dr. Stewart Alexander returned to his family practice in New Jersey, located in the small stone house built by his father, and was a beloved physician and cardiologist for more than thirty years.

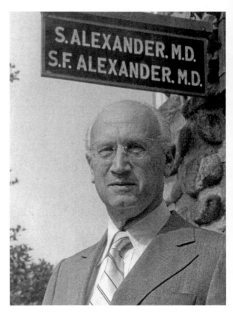

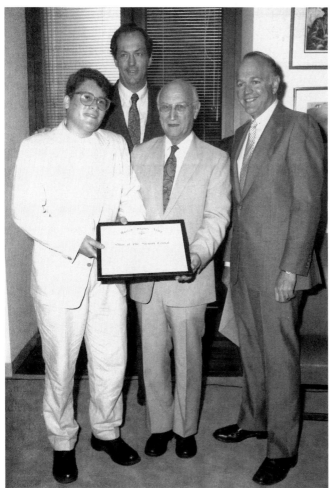

On May 20, 1988, thanks to the efforts of Tucson high school student Nicholas Spark (left), and the persistence of Senators Dennis DeConcini (right) and Bill Bradley (rear), Dr. Alexander (center) was belatedly honored by the US Army Surgeon General for his classified service to the military and to medical science.

Within a week, the team was preparing to treat its first patient, a forty-seven-year-old New York factory worker dying of lymphosarcoma, a cancer of the lymph glands, for whom all other therapeutic options had been exhausted. "JD," as he is identified in the Yale clinical records, was an unmarried Polish immigrant who had worked for a Connecticut ball-bearing plant until his illness began in 1940.* He had been in pain for months by the time he was first admitted to New Haven Hospital on February 24, 1941, with a massive tumor of the neck and tonsils as well as smaller masses in the cervical region. Multiple radiation treatments were at first successful, but by year's end they were having no effect. In May of 1942, the tumor masses had enlarged and spread, and subsequent courses of radiation were unable to control the cancerous growths. Now judged to be radiation resistant, JD was losing weight because of the difficulty of chewing and swallowing, and he was in great distress. Surgery was out of the question, and the malignancy could only have a fatal outcome.

When his case was presented to the tumor conference on August 25, the case notes record the moment when it was decided JD would make history as the first subject of cancer chemotherapy:

> The patient's outlook is utterly hopeless on the present regimen. Because the end seems near he should be in the hospital. Dr. Lindskog will investigate the possibility of obtaining one of the newer chemicals which are lymphocidal. Immediate admission arranged.

---

* The personal and medical histories of the patient presented as JD in all the scientific publications after 1946 were unknown for sixty-four years. The long-lost medical chart of the first nitrogen mustard patient was only recovered and presented for the first time in 2011 by two Yale surgeons, Drs. John Fenn and Robert Udelsman, who sought to clear up some of the mystery surrounding the origin of chemotherapy and its first use at Yale during World War II.

At 10 a.m. on August 27, the first of ten consecutive daily doses of intravenous *tris* nitrogen mustard was administered. Selecting the appropriate dosage of the highly toxic agent was tricky, to say the least—there was no precedent for using poison gas as a medication. The doctors had to rely on guesswork, extrapolating from their studies on rabbits. They settled on a sublethal dose delivered at the rate of 0.1 milligram per kilogram of body weight. Their plan was to deliver as many injections as the patient could tolerate before the white blood cell count dropped below five thousand, with a normal count being between seven and eight thousand. They went ahead with "unwarranted confidence," Gilman later admitted, bolstered by the knowledge that the pharmacology department had developed an antidote, thiosulfate, to the systemic effects of the nitrogen mustards. Moreover, there was a fairly wide margin between a dose of nitrogen mustard that was acutely lethal and that was required to affect the lymphoid tissue. Under these circumstances, they believed the experiment to be manageable, as the suppression of bone-marrow function was completely reversible.

Within forty-eight hours of the first injection, the doctors detected a "softening" of the tumor masses. Four days later, JD stated that he was feeling better. He was able to swallow and move his head with greater ease, and, for two consecutive nights, he had managed to sleep in bed for four hours—something he had been unable to do for weeks. By the tenth and last day of treatment, his condition had improved markedly, and the masses were no longer palpable. On September 27, "all cervical and axillary nodes were gone." All signs and symptoms of the cancer had disappeared. "For a short period of time the patient was delighted," noted Gilman. "But it was a short period of time." JD's white blood cell and lymphocyte counts had already begun to drop.

By mid-October, one month after the last injection, JD's white blood cell count had plummeted to two hundred. The nitrogen mustard had attacked not only the proliferating cancer cells but also the bone marrow that normally produces new cells as needed. This resulted in gingival bleeding, and he required blood transfusions to boost his falling white blood cell count. But in man as in mouse, the tumors reoccurred as the bone marrow recovered. The lymphosarcoma returned with a vengeance. By day forty-nine, the tumors were back. A shorter, second cycle of the intravenous mustard had only a transient effect, indicating the cancer cells were beginning to develop resistance. The third and final six-day cycle was begun on November 6, but by then the doctors knew their patient was on an inexorable downhill course. JD died on December 1, 1942, after ninety-six days in the hospital. Sadly, the intravenous chemotherapeutic treatment was not advanced enough to save their brave patient. The experimental drug had extended his life, though its toxicity and unpleasant side effects—nausea and vomiting—were cause for concern. Above all, it had proved effective in a patient who was no longer responsive to radiation, and one for whom all available therapies had failed.

Elated by the response of JD, the doctors became overconfident. They made what Gilman later admitted was a "serious error in judgment." Before JD's initial series of injections was completed, they started another patient on the ten-day regimen. By the time they recognized the extent of the bone marrow depression in their first patient, the second course had been completed, and it was too late to modify the treatment. In retrospect, their calculation of the dosage had been a "fortunate guess," Gilman wrote, "but our acumen as to the duration of therapy left much to be desired."

Still, the Yale team remained upbeat. Clinical trials on "compound X" continued at New Haven Hospital during the first months of 1943. Five additional patients suffering from a variety of terminal cancers were treated with more conservative regimens of intravenous mustard. Many experienced temporary remissions, though the results of the subsequent cases were less favorable than that of the first patient. But they had shown that an intravenous treatment could result in tumor regression. They had also seen that it could induce profound bone marrow suppression, immunosuppression, and death. The margin for safety in the use of these toxic chemicals was "very narrow." The greater the dose, the greater the chances of curing the cancer, but it also increased the likelihood that the attacking chemical would kill the patient. They were a long way from knowing how to achieve the right balance. The challenge was to establish a regimen that would wipe out the cancer cells completely yet would preserve enough of the bone marrow to regenerate needed healthy cells.

In June 1943, the study was terminated and the Yale team was dispersed. Drs. Lindskog and Gilman entered military service, the latter going to work for the Chemical Warfare Service at Edgewood. Goodman moved to the University of Vermont and pursued an even more extensive study. Bound by military secrecy, the dramatic results of the Yale study could not be published, but Dusty Rhoads received a summary that spring, just six months before the Bari disaster. Although ultimately disappointing, the Yale clinical trial demonstrated for the first time in history that a medicinal agent had corralled cancer. Seven cases were not conclusive, but they provided proof of the concept that the chemical warfare agent could cause tumors to "melt away"—just as Alexander had observed when he tested the nitrogen mustards on rabbits in 1942. The early indications offered a glimmer of hope that an untreatable disease might become treatable. Radiation and radical surgery would no longer be the only available options.

For Rhoads, the Bari report brought the Yale findings into sharp focus and convinced him that the important research being done on the therapeutic value of these compounds could not be allowed to lapse. It was imperative they understood more about the poisonous properties of the nitrogen mustards as they were metabolized by the body, their impact upon essential bodily constituents, and their pharmacological effects. He immediately began making plans to start a therapeutic trial at Memorial Hospital. The only problem was that the best one of these nitrogen mustards, the methyl-*bis* compound, or HN2, was still under the strict control of the US Army. Before the next phase of cancer research could begin, that bureaucratic roadblock would need to be removed. He would have to find a way to cut through the military red tape and make the compounds available to civilian doctors and scientists.

As a result of his behind-the-scenes lobbying, in June 1944 the OSRD approved the creation of the Committee on Atypical Growth of the National Research Council (NRC), with Rhoads as chairman, to advise the Army on the distribution of the nitrogen mustards for study. In short order, the committee chose three institutions to carry out the investigations on HN2: Memorial Hospital, the University of Chicago Medical School, and the University of Utah Medical School. Other qualified medical schools could apply to participate in the study. Merck & Co. was authorized to ship the agent, trademarked Mustargen, and would be distributing treatment units consisting of four 10-milligram vials of HN2 to the approved institutions. In August, Rhoads obtained permission from the NRC for Memorial to embark on a series of groundbreaking experiments with nitrogen mustard on cancer patients, "to obtain data on the therapeutic value of the compounds in different types of neoplastic disease."

Armed with the Bari report and the Yale study, Rhoads was convinced that nitrogen mustards provided physicians with a new way forward—cancer chemotherapy. Even though they were not there yet, he believed there was enough information to justify the belief that an effective treatment was within their grasp. He saw this as an opportunity to re-energize and accelerate the development of a chemical cure for cancer. It might not constitute Ehrlich's "magic bullet," but it would carry them a long way toward controlling or arresting the disease while they worked to better understand it. The new compounds offered enormous opportunities for the advancement of knowledge in the field of cell dynamics, chemical genetics, pharmacology, and the clinical care of cancer patients. At the time, only two kinds of nitrogen mustards had been clinically investigated, and they were the product of a screening program for chemical warfare agents rather than chemotherapeutic agents designed for treatment purposes. Rhoads knew that any chemist with an ounce of imagination would be able to synthesize literally thousands of derivatives of the original nitrogen mustards to be tested. It was going to take an army of mice and men to conduct the intensive trial-and-error search for the most effective compounds, along with other types of alkylating agents. Given the enormity of the task, Memorial would need to recruit a great many skilled clinical investigators. His chief concern now was finding the ways and means to expedite this progress.

With the stunning success of the D-day invasion, and Allied forces on the ground and fanning out across France, there was talk the conflict would soon be over. Rhoads began looking just over the horizon—toward returning to Memorial and figuring out how to duplicate the success of the American war effort in medicine. The tremendous mobilization of men and resources had enabled them to score a decisive victory against the most powerful enemy in the world. They had the Nazis on the run and would not rest until they had overcome their last defenses in Germany. Rhoads's war work had made a deep impression on him. During his time at the CWS, he had seen high-pressure wartime science accomplish in only a few years what would have taken decades at a sauntering peacetime pace. He had come away with a new respect for what could be accomplished when scientists, a notoriously egocentric breed, put aside their usual jealousies and rivalries, submerged their temperaments, and worked together toward a common goal.

Testifying before the Senate Subcommittee on Wartime Health on January 5, 1945, Rhoads declared that the CWS had developed such effective protective and remedial measures in case of gas attacks that "the enemy dared not use them." He stated forcefully that by employing the "same wartime system," they could make similar progress in the nation's major civilian health issues. Pointing to the way the OSRD organized scientists and physicians to find solutions to battlefield problems—such as the successful development of antimalarial agents that saved the lives of countless Allied troops serving in the Far East— he argued that a similar coordinated attack on certain diseases could propel medical research to new heights after the war.

Rhoads believed that a crash program to beat cancer, urgent and vast in scope, in which hospitals and research laboratories and pharmaceutical companies merged their efforts, could make rapid progress in the new field of chemotherapy. Joseph Burchenal, a young oncologist who joined the staff of Memorial after he was discharged from the US Army, remembered Rhoads talking about his idea for an institute in which a concentrated attack could be made on cancer:

> He dreamed of an approach to the cancer problem wherein fundamental differences between cancer cells and the normal cells and differences in the endocrine metabolism of cancer-bearing individuals would be sought, where empirical attempts would be made to find drugs that would selectively damage cancer cells without damaging normal cells and where biochemical and animal studies could be immediately translated to practical application in the patient.

Rhoads's ideal was "bench-to-bedside research," which would allow Memorial's physicians to draw constantly on the latest clinical studies and garner new ideas, new tools, and new ways to handle the disease more effectively. Conversely, the clinicians who were generally focused on scientific method could learn from the physicians' actual experiences with patients and come away with suggestions that could give rise to crucial insights.

Rhoads wrote to Stewart Alexander, who was still in Algiers, informing him of the latest developments with nitrogen mustards and his ambitious plans for Memorial. "Rhoads envisioned a new, multi-disciplined approach to cancer therapy," recalled Alexander, who was captivated by his idea for a modern cancer center that would unite a diverse group of physicians, clinical investigators, and research scientists under a single roof—one where they could pool their talents and attack problems cooperatively and from every possible angle. Alexander was pleased to hear something positive might come out of the tragic Bari incident, and proud that a man like Rhoads felt his report had played an important part in making it happen. He told Rhoads: "This may be the key to unlock the door on what mustard gas derivatives can do and what their potentials are in treating illness."

Looking back on that extraordinary time years later, he reflected: "That the Bari Harbor contribution was a focal point in initiating this chain of events comforts me."

CHAPTER TEN

"Frontal Attack"

On the sultry afternoon of Tuesday, August 7, 1945, a group of harried reporters waited impatiently in the sublime chill of the conference room atop the General Motors Building in midtown Manhattan for what had been billed as a major announcement. Despite the reprieve from the oppressive heat outside, Dusty Rhoads could tell that none of them wanted to be there. At least half of the invited science writers had not even bothered to show up. But he could hardly hold it against them—it would probably go down as the biggest news day of the war. That morning's *New York Times* carried the banner headline: First Atomic Bomb Dropped on Japan. The front page of every paper in the country carried the story that Allied scientists, working on the secret Manhattan Project under the direction of the United States Army, had created the most powerful bomb in history—a cosmic weapon that "harnessed the basic power of the universe." An American plane had dropped a single bomb, equivalent to the force of twenty thousand tons of TNT, on the city of Hiroshima, and more would follow unless Japan quickly sued for peace. This technical triumph—"a marvel," in the words of President Harry Truman—was expected to bring the war to an end.

Rhoads would not have picked such a momentous day to unveil his grand plans to make Memorial the largest, most advanced cancer center in the world, but in a way it was oddly appropriate. President Truman hailed "organized science" for winning the race of discovery, beating the enemy to the bomb, and pulling off this great achievement under pressure and in an incredibly short time. This was exactly what Rhoads had in mind in launching his own crash research program to discover cancer-killing agents and eventually to add a potent chemical weapon to their medical arsenal. Op-Ed writers and social commentators were insisting that "a fresh page had been turned in the book of human history; that human existence was about to be radically altered." In the era of the atom, the next great challenge was the conquest of cancer.

Buoyed by the giddy atmosphere in the room, Rhoads, lean and vigorous, his hair still shorn in an army crew cut, walked to the front flanked by Alfred P. Sloan Jr., the tall, stern-faced chairman of General Motors, and the taller, owlish, and affable Charles F. Kettering, a wizard engineer who was director of research and vice president of the company. The two lanky tycoons, known as the "dream team" of the automobile industry, stood awkwardly before an artist's rendering of the palatial new hospital building as they presented a $4 million grant to create the Sloan Kettering Institute for Cancer Research (SKI). The new institute would be devoted exclusively to applying "American industrial research techniques," as practiced by their own highly successful business, to the cancer problem.

Sloan, whose managerial genius had turned GM into a powerhouse during his twenty-five-year tenure, emphasized "the amazing possibilities of research when organized on a broad and comprehensive scale." He pointed to the stunning news of the atomic bomb—brainchild of the country's top physicists and product of a $2 billion research program—as a graphic illustration of what could be accomplished in medicine by a determined all-out effort: "Very rapid progress against this mysterious scourge could be made possible if the problem got the same amount of money, brains and planning that was devoted to developing the atomic bomb."

Always colorful and quotable, "Boss" Kettering, one of the nation's best-known inventors, did most of the talking. Explaining that because he and Sloan had put their heads together over the years on many "apparently hopeless" industrial problems that ultimately turned out to have simple solutions, he was inclined to think they could "apply some of our time-tried techniques to this age-old problem." Confident in the technological entrepreneurship that had forged the thriving automobile industry "from nothing," Kettering said he had developed certain research procedures that had proven extremely versatile, allowing him to contribute major innovations in a wide variety of fields—from the electric self-starter for cars and the two-cycle diesel engine to cash registers and automated inventory control systems. Peering out over thick gold-rimmed spectacles like an old-fashioned college professor, he observed in his distinctive, folksy manner, "I cannot help but feel that we call a problem difficult simply because we don't know how to solve it."

The two men made it clear that this was a strictly private venture. The money would come entirely from the Alfred P. Sloan Foundation, not the General Motors Corporation. The foundation would provide $2 million to erect the new building, and another $200,000 a year for ten years toward operating costs, which would permit them to attract the very best in the field and to plan an intensive research program with the assurance it could be carried through to completion. At the same time, the pair urged a broader, more intense national effort in the struggle against cancer, saying that Memorial would be kicking off a public campaign to raise an additional $4 million. Kettering surprised Rhoads by announcing that he intended to "direct" the research himself, taking charge of translating their industrial techniques to medicine and finding ways these methods could be used advantageously to uncover new facts to "help to conquer this so-called 'incurable' disease."

All things considered, Rhoads thought the press conference could not have gone any better. Despite the fact that the birth of the new institute was overshadowed by the bomb, when he checked the paper the following morning he was delighted to see they nonetheless had made the front page of the *New York Times*. Ironically, an editorial in the *New York Herald Tribune* even applauded the project's timeliness: "There is something steadying and heartening in the announcement that a ten-year campaign against cancer will be financed by the Alfred P. Sloan Foundation. We are assured that even as men learn to destroy life with terrifying efficiency, they are concerned also about how to save it."

It had not been easy to corral the two GM executives as cosponsors of the new institute. In 1939, Frank Howard, the vice president of Standard Oil, joined the board of managers of Memorial Hospital and approached Sloan, a close friend and business partner, about helping to establish a cancer research center. Six years later, Sloan, who had made only a token contribution to the small program that had existed during the war years, was still mulling it over. As soon as Rhoads returned to Memorial full time in April of 1945, Howard arranged an introduction in hopes of convincing the GM boss to underwrite the new effort. Even with Rhoads's "persuasive tongue," as one colleague put it, and unparalleled gift for wringing dollars out of wealthy patrons, Howard warned that the hard-nosed industrialist would be no pushover. Known for his tightly run, efficiently managed business, Sloan was not easily parted from his money. He did not feel any need to buff his reputation as one of the country's leading businessmen by making the rounds of the New York charity circuit. "He's no Scrooge," a friend observed, "but he still knows the value of a dollar."

As is so often the case, it took a scandal—and a subsequent desire to repair the damage—to pry open his wallet. His first substantial foray into philanthropy came in 1937, when he endowed the Alfred P. Sloan Foundation with $10 million following an embarrassing accusation of tax evasion. In June of that year, the Treasury Department charged Sloan and his wife with "moral fraud," reporting to a congressional committee that they had avoided payment of $1,921,587 in income taxes over a three-year period through a personal holding company set up to buy their yacht. While this tax scheme was not illegal, and brought no government charge or penalty, the headlines were unflattering. Coming at the height of the Roosevelt administration's assault on the "economic royalists" who opposed the New Deal, Sloan was excoriated in the press as a greedy corporate fat cat. FDR sent a message to Congress lambasting the loopholes by which wealthy Americans wriggled out of paying their fair share of taxes: "All are alike in that failure to pay results in shifting the tax load to the shoulders of others less able to pay and in mulcting [defrauding] the Treasury of the Government's just due."

Outraged and on the defensive, the normally private tycoon was forced to issue a public statement denying he had ever attempted to dodge his tax burden. To silence the sniping New Deal critics, he unveiled his eponymous foundation, announcing that it seemed "eminently proper" that he should give back some of the proceeds of his immense good fortune. He would use the money to promote his gospel of free enterprise—or, as he put it in the press release, provide "a better understanding of the economic principles and national policies which have characterized American enterprise down through the years." The humiliating ordeal taught him that he had ignored corporate public relations at his own peril. He excelled at selling cars and would have to learn to excel at selling GM's corporate image. As he wrote Kettering, "Our attention has been so concentrated on building up business that [we] have not given sufficient thought to simultaneous development of our relations with the public."

Sloan ran his foundation much the same way he ran his company, personally choosing every project and approving each grant. So that's why, in late May, Rhoads was invited to the formal lunch at the tall, gray GM building, where he delivered his pitch about what American scientific know-how could accomplish if applied to the cancer problem in a "frontal attack," an orderly, military-style project rather than the scattered, uncoordinated peacetime approach. In the seventy-year-old GM chairman, Rhoads found a kindred spirit. Having been immersed in industry his whole life, Sloan liked bold, innovative thinkers. He understood the high cost of expansion and moving into new, unproven fields, and he knew it could pay off. Rhoads's technical, organized approach aiming at producing maximum results also resonated—after all, it was the same model Sloan himself had used to guide GM to new heights. American prosperity was transforming people's daily lives, and harnessing technology and science to banish a centuries-old killer like cancer made sense to him.

After asking a series of rapid-fire questions about the size and scale of the proposed institute and the operating budget required to get the job done properly, Sloan pronounced himself satisfied. Rhoads was astounded that by the end of the meal they were well on their way to developing a "skeleton plan." Their conversation concluded with Sloan posing two last questions: "[W]hether the whole arrangement discussed was likely to result in substantial advances toward the better control of cancer in human beings; and whether it would provide something which did not already exist?" Rhoads's answers to both were affirmative.

Unlike Sloan, Kettering had a personal connection to cancer, having lost his sister, Emma, to a neck tumor the previous winter. Her death had been particularly painful, he confided, as he had been stranded by a last-minute snowstorm and was unable to attend her funeral service. Well-informed about the scientific fundamentals, he had endowed his own foundation to subsidize medical studies at a number of hospitals, where he reportedly was not shy about telling the physicians he funded how to go about their work. While a great believer in advanced research—he called it the "tomorrow" mindset—he was also practical, and he liked to have a concrete plan of action. A self-described "screwdriver and pliers" inventor, he was not interested in theoretical discussions. He knew Rhoads was looking for an ally, but as the longtime head of General Motors Research Laboratories, he had always played a key role in selecting projects, and he was troubled by Rhoads's proposal that they underwrite a ten-year program of research that did not appear to have "well-defined, attainable objectives." He was fearful that it was "too diffuse," and their investment might go down the drain.

Rhoads tried to explain that in coming up with the ten-year figure, he had only been thinking of the long, frustrating search for the new chemotherapeutic agents—"the interminable labor, unending disappointments, and legions of false leads followed and discarded." He wanted to be careful that there should not be "any expectation or assurance, or even discussion of the possibility, that a cancer remedy would be had within the first decade of operation." Success was not guaranteed. He could make no promises. Kettering went away unconvinced.

In the end, Sloan persuaded Kettering to be his partner in the undertaking, assuring him they wanted his brains and not his money. In-house, it was understood confidentially that it was really the Sloan Institute, and Kettering's involvement was incidental. Frank Howard would be the president of the Board of Trustees and chairman of the Committee on Scientific Policy. The other early members of this committee were the two leaders of the Manhattan Project, Karl Compton and James B. Conant, the presidents of MIT and Harvard, respectively, and among the country's most influential scientists. After that, administrative and legal matters, as well as the design for the new building, were settled with dizzying speed. By the end of July 1945, they had reached agreement on all the essential details and were drafting the press release. In the remarkably short span of two months, Rhoads's dream of building the world's greatest cancer research hospital had materialized.

IF HE HAD NOT BEEN SO DAZZLED by GM's gold, and so preoccupied with getting his new institute off the ground, Rhoads might have paused to wonder why Sloan was suddenly so eager to make his benefaction. Sloan had never suffered personally from cancer, and there was no history of it in his immediate family. Prior to this, most of the old man's money had gone to his alma mater, the Massachusetts Institute of Technology, where he had made a series of large grants to establish a laboratory to study engines and an industrial leadership program with an eye to minting better-trained GM managers for the future. His gift to Memorial was an extraordinarily generous, if uncharacteristic, humanitarian gesture.

If Rhoads had ever thought to ask, Frank Howard probably could have enlightened him about the need for this latest public relations initiative, as his company was experiencing image problems of its own. Both Standard Oil and General Motors had had extensive business interests in Germany in the 1930s. They had partnered with the German chemical firm IG Farben to build plants that produced tetraethyl lead (TEL), an essential petroleum additive in the fuel that powered Luftwaffe airplanes—and, as a consequence, they were among a number of big American companies that found themselves fending off accusations that they had contributed to the Nazi war effort. Now, with Germany's defeat and his own imminent retirement as chief executive officer, Sloan was determined to gloss over that dark chapter in the company's history and instead shine a light on his philanthropy and corporate citizenship.

Long before GM earned a reputation for itself as a proud participant in Roosevelt's "Arsenal of Democracy" by converting its production plants to manufacture airplanes, tanks, and trucks for the Allied armies, it was one of the largest businesses in Nazi Germany. Wittingly or unwittingly, according to its critics, this led GM to also become part of Hitler's "Arsenal of Fascism." In 1933, when Hitler became chancellor, GM was the biggest automobile manufacturer in Germany—indeed, in all of Europe—and was actively expanding its overseas sales, merchandising operations, and assembly plants. Four years earlier, GM had acquired the venerable German firm Adam Opel AG, which then dominated the German car market. Stimulated by the Nazi regime's measures, the Germany economy began to recover, and orders poured in for trucks and cars. Over the next two years, Opel, under GM's management and infused with American dollars, outstripped not only its German competitors but also GM's weak performance in the Depression-weary United States.

Even as the international situation deteriorated, GM's Opel operations proceeded at full throttle. By the end of 1937, Opel had grown to almost three times the size of the next largest auto firm, Daimler-Benz, and it was four times the size of the Ford Motor Company's fledgling German branch, Ford-Werke. GM's internal review in 1940 showed that Opel had ballooned in value to $86.7 million, more than double their initial investment. Unfortunately, the Nazi currency controls made it impossible for GM to extract its earnings, forcing them to use the money to purchase shares of other German industrial firms. Predicting that "a strong virile nation" like Germany would inevitably find its "place in the sun," Sloan was confident GM would soon reap the rewards and "be in a position to take advantage of the hard work and progress which has been made during the past seven or eight years in the form of profits which are transferable to America."

Despite receiving criticism from stockholders, and pressure from the Roosevelt administration to cooperate with its war-preparedness efforts, Sloan argued that maintaining good relations with a powerful rearmed

Germany was good business. Much too good to walk away from. In a private letter to a concerned stockholder in April 1939, he was adamant that GM's overseas activities be judged only by their impact on the bottom line:

> Now I believe that if an international business such as General Motors engages in the commercial activity of any country with the idea of making a profit ... it has an obligation to that country, both in an economic sense as well perhaps as in a social sense. It should attempt to attune itself to the general business of the community; make itself a part of the same; conduct its operations in relation to the customs, and design its products so as to meet the needs and viewpoint of each community, so far as it can. I believe further, that that should be its position, even if, as is likely to happen and particularly as was the case during the past few years, the management of the Corporation might not wholly agree with many things that are done in certain of these countries.

Sloan added further that it made no sense for GM to risk a lucrative business arrangement by offending its German hosts by questioning their political beliefs. "In other words, to put the proposition rather bluntly," he wrote, "such matters should not be considered the business of the management of General Motors."

In the fall of 1939, Sloan watched the Nazis take Europe, knowing full well that the blitzkrieg rolling over Norway, Luxembourg, the Netherlands, Belgium, and France was transporting soldiers in three-ton trucks built by GM's German subsidiary. But the United States and Germany were not at war, and supplying Hitler's army was generating hefty sales. When John Pratt, a former GM executive who went to work for the government, wrote and asked him to hold off on retooling the US factories for the 1941 year models in case Washington needed them for the defense mobilization program, Sloan turned him down, effectively telling him it was too late. The Allies were "outclassed on mechanical equipment," he wrote, and it was "foolish to talk about modernizing their armies in times like these." Like many other American businessmen, Sloan assumed the combined strength of Germany and its then-ally, the Soviet Union, far outweighed that of England and the European democracies. The war was rapidly moving toward a conclusion, they thought, and it was better to be on good terms with the victor. Like Standard Oil and other American companies with operations in Germany, GM hoped the war would be short-lived and that they could recoup their investment in better times. There was every reason to believe the hardy "Blitz truck," as it was known, would become a mainstay in the postwar market.

As the Nazis imposed their nationalistic ideology on all aspects of Opel's factory life and employees, GM's local managers dealt with the increasingly repressive, anti-Semitic, and antiforeign atmosphere through a policy they called "camouflage," a strategy designed to conceal American control of the company behind a false façade of local management. While GM has consistently asserted that the company lost day-to-day control over its German plants in September 1939 and "did not assist the Nazis in any way during World War II," contemporaneous German documents and postwar investigations by the US Army indicate otherwise. Two weeks after the German invasion of Poland, James D. Mooney, GM's director of overseas operations, met with Hermann Göring, the leader of the Nazi Party, and offered to lobby for the economic appeasement of Germany in Washington. In his misguided role as mediator, he then held amicable discussions with Hitler in Berlin on March 4, 1940, unaware that plans were already in place for the invasion of Denmark and Norway a month later.

Mooney's own typewritten notes show that, following Sloan's orders, he continued to try to placate Nazi officials while at the same time doing his best to protect GM from being directly involved in the production of war matériel. In an effort to keep GM's large Rüsselsheim factory from being conscripted for the Nazi war effort, Mooney helped negotiate a compromise arrangement by which a portion of the plant would be given over to producing engines and components for the German aircraft firm, Junkers, and their versatile new bomber, the Ju-88.

By dividing the plant and going along with the conversion of part of their plant to military production, Mooney hoped to free the rest of Opel from making munitions. But, as Yale historian Henry Ashby Turner Jr. found in his examination of internal company records, it proved impossible to hold the line under the pressure of wartime conditions. Threatened with a takeover by Junkers, GM's American managers dropped the leasing arrangement and agreed to manufacture components for the Ju-88s as long as the parent company was shielded by transferring Opel entirely to a German directorate comprising prominent businessmen and Nazi Party officials. In a formal report on its overseas operations, Mooney attempted to discount the significance of their growing contribution to the German military machine, stating only that "a plan has been worked out whereby Opel will produce non-automotive parts (mostly miscellaneous airplane parts)" at their Rüsselsheim facility.

The truth was that GM had lost control of Opel and the firm had become "a hostage of Hitler's regime." By the end of 1940, according to evidence uncovered by Professor Turner in the wartime archives, "more than ten thousand employees at Opel's Rüsselsheim plant were engaged in producing parts for the Junkers bombers heavily used in raining death and destruction on London and other British cities during the air attacks of the Battle of Britain." The same Ju-88s that would later make up the entire strike force that wreaked havoc on Bari.

Mooney did such a good job of ingratiating himself with the Nazi regime that Hitler awarded him the German Eagle, First Class, for his "distinguished services to the Reich." The hero aviator and America First spokesman Charles Lindbergh was similarly honored, along with the rabid isolationist Henry Ford, whom Hitler referred to as his "inspiration" in an interview with a *Detroit News* reporter. On the home front, however, the high-profile GM executive's efforts to broker a peace with the barbarous regime were less well received. After the *Saturday Evening Post* published an article in August 1940 expounding his unrealistic view that if the hostilities were called off, political and economic order could quickly be restored, Mooney found himself embroiled in controversy. A left-leaning New York newspaper, *PM,* accused him and Lindbergh of belonging to a "League of Benedict Arnolds" and conducting a "treasonable undeclared war against the United States." When other publications joined in the attacks on Hitler's carmaker, Mooney's name—and GM's—was muddied.

Sloan was aware of the gist of Mooney's overtures to the Nazis. While skeptical his employee's meddling would amount to anything, and telling a colleague that Mooney was "wasting his time dealing with that crowd," Sloan did nothing to curtail his activities. What GM's chairman failed to consider was that because of Mooney's stature as the international representative of the automobile giant, his outspoken views might reflect poorly on the company—and, worse, could be construed as meaning GM was aligned with or sympathetic to the Nazi cause. At the very least, he was providing ample fodder for the German press. Much of GM's reputation as an early supporter of the Reich dates back to Mooney's naïve, ill-considered statements and deluded diplomacy. By 1940, even Sloan realized Hitler was "an outlaw" and would never respond to "anything but force." With Opel now being run by the Germans, Sloan reassigned Mooney to a key job stateside as liaison with the defense program. A watchdog group, the Non-Sectarian Anti-Nazi League, immediately objected, writing to President Roosevelt to warn him that he was placing "a Nazi sympathizer and a Hitler servant (one must render service to the Reich to deserve such a medal) at the throttle of our defense program."

For someone so intuitive about the concerns of American consumers, Sloan remained deaf as ever to the way GM's actions might be regarded from a patriotic and public relations standpoint. When Sloan wrote to DuPont's president, Walter Carpenter, in April 1941 to complain about State Department demands that GM sever its relationship with pro-Fascist auto dealers in Latin America, the chemical executive cautioned him that if he did not heed their instructions, "there will be a blast of some form from Washington. The effect of this will be to associate General Motors with Nazi or Fascist propaganda against the interests of the United States." Carpenter, a GM board member, added prophetically, "[T]he effect on the General Motors corporation might be a very serious matter and the feeling might last for years." Sloan stubbornly refused to listen. He loathed Roosevelt and continued to resist calls by FDR's administration to toe the line on national security issues.

While Sloan tried to avoid being drawn into the war as long as possible, "Boss" Kettering threw himself into the preparedness program. As soon as the Nazi drumbeat began, he volunteered his technical expertise to the US military, where he had retained close contacts from World War I through his work on various aviation and naval committees. He contributed innumerable innovations, some better than others. In 1939, he wrote to General Henry "Hap" Arnold, chief of the Air Corps, saying that the flying bomb he had developed under the sponsorship of the US Army in 1917 could be an important addition to the Allied forces. The Kettering "bug" was a pilotless biplane designed to deliver a three-hundred-pound bomb to targets behind enemy lines, but there had been problems with the accuracy of its controls, and the Armistice occurred before all the kinks were resolved. Kettering immediately set to work improving the weapon, adding radio controls and obtaining a $250,000 appropriation from the Army Air Corps for the design and construction of a sleek new monoplane with a five-hundred-pound payload capacity.

In late December 1941, Gen. Arnold, who had been a young colonel during the flight trials of the original model, called a meeting to discuss the new torpedo's viability as a weapon, but the conclusion was that its range was too limited. Even if they used bases in England as launching sites, the bug could not reach the enemy—the interior of Germany itself. Plans for the bug were scrapped. Exactly one week after Eisenhower's forces landed on the beaches of Normandy, the Germans sought retribution by launching their terrifying pilotless buzz bombs over London. Writing to "Ket" that Christmas, Arnold reflected that his "flying bug" had anticipated the V-1s, and as always he had been "on the right track."

Insisting that in battle "horsepower is war power," Kettering, who had made significant advances in aviation fuel during World War I, began experimenting with a new "super fuel" called triptane. Discovered by chemists at GM and at the Ethyl Corporation—the latter formed jointly by GM and Standard Oil—blends of triptane and tetraethyl lead (TEL) greatly improved performance and knock resistance, or "pinging," and withstood high-compression engines. Most important, the supercharged pressure promised to help with the takeoff of heavily loaded military aircraft. Kettering also foresaw the possibility that it could be used as a gasoline extender in case of fuel shortages. Sloan approved the construction of a half-million-dollar pilot plant, but the high cost of triptane ultimately made it unprofitable, and it never went into full production.

Kettering toured GM's tetraethyl lead production plants in Germany in 1938, but it is unclear how much attention he paid to the precarious political situation and the possibility that the Nazis might want to use the high-octane aviation fuel for their own war planes.* Because of his distaste for administrative matters, he rarely attended board meetings and had little patience for corporate strategy. "He is so engrossed with technical matters . . . the meetings become one of

---

* When the US government later instituted antitrust proceedings against Standard Oil for conspiring with IG Farben, General Motors, a passive partner until 1939, when it sold its holdings in Ethyl, was not included in the suit.

listening rather than doing business," Sloan conceded to a board member who vetoed Kettering's presence on a postwar policy committee, fearing he would drown out all planning discussions with a torrent of anecdotes about his latest inventions. "It is probably good for us and we profit thereby, but business must be carried on."

On December 7, 1941, Pearl Harbor was bombed and America entered the war. GM severed its relationship with Opel and, along with Ford and the rest of the auto industry, had no choice but to cooperate with Washington's demands to fully mobilize. As part of the crash militarization program, GM converted its US factories to produce war matériel and went on to become the country's top defense contractor, operating some $900 million ($120 billion in today's dollars) worth of manufacturing facilities paid for by the government. Many GM workers proudly participated in the war effort. But in his diary, Secretary of War Henry Stimson gave a frank assessment of what it took to get American industry on board: "If you are going to try to go to war or prepare for war in a capitalist country, you have got to let business make money out of the process, or business won't work." From February 1942 to September 1945, GM did not produce a single passenger car. During that same period, the company spent millions on advertising, reminding the American public of their can-do attitude. The new ads boasted that GM plants were rolling out everything from tanks and machine guns to airplane propellers; they ended with the bullish slogan "Victory Is Our Business."

In 1942, Opel's facilities were completely taken over by the Reich, and its American personnel were barred from the country. GM continued to benefit handsomely from its German subsidiary, however, and, taking advantage of a special tax law enacted by Congress, declared Opel a total wartime loss that year. The write-off of the nearly $35 million investment created a tax reduction of "approximately $22.7 million," according to an internal Opel document. Even though GM and Opel had ostensibly cut all ties, the Reich preserved GM's 100 percent stock ownership in Opel, keeping it safe for the American firm until after the war.* GM also collected another $33 million in "war reparations" as a result of Allied bombing of Opel's factories. The company would maintain that it was "unaware of any forced labor being used at the Opel facilities while American personnel had operating control of them" but was aware of reports that may have occurred after the Nazis confiscated the plants.

GM may not have intentionally colluded with Hitler's regime, as some of its harshest critics alleged, but Sloan and GM's top executives cynically profited from the conflict and made a series of errors in judgment before and after war was declared. Their actions raised serious questions about the extent to which they aided Hitler's rearmament juggernaut by allowing Opel to become an important source of war matériel. As DuPont's Carpenter had tried to warn Sloan, GM's unpatriotic and unseemly pursuit of profit would be remembered, and it would do lasting damage to the company's reputation.

"Corporate officials are not only businessmen, they are citizens of the world," the *New York Times* wrote in an Op-Ed piece after the extent of GM's corporate entanglements with the Reich emerged as part of class-action suits on behalf of former prisoners of war in 1998. "Some regimes are so heinous that simply to continue making profits under them is reprehensible. Nazi Germany was surely one."

Imagine their surprise when American troops fought their way across France to Germany in the spring of 1944, only to discover that the Nazis rode to war on Opel trucks and flew Opel-powered

---

* After the war, beginning in 1948, GM resumed control of Opel and reclaimed its prewar dividend that had been frozen by the currency controls. Yale historian Henry Ashby Turner Jr. was given full access to GM records as part of the company's response to class-action suits on behalf of victims of forced labor against American corporations that had owned German firms during the Third Reich. He concluded that while he found no evidence of collusion with the Nazis, the management's decision to claim the tainted money "rendered GM guilty, after the fact, of deriving profit from war production."

bombers—all courtesy of their very own GM. Countless Allied ships sunk in the Atlantic were struck by German torpedoes equipped with Opel detonators. Many of the Allied ground troops in Europe in the last months of the conflict were killed or maimed by Opel-built land mines. On August 27, 1944, the *New York Times* reported that Opel was the "principal target" of a fourteen-hundred-plane RAF bombing mission because its thirty-five-thousand-worker Rüsselsheim plant was turning out aircraft and crucial military transport and was "known to have been developing rocket missiles."

Small wonder then, that after victory in Europe was achieved in May of 1945, Alfred Sloan felt a twinge of conscience over his willingness to do business with the Nazis. He must have hoped that by joining Rhoads's "war on cancer" he would put an end to the moralizing over GM's dealings with the evil regime. Once again, he sought to quiet his detractors with his largesse, and he would pay whatever it cost to defeat what he called "the greatest curse nature has leveled against man." If a cure for cancer could be found using his industrial organizational methods, it would further validate the corporate system he had done so much to create and develop. It is a bitter irony, however, that he sowed the seeds of his philanthropic legacy in the ashes of Bari.

BEFORE THE INK WAS DRY on the *Times* article announcing the new institute, Dusty Rhoads began dealing with the fallout. Versions of the story appeared in newspapers across the country, all emphasizing the merits of GM's methods and creating the unfortunate impression that Sloan and Kettering planned to operate SKI along the inflexible, overcategorized lines of an industrial R&D lab. In one widely read newspaper, the headline KETTERING WILL DIRECT only compounded the problem. When Rhoads began interviewing prospective staff members, he quickly discovered that the "scientific community regarded the new enterprise with suspicion." Gossip quickly spread that those who worked at Sloan Kettering would not be permitted to publish research papers under their own names. Investigators feared important information would be withheld, pending the development of patent rights. Inevitably this gave rise to a great deal of opposition. There was also considerable skepticism at the idea of a "professional amateur," as Kettering liked to call himself, leading the most advanced cancer research center in the world. There was so much unnecessary confusion and controversy that, at a meeting on October 5, 1945, the trustees decided to clarify the situation and formally appointed Rhoads director of the Sloan Kettering Institute.

With the launch of Memorial's major fundraising campaign that fall, Rhoads quickly gained national fame as the leader of the war on cancer. He traveled the country giving lectures, making appearances on local radio shows, and giving newspaper interviews. Realizing that early detection was half the battle, he worked to educate the public about cancer prevention and treatment. He beat the drum for research and more research, both basic and clinical. He always cast his mission in martial terms, the language and imagery conjuring up a struggle between life and death. The statistics were dire, he informed audiences: Between Pearl Harbor and V-J Day, cancer killed more Americans than the Germans and Japanese combined. Unless something was done about it, twelve million Americans now living would die of the disease. "As such," he would finish with a characteristic flourish, "it now ranks as our number one enemy."

Rhoads defined cancer as a war between the body and its rebel cells. Worse yet, it was a particularly nasty civil war, where the body was singularly ill equipped to defend itself. "The Nazis were rather like cancer," he told one reporter, his blue eyes burning bright behind steel-rimmed glasses. "Starting with a variant cell, Hitler, the Nazis multiplied throughout the German nation, bringing it to destruction.

It took external forces to kill the Nazis." The external forces he planned to bring to bear on cancer were a staff of several hundred of the very best biologists, bacteriologists, chemists, statisticians, and laboratory technicians in the country, working together to defeat a common foe. "All I can do," he said, "is pick good men, give them opportunities, and help keep them pointed at the target." He also recruited talented women such as Marguerite Sykes, who became one of the first leading female chemotherapists.

In August 1945, Rhoads and more than a hundred cancer researchers had convened at a symposium on tumor chemotherapy held during the annual summer meeting of the American Association for the Advancement of Science. In a nod to the daring of the clinicians who came out of the wartime generation, Dr. Jacob Furth of Cornell University Medical School observed, "There is a tendency for scholarly men to keep aloof from experimental cancer therapy altogether, regarding it as a hopeless task." In contrast, the clinicians forged ahead and were willing to try almost anything because they faced "pressure on the part of the patients to do something." He applauded the new method of attack on cancer research problems and urged the chemotherapists to seek scientific evidence of treatment success.

This was an endorsement of Rhoads's approach, and it became his battle cry. In an address that fall, Rhoads argued that the only way to maintain progress "in the war of science against disease" was to organize a national program that would continue in the future the work that had been done by the military in medicine. "Coordinated research solved the scientific problems of the war, demonstrated by the development of the atomic bomb," Rhoads explained. While it was reasonable to assume similar methods applied to the problems of disease would yield similar results, he warned that cancer presented a much bigger challenge because researchers did not begin to have the same store of "fundamental knowledge." The disease could not be conquered until more basic work was done in the related fields of biology, chemistry, and physics. Rhoads announced that the American Cancer Society had pledged $500,000 in privately raised funds for cancer research, but they would raise nearly $1 million, and within two years the sum rose to $14.5 million. His recently rechristened Committee on Growth would serve as an advisory board for how the money should be expended. At least $50,000 would go immediately to fellowships for experienced research scientists as they were released by the armed forces.

While he waited for the new SKI building to be completed, Rhoads started recruiting his chemical warfare colleagues to begin work on the science of chemotherapy. These experts—who had spent years under military contracts studying the effects of an array of chemical toxins— would form the nucleus of the cancer institute "brain trust" and allow him to swiftly expand their research program once the new facilities were ready. Before he was done, nearly the entire core staff of the Chemical Warfare Service's Medical Research Division would be reassembled at Sloan Kettering. Rhoads invited Alexander, who had recently been promoted to full colonel, to join him as his assistant at the new institute. There they could work together to take his "important observation" of nitrogen mustard's systemic effects to the next level—and possibly all the way to a treatment for cancer. He expected their first point of attack would be leukemia, in which the bone marrow produced too many white blood cells.

Alexander was sorely tempted by the offer. He briefly allowed himself to imagine what it would be like to enter the ranks of the country's top cancer researchers and work on developing a new chemotherapeutic agent that could "lead to a cure or major remission." It was an alluring prospect, but he had promised his father that he would carry on their family medical practice after the war. The old man had waited five long years for his return. It would not be fair to keep him waiting any longer.

It was with real regret that Alexander informed Rhoads that he would not be able to accept the job at Sloan Kettering. "Stewart had many excellent opportunities before him, but he chose to return to Park Ridge to assist his father in his country practice," recalled Dr. Michael Nevins, a close friend and colleague. Nevins, a Bergen County cardiologist, always felt that Alexander was secure enough in his own abilities, and at the same time loyal enough to his father, to welcome rather than resent the challenge of carrying on the family tradition. "Perhaps more than any single action, it was characteristic of the man," Nevins reflected. "He had a very strong sense of roots and responsibility to family and community, qualities which superseded any ambitions for a glamorous career in the big time."

There was also Bunny to consider. They had both followed Eisenhower's forces into France, but she had supervised the care of the thousands of wounded Allied soldiers and he had scarcely seen her. Three days after the June 1944 invasion, she had made news again when a group of American war correspondents she was guiding to the front came under fire from the Germans. Seeing that a number of soldiers were seriously injured in the attack and needed immediate transfusions, she had pressed the reluctant reporters into donating blood then and there. Alexander had chuckled at the AP story about her "volunteering" the arms of the war correspondents, but then he sat down and wrote her a letter begging her to be careful. A few weeks later, she narrowly escaped injury when an enemy plane strafed the jeep in which she was riding, forcing her and the driver to take cover under the vehicle. He was greatly relieved in October 1944 when the Army sent Bunny, who was expecting their first child, back to the United States and assigned her to the Office of the Surgeon General in Washington. Wearing six gold battle stripes and an array of ribbons, including the Legion of Merit awarded for valor and her outstanding contributions to the Army Nurse Corps in the Mediterranean, she spent her last month in the service as the spokeswoman for another public relations campaign aimed at recruiting nurses for overseas duty.

When he was discharged in June of 1945, Alexander hurried home to Park Ridge, where his wife was already installed with their six-month-old daughter Diane in the small stone house where he had been born. When he folded his little girl in his arms for the first time, he knew with certainty that he was not leaving home again. Before the summer was over, Bunny was pregnant with their second child, and another daughter, Judith, was born the following spring. As much as he had been flattered by Rhoads's offer, Alexander did not see how he could support a family in New York on the modest stipend of $3,000 a year provided by the fledgling institute. He wanted to settle down, build up his practice, and raise the "army of children" Bunny told him she wanted.

Alexander put Bari and chemical weapons behind him. He picked up his black doctor's bag and went back to work, specializing in internal medicine and cardiology. He made house calls every morning, saw patients at his small surgery in the afternoon, and did hospital rounds until 8 p.m. It was a busy life that left little time for thoughts of what might have been. "I was young and alive," he recalled. "I really forgot about the whole thing."

———— ·◆· ————

CHAPTER ELEVEN

Trials and Tribulations

As Dusty Rhoads became famous for his crusade against cancer, he became even more famous in medical circles for his zeal and consuming ambition. There were complaints that, as director of both Memorial Hospital and the Sloan Kettering Institute, in addition to sitting on a wide variety of boards of local, state, and national significance, he exercised, as *Time* put it, "too much power over cancer research." He was accused of being "arbitrary and autocratic," regimenting his army of elite researchers and their supporting forces, and requiring that every responsible person report directly to him. Even more unforgivable, he actively courted the press in the belief that the public must understand cancer research in order to support it, which earned him a reputation among his peers for "publicity seeking." While overseeing the vast empire he had created, Rhoads conceded he could be heavy-handed at times, but he argued that allowances should be made for his urgent mission and critical patients, comparing the situation to a "wartime emergency."

No one questioned his selfless dedication to the job or his lack of concern for personal remuneration. Rhoads worked ten-hour days at the hospital and put in another two to three hours of fundraising most nights with trustees and deep-pocketed patrons. He lived "above the store," occupying an apartment on the top floor of the new fourteen-story Sloan Kettering building that he called "a tower of hope." He and his wife, Katherine, an attractive former medical secretary, had no children, and his grueling schedule left room for few friends or diversions. Rumor had it that on weekend getaways to their country home in Stonington, Connecticut, she spent the drive taking dictation. Forced by administrative duties to forgo the lab work that was his first passion, Rhoads characteristically went a step further and once volunteered his own back to an associate who was conducting an experiment to see whether tobacco tar applied to the skin could cause cancer cells to grow. For a period of weeks, he served as a "human guinea pig," recalled Dr. Ernst Wynder, who said Rhoads swore him to secrecy about his medical martyrdom.

So intense was his commitment to finding a cure that Rhoads made no secret of his contempt for scientists who were inclined solely toward "pure research," which he regarded as of "no necessary, immediate pertinence to the interests of anyone else," and he frequently denigrated it as "rather irresponsible or even selfish." Among the tight coterie of "purposeful"—in his words—physicians and clinical investigators he brought to Memorial and Sloan Kettering, he generated deep loyalty. There was, however, a long line of older colleagues who did not care to have Rhoads's sense of purpose imposed on them. They flinched under his predatory "hawk-like eyes," and they felt bruised by his "outspoken, frequently blunt, comments," noted the *New York Times*, adding, "He has stepped on a lot of toes." Rhoads's unadorned manner of speaking could be curt to the point of insulting, and the mounting pressures of the job triggered his impatience. He tried hard to conceal the inner demons that drove him, but one episode in his past continued to haunt him and always lurked in the background, threatening to undo his reputation and everything he had worked so hard to accomplish.

It had started out as a chance to do an interesting study of pernicious anemia in Puerto Rico for six months in 1931. Not only would it keep him out of the ordinary postmortem work that was the lot of most pathologists, but if everything went well, it might even produce an important paper that would help boost his career as a research scientist. The thirty-three-year-old Rhoads, then an associate at the Rockefeller Institute, had accepted with alacrity when Harvard hematologist Dr. William Castle told him he had snagged a generous Rockefeller Foundation grant, and he invited him to partake in the study and extend the benefits of Western medicine to the poor and sick on the island.

John D. Rockefeller, the cofounder of Standard Oil and reportedly the richest man in the world, had run into trouble over unethical business practices, and in 1901 he decided to improve his image by donating large sums to medical charities. First he founded the Rockefeller Institute for Medical Research, whose sole purpose was experimental medicine, which at the time included experimental studies on human subjects. Then in 1909, he created the Rockefeller Sanitary Commission to eradicate hookworm in the South, and four years later he endowed the Rockefeller Foundation to continue that work and expand the scope of its public health work abroad. Physicians and scientists, eager to explore the burgeoning fields of microbiology and nutrition, took advantage of America's new colonies—Cuba, Puerto Rico, Guam, and the Philippines—to carry out their research in the name of doing good.

Under the terms of the newly formed Rockefeller Anemia Commission, headed by Dr. Castle, the researchers were supposed to concentrate on finding the best methods of prevention and possibly a cure for hookworm-caused anemia and sprue, two common and often fatal tropical diseases. Rhoads immediately started getting "big ideas," recalled Castle. Before he knew it, Rhoads had rapidly acquired additional research beds in the local Presbyterian Hospital and even more in the Municipal Hospital in Santurce, Puerto Rico, and they were treating far more patients than he could have ever imagined possible. At one point, they had to employ eight female technicians to help them with all the bloodwork. Numerous samples had to be taken from the ear or the veins of the arm to study the effects of the different medications, and just as many intramuscular injections of special preparations of liver extract had to be administered. Many of the patients were peasants from rural areas who had never been in a clinic and could not afford one, so they had to be persuaded that the medicine and fees would all be paid for with Rockefeller money. To what extent they understood they were giving their consent to be subjected to experiments is unclear.

The team set up a careful screening process, and only individuals with half the normal number of red blood cells or normal hemoglobin value were considered suitable candidates for study and "of scientific value." Those who appeared in relatively good condition were referred to another clinic. Inevitably, many of the patients brought to the commission were in very poor condition, rundown and emaciated, but the clinic could not accept cases complicated by other disorders such as chronic infections or cancer. The majority of the 257 treated patients showed "prompt clinical improvement," Castle reported, and attained "a sense of wellbeing and high blood values not enjoyed for years." Thirteen deaths occurred, all unrelated to the anemia, and "by the unexpected nature of the complication rendered successful treatment impossible." All in all, Castle concluded, "the gratifying results" of the study confirmed the curative value of liver and iron for anemia, the treatment developed by the Harvard Medical Services.

In September, Rhoads wrote to his boss Dr. Simon Flexner, director of the Rockefeller Institute, about an "exciting experiment." He was attempting "to cause experimental sprue in humans." Just as debilitating as anemia, tropical sprue was an obscure disease and not well understood, so any progress he could notch would be noteworthy. "We now have only two 'experimental animals,'" he reported, "and will increase the number to ten in a week or so." Rhoads hoped to induce sprue in his Puerto Rican test "animals" by placing them on a "characteristic native diet, which generally consisted of carbohydrates and fat, very little protein (only 30 grams a day) and almost no vitamins." As he told Flexner, "If they don't develop something they certainly have the constitutions of oxen." The researchers studied ninety-two sprue subjects, the majority of whom were already affected by the disease, but they were unable to reach any firm conclusions.

Rhoads's research project in Puerto Rico was nearly finished when things went horribly wrong. By that fall, he had begun to chafe at the working conditions and admittedly found it difficult to accommodate himself to life in the tropics. After a long, wearing week of dealing with patients, he attended a party on November 10 in the small town of Cidra, thirty miles outside San Juan. When he emerged somewhat inebriated, Rhoads discovered his Ford roadster had been vandalized, and the thieves had made off with everything that could be pried loose and left the tires flat. Still angry about the damage when he reached home, he fired off a letter to a fellow pathologist in the United States, Fred "Ferdie" Stewart, venting his fury at the local villains. Afterward, he felt better and forgot all about it. The next day, the commission's Puerto Rican stenographer found the handwritten note denouncing her countrymen. She shared it with her friends, including a twenty-year-old lab technician named Luis Baldoni. Disturbed by the contents of the letter, which was signed "Dusty," Baldoni immediately made copies and distributed them among the staff.

When the director of Presbyterian Hospital, Dr. William Galbreath, received a copy three days later, he immediately called Rhoads to account. The Rockefeller researcher appeared "very much surprised" by the uproar caused by the letter, according to Galbreath, as he thought he had thrown it away.

Rhoads then gathered the laboratory employees together and made a short speech of apology. Admitting that he wrote the letter in a moment of rage but never sent it, he said he hoped he had not offended anyone. He assured them of the "high regard and esteem" in which he held the Puerto

Rican people, adding that no one who knew of the work he had done on behalf of the sick and needy patients in the hospital could possibly believe that what was in the letter was true, and that it was "all a joke." The following Monday, November 16, Rhoads personally apologized to Baldoni, who had kept the original letter in hopes of persuading someone to discipline the American doctor. The two shook hands, and Rhoads expressed the hope that the technician bore him no ill will. To placate Rhoads and the senior members of the commission, Baldoni, who was understandably filled with "fear" and "distrust," told them he had destroyed the letter.

If Rhoads thought that was the end of it, he could not have been more wrong. When he learned a few weeks later that copies of his letter had been sent to the Puerto Rico Medical Association, which was debating whether or not to take action against him, he realized the situation had spiraled out of control. Advised that partisan feeling on the island was running high, he decided it would be best if he left, so he sailed for New York on December 10. On his return to the Rockefeller Institute, Rhoads downplayed the episode to his superiors and gave them the impression that he "considered the matter closed."

On the afternoon of January 29, 1932, Rhoads received a phone call from a tabloid reporter informing him that the controversy that had been simmering in Puerto Rico since his departure had spilled onto the front pages of all the local newspapers. Copies of his now-infamous letter had been reprinted in full in both English and Spanish for all to read. The damning passage appeared in the second paragraph, when Rhoads wrote to his friend Ferdie that he might be able to get a permanent job at Presbyterian Hospital in San Juan, adding that "it would be ideal except for the Porto Ricans [the Anglicized spelling then in use]." He continued:

They are beyond doubt the dirtiest, laziest, most degenerate and thievish race of men ever inhabiting this sphere. It makes you sick to inhabit the same island with them. They are even lower than

Italians. What the island needs is not public health work but a tidal wave or something to totally exterminate the population. It might then be livable. I have done my best to further the process of extermination by killing off 8 and transplanting cancer into several more. The latter has not resulted in any fatalities so far. . . . The matter of consideration for the patients' welfare plays no role here—in fact all physicians take delight in the abuse and torture of the unfortunate subjects.

After Rhoads left, Baldoni had passed the original letter to Pedro Albizu Campos, leader of the Puerto Rican Nationalist Party, which was dedicated to securing the island's independence from the United States. A shrewd political operative, Albizu Campos seized the opportunity to use the rich, white, Rockefeller doctor's derogatory tirade as a way to rally local sentiment against the American government on the eve of his party's annual convention. He saw to it that Rhoads's screed got the widest possible circulation, sending copies to newspapers all over America and Europe, as well as to the League of Nations, the Pan-American Union, and the American Civil Liberties Union. Even the Vatican received a copy. The nationalists enclosed a cover letter stating that Rhoads's comments confirmed the genocidal nature of the American occupation—the United States had invaded and seized Puerto Rico in 1898—and compared Rhoads's plan to "inoculate" islanders with cancer to the "system of extermination" of the American "Indian race," as well as the natives of Hawaii, by exposing them to "tuberculosis and other devastating diseases." The governor of Puerto Rico, James Beverley, called Rhoads's letter tantamount to a "confession of murder" and a "libel against the people from Puerto Rico," and ordered an investigation.

A nervous Rhoads called his superiors to warn them that reporters were seeking a statement from him about the letter. He was instructed to sit tight and say nothing. Flexner arranged for him to meet with Ivy

Ledbetter Lee, a savvy former newspaperman turned public relations expert who had been handling publicity for the Rockefellers for two decades. Lee had been brought in during the 1914 Ludlow Massacre, when twenty-four men, women, and children were killed during a labor riot at a Rockefeller-owned Colorado mine. Not only did he stop the flow of negative print, he succeeded in transforming Rockefeller's reputation from that of a ruthless and reclusive tyrant to a benevolent employer and philanthropist. Dubbed "poison Ivy" by critics who considered him little more than a highly paid liar, he was a forerunner of the modern "spin doctor," and certainly the man to call in a crisis.

Lee, with help from Flexner, crafted the glib message of apology Rhoads cabled to the governor:

```
Regret very much that fantastic composition written
entirely for my own diversion and intended as parody
of supposed attitude of American minds in Porto Rico
should have become public document and taken liter-
ally by anyone. Of course, nothing in the document
was ever intended to mean other than the opposite of
what was stated.
```

Rhoads went on to assure the governor that if the "slightest seriousness" was attached to any aspect of the subject, he would be glad to return to Puerto Rico at once and help clear up any misunderstanding.

The following day, the *New York Times* broke the sensational story that the governor of Puerto Rico had ordered an inquiry into Rhoads's murderous missive. The subhead, in all capital letters, stated: IT TELLS OF EIGHT KILLINGS. Again Ivy Lee managed to do some damage control: The *Times* story quoted a sympathetic "friend" who described the hostility Rhoads and the other members of the Rockefeller Commission had encountered throughout their six-month stay on the island, and the way they were repeatedly depicted by the nationalist press as "arrogant and contemptuous" of Puerto Ricans. The friend went on to offer yet another explanation for Rhoads's letter, stating that it was penned in a moment of despair after a patient died, despite the staff's best efforts to save him, and it was meant to be a "parody" of his idea of "what a nationalist sympathizer, obsessed with anti-American beliefs, might suppose to be the sentiments of the doctor who had treated him."

The "parody" spin was not well received in Puerto Rico. Dr. George Payne, the resident representative of the Rockefeller Foundation, warned officials in New York that no one on the island believed Rhoads's story. But given the endemic racism at the time toward the inhabitants of new territories, most of their American colleagues were inclined to dismiss the incident. It was viewed as a moment of private folly that should never have become public. Flexner and the other Rockefeller administrators stood by Rhoads, though behind closed doors they conceded that his gallows humor—typically regarded as an acceptable "safety valve" by most doctors and medical insiders—was in very poor taste. However, his career was regarded as too promising to allow it to be derailed because of a political stunt by a bunch of nationalist agitators.

Rhoads was not the first, and would not be the last, Rockefeller scientist to run afoul of the locals in a developing country. According to University of Wisconsin medical historian and bioethicist Susan Lederer, "Only a few years before the Puerto Rico incident, Rockefeller researcher Hideyo Noguchi also encountered problems in working with 'native' technicians as part of the Rockefeller yellow fever commission in West Africa." When Noguchi contracted yellow fever and died under mysterious circumstances in 1928, the African technicians were held responsible for the mistakes that may have played a part in the project leader's demise. All too aware of the obstacles and potential pitfalls their researchers faced in these primitive settings, Rhoads's superiors were inclined to give him the benefit of the doubt, and they accepted his explanation of the letter as a private exercise in venting his frustration at the Puerto Rican staff.

Reflecting an imperial condescension toward the colonies, *Time* magazine publisher Henry Luce told Rockefeller's publicist in a telegram not to worry:

> The incident casts no reflection on anyone or any-
> thing except native ignorance. Would describe it not
> as frivolous, but as very human.

Luce had every intention of covering the medical scandal because it was "news," but he assured Lee it was unlikely their story would harm the foundation's important work—the magazine helpfully agreed to delete several objectionable sentences from the original letter—and he hoped everyone would "agree in two or three months hence that no damage has been done."

Indeed, the February 15, 1932, issue of *Time* headlined the affair as Porto Ricochet, the wordplay implying it was a typical example of local ingratitude, and Rhoads's noble efforts to introduce medical advances to the island had backfired on him. "He and Dr. Castle developed a thoroughgoing and inexpensive remedy for pernicious anemia," the article stressed, noting that it would have enormous ramifications for the treatment of tropical diseases and "promises to be one of the best things that ever happened to the populace there." The story included a photograph of a buttoned-down, sober-looking Rhoads, accompanied by the caption, "His parody was taken seriously."

Castle, who had remained behind in Puerto Rico to assist with the investigation, publicly defended Rhoads. In an extremely detailed statement, Castle presented a case-by-case review of the thirteen deaths in the study, all of whom were seen personally by him, with nine also examined by Rhoads, "acting on my instructions." In three cases, one of which Rhoads never saw, preexisting cancers were discovered shortly after treatment began. One was an "unsuspected neoplasm of the kidney" discovered in the postmortem; the other two cases involved "tumors of the breast and bladder," and the patients were referred to other physicians for treatment. Castle emphasized that the techniques for taking blood, along with those used to administer drugs, as well as the sterilization of needles, were all done in accordance with approved methods and were identical to those in use in Boston hospitals for many years. Finally, he explained how, in the absence of blood donors, commission doctors valiantly offered to fill the void, and "Dr. Rhoads, in particular, gave blood for several transfusions" when emergencies arose in the hospital. He maintained Rhoads's work had been of the highest order: "I have never had the slightest doubt of his total lack of inclination or opportunity for any actions jeopardizing the welfare of the patients under my charge."

It was a measure of the Rockefeller Foundation's clout that the investigation was wrapped up in two weeks. The prosecutor, Special Attorney José Ramón Quiñones, found no corroborating evidence that Rhoads deliberately gave cancer to any patients "by direct or indirect action," or caused any illegal deaths. While he did not absolve the American doctor of writing the "untrue and injurious statements" about Puerto Ricans, and he could only conclude he was "a mental case or unscrupulous person," because Rhoads never actually mailed the letter, he committed no crime under the law. DR. RHOADS CLEARED OF PORTO RICO PLOT, declared the *New York Times*, explaining that the nationalists had failed in their attempt to turn the purloined letter into a race-extermination plot.

On February 17, Governor Beverley reported to Rockefeller Foundation officials that he was "very happy that the investigation resulted as it did." Then, in the spirit of altruism, he let them know the full extent of his efforts on their behalf: "Incidentally, another letter in Dr. Rhoads's handwriting turned up during the course of the investigation, but it was suppressed by the government, and no publication was given to it. The second letter seemed to me to be even worse than the first." No doubt, the Rockefeller Foundation found a way to show its gratitude for his discretion. Their own internal probe was also unable to confirm Rhoads had acted on his bizarre boast that he had injected patients with cancer cells. In the end, the Rockefeller administrators decided to put Rhoads's temporary lapse in judgment down to strain. "I think we have enough evidence of an emotional upset without going deeper into the details," Payne wrote on February 25, noting that he was not going to pursue the matter further.

During the investigation, witnesses were profuse in their praise of Rhoads and testified that he had saved many lives. In a letter to the editor of *La Correspondencia de Puerto Rico*, a conservative daily, a grateful patient, Rafael Arroyo Zeppenfeldt, wrote that he found the charges against Rhoads to be completely at odds with the man he knew. "To him and to his colleague, Dr. Castle, I owe my life," he asserted, adding that Rhoads never treated him with the cold indifference Baldoni described in his testimony, and in his presence "never treated anyone brusquely or rudely." He also disputed Baldoni's account of dirty needles being used on Puerto Rican patients, stating that he observed the syringes being washed in a solution that was "always within reach." If anything, Zeppenfeldt had been touched by the "genuine interest" Rhoads always showed in his case, "which was clearly reflected in the joy with which he received the news that my system was responding to the treatment."

At the same time, Zeppenfeldt suggested that by virtue of his single-minded focus, and willful ignorance of the economic and political tensions on the island, the American doctor might have brought some of the trouble upon himself. "No patients [sic] can avoid forming in his mind an idea of the physician who treats him," he wrote. "I always saw in Dr. Rhoads a man whose enthusiasm and whose love for his profession blinded him to ulterior considerations."

Rhoads weathered the storm. Despite the widespread publicity, his reputation remained untarnished. The old-boy network that ruled medicine in those days was unperturbed. Only a few years later, several prominent Boston institutions tried to woo him away, forcing Flexner and Rockefeller Institute administrators to increase his salary and offer other incentives to persuade him to stay. "The work he began with Dr. Castle in Porto Rico led to his outstanding contributions in the past few years," wrote Dr. George Minot, head of the Thorndike Memorial Laboratory of Boston City Hospital, who a year earlier had shared the 1934 Nobel Prize for his work on pernicious anemia. Minot had already hired Dr. Castle and had set his sights on Rhoads, who he predicted had a brilliant future in store: "His work is of the sort that will be profitable to the world at large and an honor to the institution where it is conducted." Rhoads remained in New York and in 1939 was lured away by Memorial Hospital, where he succeeded the revered pathologist Dr. James Ewing as director of the world's preeminent private cancer hospital. An official history of the Rockefeller Institute that ran to biblical proportions stated that Rhoads was known for his devotion to his patients, "and his skill and kindness as a physician were much appreciated."

The Rhoads scandal never completely disappeared, however. Over the years, it would crop up again and again, and he could never be sure when it might resurface. In March of 1942, just before beginning his military service, he contacted the Rockefeller Institute and asked them to send him the confidential file on the "Porto Rican episode." He may have been anxious that something incriminating from that period could prevent him from receiving the high-level clearance required by the Chemical Warfare Service. But there was no cause for concern. Ivy Lee had done a good job of polishing his image, and the security check turned up nothing problematic. Rhoads would go on to have an exemplary military career, and he was awarded the Legion of Merit in 1945 for his work with the Chemical Warfare Service. He championed the use of nitrogen mustards as a treatment for cancer, ushering in the modern age of chemotherapy. But the trials and tribulations of the Puerto Rico expedition had been mortifying, and Rhoads was a man in search of redemption. His blunder served to drive his intense interest in alleviating the pain and misery caused by malignant disease. Finding a cure became almost an obsession.

———— ·◆· ————

CHAPTER TWELVE

"The Sword and the Ploughshare"

On October 2, 1946, almost three years after the Bari incident, Dusty Rhoads gave a rousing speech to an audience of physicians at New York's Mount Sinai Hospital, openly discussing for the first time the secret wartime research on poison gas and its peacetime benefits as a treatment for cancer. The Office of Scientific Research and Development had recently lifted the security restrictions on the clinical studies of the toxic agents, allowing the results to be published. The details of the Bari disaster, however, were still classified when Rhoads decided to divulge the true story of the chemical-weapons accident and Stewart Alexander's investigative saga in order to highlight the connection between military research and the medical discovery of chemotherapy.

"For a moment, I would like you to relive the dark days of the winter months of 1943," Rhoads began, pausing a beat to make certain he had their full attention before launching into his vivid account of the German air raid that sank seventeen Allied ships, including the *John Harvey* and its cargo of mustard bombs, and resulted in more than a thousand men being plunged into the blazing, oil-covered sea. He explained how the shipwrecked men were "routinely wrapped in blankets, without the removal of oil." His account was simple and eloquent and did not attempt to allocate blame. After listing the victims' curious symptoms—from the weak, apathetic state that failed to respond to the usual therapeutic measures for immersion shock to the terrible conjunctivitis and generalized brawny edema of the skin and subcutaneous tissue—he described the characteristic syndrome that led to a depressed leukocyte count and then death. The cavernous auditorium was still. His listeners, leaning forward in their seats, were spellbound.

"A medical officer trained in the Chemical Warfare Service," Rhoads continued, his voice rising, "realized the true situation: that the casualties were not shocked from immersion or blast but were dying from the late results of mustard gas poisoning. Col. Alexander wrote a most detailed, indeed, a classic report. He did more, he saved tissue in a hastily improvised fixative and sent the specimens with a personal letter to the medical laboratories of the Chemical Warfare Service in this country. All this was done in anticipation of the reports which would follow. . . ." His clinical observations of forty cases "illustrated as adequately as any example can, the effects of the mustard compounds on blood formation." Rhoads emphasized the importance of Alexander's report in providing the "first confirmation" of the agent's profound and almost specific effect on lymphoid tissue, which he credited with infusing momentum into their research into nitrogen mustard as a treatment for neoplastic disease.

The dramatic introduction was designed to soften the blow of what came next—Rhoads's acknowledgment that the present therapeutic status of the nitrogen mustards was not quite as promising as first hoped. He went on to summarize the results of the preliminary experiments carried out by Memorial Hospital, the University of Chicago, and the University of Utah over the previous two years. The three groups of researchers studied a total of 160 patients, suffering from various types of cancer, who were treated with intravenous nitrogen mustard, HN2.

Rhoads's Memorial team injected nitrogen mustard into the veins of sixty men and women, most of whom suffered from blood diseases such as leukemia and lymphomas. Therapeutically, their aim was "to produce more severe injury to the tumour than to the host." They found that the compounds were capable of injuring many types of tissue, and they appeared to exert their greatest effect on the fastest-growing cells, whether normal or neoplastic. They produced regressions of "striking proportions" in some patients, as well as gratifying palliative effects in others. But even in tiny, carefully monitored doses, the chemotherapeutic agent caused nausea, vomiting, fatigue, and weight loss. The toxicity was a definite liability. The dosage required to destroy tumors was often more than the patient could bear. And, inevitably, the cancer came back. The inhibitory effect of the mustard failed to last, rarely enduring beyond a few months.

Rhoads could claim only an incremental advance in cancer medicine. Nitrogen mustards had emerged as a "chemical tool" to treat Hodgkin's disease and some patients with lymphosarcoma and leukemia. They produced results "about as good as, and not much better than," those obtained by standard X-ray therapy. In some respects, radiation still had the advantage in that it could be applied locally to target one area rather than affecting the entire body. In rare cases where radiation did not work, the nitrogen mustards had been shown to have some effect. Like radiation, they constituted a treatment, not a cure. The researchers' work on this "unique group of chemicals" was just beginning.

Despite his restrained appraisal of their usefulness, Rhoads insisted nitrogen mustards continued to be a fertile field of investigation. Their selective toxic action on certain cell types was spurring the search for better chemotherapeutic agents against cancer. "It is quite true that the mouse is not a very large one, and the mountain was of very considerable size," he observed, referencing one of Aesop's fables in which a mountain shudders and quakes as if in labor, raising expectations all over the land, only to deliver the tiniest of creatures. "The important question, however, is how much the mouse will be able to grow in the future. This is the first mouse of this type that has ever been produced, and it might very well become the parent of a great race of new chemical compounds." By the time he had finished, Rhoads's unwavering faith in progress had won over the crowd of civilian doctors filling the large auditorium. Applause resounded from every corner of the room. There was a palpable sense of excitement about the new chemical approach, a surge of optimism that keeping up a concentrated, well-financed attack on cancer would yield positive results.

Although Rhoads would continue to enthrall audiences with his tale of a young doctor's Sherlock Holmesian detective work in solving the baffling mystery of the Bari victims, it did not spread beyond medical circles. The war was full of tragic stories, and the war was in the past. People were looking to the future and were hungry for scientific break-throughs that would improve their lives. If physicists had unlocked the power of the atom—and with it the unlimited potential of radioactive isotopes—then surely chemical warfare physicians had opened a locked chest of untold wonders that could be used to treat hitherto-incurable diseases and end suffering and premature death. The postwar belief in the bright promise of military developments to revolutionize medicine made it easy for the public to accept the crude chemicals and to ignore the undercurrent of doubt about the dangerous side effects. Relentlessly upbeat, Rhoads told reporters that the spoils of war offered science opportunities for research "undreamed of only a few years ago."

The press pounced on the more tangible results of the wartime can-cer trials, and in all the hoopla that followed, a new pair of white-coated heroes was anointed. The laurels went to Louis S. Goodman and Alfred Gilman Sr., who were hailed as pioneers in chemotherapy for conduct-ing the first therapeutic cancer trial in America, and their achievement of a remarkable—if temporary—remission. Their reputation was sealed with the publication of their seminal investigations of the nitrogen mustards. Gilman coauthored a lengthy article with Frederick S. Philips in *Science* magazine, and another comprehensive study with Goodman and a group of research scientists in the *Journal of the American Medical Association (JAMA)*. The *New York Times* noted that the Yale group was "prompted" to begin studying the effects of nitrogen mustard gas on the body by "the experience of shipwrecked men in Bari." This created the widespread misapprehension that the disaster preceded the first clinical trial, when in fact the reverse was true, but the wealth of information from the Bari victims provided further proof that they were on the right track. (The *Times* story clarified the timeline in a later paragraph, but the confusion continues to the present day.)

After reading the articles, Alexander wrote to the War Department in December, asking to be allowed to publish his account of the Bari incident. By the time he received permission six months later and submitted his report, *JAMA* felt his findings had been eclipsed by the Yale studies and rejected it. Alexander's "Report of the Bari Harbor Mustard Casualties" eventually appeared in a specialized periodical, the *Military Surgeon*, in July 1947.

Rhoads's revelation that the Army's chemical warfare experts had discovered a weapon in their "deadly artillery" that could kill cancer cells precipitated dozens of newspaper and magazine stories, all bullish about the new chemical "cure." WAR GASES TRIED IN CANCER THERAPY, announced the *New York Times* four days after Rhoads's speech, revealing that the results of the first sixty-seven cancer cases treated with the nitrogen mustards at Yale, Chicago, Utah, and two dozen other hospitals showed that the chemicals did "prolong life in many instances." Gilman, now a major in the Chemical Warfare Service, was quoted as saying the treatment might extend the lifespan of patients with Hodgkin's disease "fifteen or twenty years."

MEDICINE: MUSTARD AGAINST CANCER, trumpeted *Time*, heralding "the new therapeutic possibility" and the amazing transformation of nitrogen mustard from virulent poison to potent drug. The *Time* article focused on the results from the University of Chicago group, led by Dr. Leon Jacobsen, who gave intravenous doses of the methyl-*bis* nitrogen mustard (Goodman and Gilman used *tris*) over a protracted period to fifty-nine terminally ill cancer patients. Most experienced some relief: Their fever and malaise disappeared, their tumors subsided, and they gained weight. Some even went back to work. The best results were recorded against the invariably fatal Hodgkin's disease. The researchers obtained "significant remissions" in some Hodgkin's patients, including certain cases where radiation treatments had ceased to be effective. One patient, a thirty-seven-year-old commercial artist, "had been kept in good working health for thirty-three months by periodic injections of mustard."

The results were encouraging, but the Chicago team cautioned in their report that this was still a "potentially dangerous drug," capable of severely damaging blood-forming organs. They concluded, "The efficacy of a chemotherapeutic agent in controlling a disease cannot be judged only by the period of remission it will produce, for the toxic reactions must not endanger life or delay recovery of general health." In short, the drug was not sufficiently free from risk to be released for general use anytime soon.

The excitement about mustard as the next medical marvel soon faded as it became clear that scientists had made little headway in the nascent field of cancer chemotherapy. No practical benefits could be expected in the near future. Within the conservative, tradition-bound medical profession, the prevailing attitude was one of wait-and-see. At conferences, the main topic of discussion and debate was whether the chemicals did more harm than good.

Many physicians doubted the approach could ever be made to work, and they questioned the fleeting remissions and brutal treatment. It was all very well for Dusty Rhoads to declare war on cancer, but the problem was that cancer was not one disease. As far as anyone knew, it did not have a single cause or pathogen. How could they wage war against an unknown enemy? They protested that Rhoads was diverting resources from the proven cancer treatments of surgery and radiation. The most vociferous critics felt Rhoads had misled them, promising a cure he could not deliver. They contended a medicine for cancer was Ehrlich's unsubstantiated dream, and that combating the disease with drugs was not a practical approach rooted in reality. Dr. Alfred Gellhorn, a cancer researcher at Columbia University College of Physicians and Surgeons, recalled that Dr. Robert Loeb, a legendary clinician and chairman of Columbia's Department of Medicine, strongly disapproved of the early testing of chemotherapy drugs and would often tell him, "Alfred, you belong to the lunatic fringe."

Dr. William H. Woglom, the snowy-haired dean of cancer investigators, known for his lucid analyses of the scientific problems of the day, summed up the near-impossibility of the task facing chemotherapists. "Those who have not trained in chemistry or medicine," he wrote, "may not realize how difficult the problem of treatment really is. It is almost, not quite, but almost as hard as finding some agent that will dissolve away the left ear, say, yet leave the right ear unharmed; so slight is the difference between the cancer cell and its normal ancestor."

Rhoads's defenders dismissed the sniping as envy, pointing to the fact that scientists at Memorial had already succeeded in developing leads that were being exploited as effective treatments. Joe Burchenal refused to accept that the conquest of cancer was impossible, when the conquest of infectious disease suggested that it could be accomplished. Burchenal had lost his stepmother to bone cancer during his undergraduate years at Princeton, and he passionately believed in the possibility of new drugs that could rid the body of cancer. He admired Rhoads for audaciously tackling what was considered an incurable disease, and for his willingness to put his prestige behind the effort to develop controversial new areas such as chemotherapy, virology, and immunology long before they were accepted by the mainstream.

Burchenal and the other young recruits from the CWS—including Drs. David Karnofsky, C. Chester Stock, Fred Philips, John Beasley, and Oscar Bodonsky—had all worked together in the Army, and they became the core staff of the new Experimental Chemotherapy Division of Sloan Kettering. In the 1940s, oncology was not yet recognized as a clinical specialty, and Burchenal recalled that during those early years, "neochemotherapists," as they were called, were very much a disdained minority. Whenever the fledgling group came together for scientific meetings, no more than forty would show up.

Aware of the widespread skepticism, Rhoads tempered his enthusiasm for the nitrogen mustards in his public remarks and written reports, but in practice he was chasing a cure harder than ever. He remained committed to the idea that since cancer cells were different from normal tissue, they—like bacteria—should be susceptible to selective destruction and would eventually succumb to drugs. He believed the nitrogen mustard compounds could be used in increasingly refined forms, and in combination with radiation and other drugs, in very specific dosages, in very specific cancers, to attack malignant cells. His strategy at Memorial and the newly established Sloan Kettering was to put together a crack team to facilitate advances and concentrate on "studies of a fundamental nature frankly designed to develop methods of control or cure."

During the war, he had plucked Karnofsky, a brilliant young pathologist, from the ranks of the CWS for temporary assignment to Memorial to begin translating the wealth of data from the Bari report and other wartime studies of nitrogen mustards into practical applications for patients. Karnofsky had already spent months at Camp Bushnell in Florida studying the biological effects of mustard gas on goats, and he was already disposed to doing exactly the kind of research Rhoads wanted. As soon as he was discharged from the Army, Karnofsky went straight from Edgewood Arsenal to Memorial, where he became the lead clinical investigator in a series of human experiments with the nitrogen mustards.

The wisdom of Rhoads's hire quickly became apparent when Karnofsky's research yielded more encouraging findings. In their first attempt to treat patients with inoperable lung cancer with nitrogen mustard, the Memorial team reported that of the thirty-five patients, 74 percent showed some clinical improvement. The beneficial effects usually lasted from two weeks to two months. The investigators found that the nitrogen mustards appeared to "briefly interrupt" the course of the disease, causing the tumors to shrink and alleviating symptoms ranging from coughing and spitting up blood to shortness of breath, pain, and weakness. In these rapidly growing lung cancers, nitrogen mustard seemed to be more effective, and less hazardous, than radiation therapy.

The Memorial team also made some progress treating patients with acute leukemia, which had proved unresponsive to drugs in the past. They found that some of the nitrogen mustard derivatives caused a drop in total leukocyte count and a decrease in the size of the spleen and lymph nodes. Remissions were few, however, and possibly coincidental. But in the case of chronic myelogenous leukemia, real—though transient—remissions were produced with regularity. The drug appeared to control symptoms in the early stages of the disease, enabling patients to live more comfortably and usefully during the remainder of their illness.

In keeping with their benefactor's R&D model for medical science, Karnofsky stressed the importance of the meticulous clinical evaluation of the new drugs and moved to change the reporting of the experimental chemotherapeutic results from anecdotal to a more objective, standardized format. He created the famous Karnofsky Performance Status Scale (KPS) to more accurately quantify, in terms of percentage, the subjective effects of the toxicity that were not as easily measured as survival time. The scale measured the patient's well-being during the treatment and the management of a terminal illness that was now being extended for increasingly long periods of time. The scores range from 100 (normal) to 0 (dead), with categories covering "able to carry on normal activity" to "disabled" and "very disabled/hospitalization indicated." Three decades before "quality of life" issues became part of the medical conversation, Karnofsky was attentive to the consequences of the aggressive treatment and the need for another standard for measuring patients' tolerance of the toxin that would half-kill them in order to keep them alive.

When the new Sloan Kettering Institute opened its doors for business on April 16, 1948, Rhoads, together with Karnofsky and Burchenal, started the first organized clinical cancer chemotherapy program. Memorial expanded from a single building with 242 beds into a sprawling cancer center whose various components covered an entire Manhattan block. C-DAY LANDING WON IN WAR ON CANCER, gushed the *Times*, its journalistic effusions over the new modern complex inspiring comparisons to the successful Normandy invasion. "As of today," the *Times* continued in breathless prose, "the Memorial Cancer Center will become the GHQ of the most concentrated assault on cancer so far in history."

In one of his frequent communiqués from the front, Rhoads announced that the first of the nitrogen mustards to be safe enough to be used clinically was mechlorethamine, aka Mustargen. Sloan Kettering immediately put it into use and packed it off to the FDA for approval, which was granted in 1949. The new drug exerted its anticancer effect by a process called alkylation, which damaged the DNA of cells, preventing them from dividing and causing them to die. Since it affected the multiplying malignant cells to a greater degree than healthy cells, it slowed or arrested the growth of cancer. At the time, doctors did not make a practice of telling patients they were receiving Mustargen or drugs derived from it.

Eager to develop superior treatments, Rhoads pursued an increasingly intensive trial-and-error search for agents that could induce longer remissions. Only a handful of nitrogen mustards had been used in clinical studies at this point, hundreds had already been produced in commercial labs, and thousands more were in the pipeline. The screening process was slow and expensive. Each compound with therapeutic potential had to be tested on organisms, mice, and then patients. The pace of progress depended on the generosity of the American public, as Rhoads, a master at promotion, would tell journalists while parading them through the gleaming laboratories of Sloan Kettering's Experimental Chemotherapy Division.

In temperature-controlled rooms, ceiling-high tiers of metal cages housed a massive colony of white mice that were maintained on a diet of sunflower seeds and vitamins while they awaited the next trial of an agent with anticancer activity. Each week, five hundred mice, at a cost of thirty-six cents a head, were inoculated with tissue-cultured cancer cells. After the tumor had time to "take," they were injected with a less-than-fatal dose of one of the derivatives being tested. After ten days or so, if the autopsy of the mouse revealed that the grayish-pink, thumbnail-size mass had shrunk, or even disappeared, the compound would be listed as promising and slated for further testing. "In the fight against cancer," asserted a reporter, "one of these 36-cent mice might turn out be man's best friend."

By the end of its first year in business, Sloan Kettering's Experimental Chemotherapy Division had 2,300 chemical agents on file and had already tested 1,500 of them. Only six had proved to have a "differential effect," meaning they targeted only the diseased cells without harming the healthy tissue. Several dozen had a lesser effect. Rhoads was not discouraged. Even if the next compound had only a slight effect, they were rapidly accumulating knowledge and experience and would be that much closer to finding an effective chemotherapy compound. When critics pointed to the costly, inefficient, low-yield screening process, he took to quoting Kettering, who liked to tell an anecdote about Thomas Edison's answer to an inquirer who asked whether he felt frustrated after testing more than six hundred materials to use as incandescent-bulb filaments without success. Edison's answer was no, he felt he was getting somewhere because he had eliminated six hundred substances that he would not have to test again.

Kettering, who had retired from GM by this time, had recently thrown himself into the institute's work after the unexpected death of his wife, Olive, from pancreatic cancer in April 1946, at age sixty-eight. After performing exploratory surgery in January, the doctors had informed him that nothing could be done. She was given less than three months to live. Kettering said nothing to his wife about the prognosis—cancer was still an illness that was not spoken of—but he stayed by her side as much as possible and saw to it that she was happy and surrounded by family to the end. For the grieving inventor, cancer changed from an academic puzzle to a deeply personal cause. Ironically, just as he took a more active interest in the new experimental treatments, the disease struck the family again. In October 1948, Kettering called Rhoads and told him a second sister, Daisy, had been diagnosed with a malignancy. He asked whether Rhoads would accompany him to Mansfield, Ohio, to review her case with the local physician. Once again, Kettering was told the prognosis was not good. "It was a sad occasion," Rhoads wrote of his visit to Kettering's hometown in Loudonville and the subdued supper in the old farmhouse that wet autumn night.

From then on, Kettering became Rhoads's close friend and confidant. The two talked constantly, and Kettering used his considerable influence to expand the institute's collaboration with hundreds of industrial laboratories. He would regularly fly from his home in Dayton to Birmingham, Alabama, to confer with Dr. Howard Skipper, who had worked at the CWS, and was now head of the biochemistry division of a new independent, nonprofit scientific research organization called the Southern Research Institute. Rhoads had been so impressed with his work he had tried to hire him after the war, but Skipper, who was from an old Florida family, did not like New York. So Rhoads arranged for his GM patrons to help underwrite the new lab, and Kettering would become one of Skipper's biggest supporters.

Wherever he went, Kettering rhapsodized about the importance of scientific research, giving by his own estimate four thousand talks—or, more likely, the same talk, four thousand times—on the subject, repeating his favorite mantra: "There is no place to go but forward." Already a celebrity from his days as host of NBC's *Symphony of the Air*—when Kettering, with his familiar twangy voice, would deliver short patriotic talks on the triumphs of American knowhow—he was always a big draw at cancer-society benefits. His wartime broadcasts, sponsored by GM, completed his metamorphosis from inventor to popular sage and homespun philosopher of the new technological age. "All research is 99.9 percent failure," he would tell the crowds that thronged to see him, adding that the only time he didn't expect an experiment to fail was the last time he tried it: "The price of progress is trouble, and I don't think the price is too high."

CANCER CHEMOTHERAPY RAN INTO A LOAD of trouble that same year when Dr. Sidney Farber, a pediatric pathologist at Boston Children's Hospital, decided to try using folic acid, a B vitamin found in fruits and vegetables, as a treatment for leukemia. Farber had read that the missionary physician Lucy Wills had used Marmite—a dark, yeasty English spread rich in folic acid—to treat anemia and leucopenia in impoverished, pregnant textile workers in India in the 1930s. Aware that folic acid was the essential building block of DNA, and crucial for cell division, and observing the similarities between megaloblastic anemia and acute lymphoblastic leukemia, Farber wondered whether it would also be useful in the treatment of children with advanced cancer. At the same time, researchers at Lederle Laboratories had reported that the chemical teropterin, an extract of brewer's yeast, had stimulated antitumor activity in mice. What they did not recognize at the time, however, was that it was not a folic acid but its *antagonist*, a slight variation that acted against or inhibited folic acid's absorption into the cell. Mistakenly believing they had isolated an anticancer agent, Lederle Labs synthesized the compounds and, in the summer of 1946, Farber arranged for a clinical study of ninety late-stage cancer patients.

"Devastation rather than triumph ensued," noted the medical historian Dr. Morton Meyers. The treatment had the exact reverse of the effect intended. Instead of halting the progression of leukemia, the folic acid actually *accelerated* it. All the patients died. The postmortem findings confirmed that eleven children in the study were riddled with cancerous white blood cells. Farber managed to salvage something from his terrible mistake with the insight that the reverse phenomena—depriving cells of folic acid—might suppress the growth of malignant cells. He went back to Dr. Yellapragada Subbarao, the brilliant Indian biochemist at Lederle Labs, and they began all over again, this time experimenting with folic acid antagonists, or antimetabolites, to block the folate pathway and slow or arrest the spread of cancer in the body.

Farber's shocking error outraged his fellow pediatricians at Boston Children's, but Rhoads was more sanguine than many of his peers. It was an unfortunate example of what patients had to endure as doctors struggled to find effective chemotherapeutic agents. If they did no harm, then they did not lay a glove on the cancer, either. In order to move the goal from palliation to cure, they had to experiment.

Sensitive to the need to reassure the public, Rhoads emphatically maintained the separation between Memorial Hospital and the Sloan Kettering laboratory. In truth, however, the two were not mutually exclusive. Desperately ill patients—and their parents—were usually more than willing to try a new experimental therapy even after being advised of the risks. In each case, physicians had to make a grim decision: Should they, in terminal cases when everything else had been tried, use a drug still in development that was so powerful it could hasten the patient's death? Rhoads preferred to look at the problem through the lens of a research scientist. Acute lymphoblastic leukemia (ALL) was the most voracious and common childhood cancer, typically striking two-to-five-year-olds and invariably killing them within a span of a few weeks or months. This led many doctors to view these cases as lost causes, not worth the daily needle jabs and added distress. To Rhoads, it meant the patients had nothing left to lose and everything to gain from the experimental therapy. He argued that it took great courage and compassion on the part of chemotherapists to take up the challenge of treating terminal cases, rather than resigning themselves to the idea that their efforts were futile and merely prolonging the agony.

Rhoads had closely followed the case of one of the first, and certainly the most famous, subjects of an ill-fated chemotherapy trial. In the summer of 1946, George Herman "Babe" Ruth, the legendary baseball player, was suffering from a persistent sharp pain in his left eye, his voice had become hoarse, and he had difficulty swallowing. By that fall, he could hardly speak. At French Hospital in New York, doctors first diagnosed sinusitis, then decided it was a dental problem and pulled three teeth. By December, his puzzled doctors prescribed a course of radiation for his swollen lymph glands, but his symptoms worsened. The surgeons who opened up his neck found the cancer, a rare nasopharyngeal carcinoma that had ravaged the air passages in the back of his nose and mouth. Because complete removal of the growths was impossible, Ruth was doomed. In the spring of 1947, Dr. Richard

Lewisohn, a surgeon at Mount Sinai Hospital who had been research-ing teropterin's effects on mice, offered Ruth the experimental therapy as a last chance for a reprieve. The once-powerful six-footer had been battling the disease for months, had lost eighty pounds, and was barely hanging on. He welcomed anything that might alleviate his pain and offer him a few more months of grace.

After being advised that the drug probably would not help, and could even make his condition worse, Ruth agreed to the six-week course of treatment. Even if it did not help him, he said, it would pro-vide information that could help others suffering from the same ail-ment. Over the strenuous objections of some of Lewisohn's team, who argued it was much too soon to start using it on people, Ruth began receiving the daily injections of teropterin on June 29. This was before consent forms were required for volunteers in medical research, and Ruth never signed one. Doctors often refrained from telling cancer patients their true diagnosis, and Ruth reportedly never knew much more about his condition than the description of "pulmonary compli-cations" printed in the newspapers. In his autobiography, he wrote that he "asked no questions" about his disease or the unproven drug.

At first, the fifty-two-year-old Ruth had a remarkable clinical response. His symptoms abated and the enlarged lymph nodes shriv-eled to nothing. He could eat solid food again and was gaining back some of the weight he had lost. His improvement was so marked that Lewisohn presented Ruth's case, without using his name, at an inter-national medical conference in St. Louis that September. But rumors quickly spread that the baseball hero's health had rebounded thanks to the novel therapy, creating a furor among the attending physicians. Citing the medical success story of a "famous national figure," the *Wall Street Journal* reported that doctors were converging on "a cure for can-cer." Teropterin was "hot news," reported the *New York Times*. In fact, it was too hot for Lederle Laboratories. In a series of advertisements and letters to a hundred twenty-five thousand physicians, the lab sought to clarify that teropterin was a treatment and not a cure for cancer.

On June 13, 1948, the Babe felt strong enough to don his old pin-stripes, bearing the legendary number 3, and take a star turn at the opening ceremonies of the twenty-fifth anniversary of Yankee Stadium, telling misty-eyed fans how glad he was to be back. A few days later, however, he was admitted to Memorial Hospital. Unfortunately, Ruth's cancer had recurred. Despite receiving additional radiation therapy, he died of pneumonia and metastatic cancer two months later.

Rhoads saw to it that Memorial Hospital's official press release made it clear that their VIP patient received "no special drug or chemical in the attempt to control his tumor" while he was under their care. Teropterin, according to the statement, was never administered to Ruth because the drug "had been previously investigated at Memorial Hospital and found to be of no value in the treatment of cancer." They could not vouch for Lewisohn's results. Rhoads later characterized the teropterin experiment as a "bold" play for what looked like victory, only it was "in the wrong direction." The clinical stumble had "complicated the struggle," he told *Newsweek*, but he added that it had proved to be enormously important because it directed their attention to related chemicals known as amines, derivatives of ammonia. "In spite of past failures, mistakes, and confusion," he assured the *Newsweek* reporter, "progress in cancer therapy is being made." Babe Ruth's contribution to cancer research extended beyond his own case. It was carried on by his charitable foundation, run by his daughter Dorothy, which funded many of Sloan Kettering's subsequent studies on the new chemotherapeutic agents.

Doctors struck out with teropterin, but within months Lederle Laboratories had synthesized a new antifolate called aminopterin. In June 1948, Farber published the results of a second clinical trial of sixteen children with acute leukemia that showed that a folic acid antagonist, or antimetabolite, did stall the disease's deadly course. Ten children experienced unprecedented remissions. Another five children in the group responded, and their young lives were extended four to six months. Although the cancer returned, the repeated remissions were a home run for Farber and a historic milestone in chemotherapy. It was proof that a simple chemical compound could be effective against acute leukemia.

In 1949, a second anticancer drug, amethopterin (methotrexate), a safer antifolate, was introduced, and it is still in use today. Methotrexate remains a standard component of the treatment of acute lymphoblastic leukemia as well as a key agent, in combination with other drugs, for many other cancers. These laboratory triumphs raised hopes that research scientists had at last found a way to beat the dread disease.

News of Sidney Farber's repeated remissions with leukemic patients reverberated in laboratories across the country and changed the field of chemotherapy almost overnight. Rhoads immediately dispatched Joe Burchenal to Boston to see the results with his own eyes, not convinced the forty-five-year-old Boston pathologist could have made such a major breakthrough on his own. The children under Farber's care had responded positively. Not only did their white blood cell counts fall, but their enlarged spleens and livers shrank and their bone marrow returned to normal for a few months. As soon as Burchenal confirmed that the remissions were genuine, Rhoads obtained some of the drug, as yet unlicensed, for trials on cancer patients. Initially, the Memorial team thought the drug might be ineffective. The first nine children they treated showed no response. But just when the doctors were about to give up, they got a result—the tenth child went into remission. Even though they only obtained a single positive response, it encouraged Rhoads and his research staff to look at other antimetabolites.

Rhoads sent Sloan Kettering's scientists back to their labs to search for more folic acid analogs that were selectively injurious to cancer cells, looking for the next lucky hit. He had long been interested in the "anti-metabolic effect"—the way certain substances interfered with the metabolism of microbes was analogous to the way sulfa drugs attacked bacteria. While the derivatives of folic acid and nitrogen mustard had little similarity in chemical configuration, the two classes of compounds acted the same way to kill cancer cells—by inhibiting the formation and use of nucleic acid. Recent studies also indicated that cancer cells contained more nucleic acid than normal ones. In addition, the agents that caused cancer were those that induced changes in normal cells because they affected the chromosomes, which are made up in large part by nucleic acids. If they could find an agent that had this "differential effect" on lawless cancer cells, selectively inhibiting the formation or action of nucleic acid in malignant cells while leaving normal cells unharmed, they might be able to discover the disease's Achilles heel.

Cell chemistry was maddeningly complicated, and Rhoads knew just the man to help. He contacted Howard Skipper. Like Alexander, Skipper's interest in cancer research had begun with his study of the captured German nitrogen mustards at Edgewood. And like Alexander, he became convinced that they had the potential to heal. He readily agreed to continue the lines of investigation they had started and to integrate his lab with Sloan Kettering and help discover new substances that could be used to attack cancer cells. Their wartime connection was a great boon to cancer research: Skipper devised quantitative animal models to evaluate the effects of chemotherapy on cells, and he worked closely with Rhoads to help choose the most auspicious compounds and the most promising areas of exploration.

In June 1949, *Time* magazine put Rhoads on the cover, hailing the country's leading "Cancer Fighter" next to an image of his mythic coat-of-arms—the symbolic crab, its carapace in the shape of a death's-head, pierced by the radiant Sword of Hope with the twin-serpent caduceus wrapped around its hilt. The iconic sword represented the crusading spirit of Rhoads's quest to eradicate the scourge on mankind. His most consistent message was his optimism that cancer could be conquered.

In the pages of the magazine, however, Rhoads's tone was more muted than triumphant. There was no magic bullet. In the endless war on cancer, scientists had scored only partial victories, no permanent cures. They had discovered nothing that could vanquish the disease, only a handful of imperfect chemical weapons they could deploy to keep a variety of human malignancies at bay. Relapse was inescapable. "We can help only 25 percent," Rhoads said solemnly, standing in the immaculate corridor outside Room 102L, where all of the pale-faced children in the neat rows of beds had leukemia. "And they have remissions only. Their disease will recur and recur, perhaps in more violent form."

He paused, his confident blue eyes momentarily clouding over. This was not a battle for the faint of heart. On a day-to-day basis, Sloan Kettering was a difficult, often depressing, place to work. Rhoads was "no callous technician," noted the magazine, in a veiled reference to the Puerto Rico episode. He was not impervious to the occupants of the building, the ever-present patients who at that very moment lay in wards fighting for their lives, their last days frayed by pain and dimmed with morphine. "Some people ask, 'Why keep them alive, if they must die eventually?'" he asked rhetorically, then hastened to answer his own question, conveying a sense of urgency. "Because we're moving faster now. Perhaps, before they exhaust their last remission, we'll have something really good." It was always a race against time. If progress continued at the ever-accelerating rate of the previous six years, he was sure that in the not-too-distant future leukemia would cease to be a death sentence for children. It was the best Rhoads could offer—a pledge to tomorrow.

DUSTY RHOADS'S DECISION TO JOIN FORCES with a remarkable pair of researchers, George Hitchings and Gertrude Elion of the pharmaceutical firm Burroughs Wellcome, would turn out to be a major turning point. In 1950, Hitchings, a balding, brilliant physician-turned-chemist, was at the forefront of research into the nucleic acids of malignant cells. Dissatisfied with the inefficient hit-or-miss attempts at drug discovery, he was looking for a more "rational" method of drug design. He decided to narrow the search to compounds closely related to teropterin known as purines—specifically, the purine bases adenine and guanine, which are building blocks of DNA.* After studying the role of purines in nucleic acid metabolism, Hitchings observed that bacterial cells require certain purines to make DNA. He hypothesized that by interfering with the natural production of DNA, it would be possible to interrupt cell growth. Hitchings assigned the purine compounds to Gertrude Elion, a thirty-year-old research chemist he had hired, for fifty dollars a week, to investigate how they worked. She soon created a purine chemical, the synthesized artificial compound 2,6-Diaminopurine, which blocked the metabolism of folic acid and adenine and had a pronounced effect on cancer.

Sure enough, in Burchenal's tests at Sloan Kettering, "2,6" prolonged the life of leukemic mice by 60 percent. It controlled or destroyed rat tumors. At first, the experimental results raised their hopes. He managed to achieve two good clinical remissions in adults with leukemia, but the patients relapsed and died. Once again, the terrible toxicity of the drug caused severe nausea and vomiting, making it unusable in humans. Elion and Hitchings went back to the drawing board and modified the compound to reduce the side effects. Within three years, they developed two new chemotherapeutic drugs—diaminopurine and thioguanine—that could interfere with the formation of cancer cells and put leukemia patients into remission. Thioguanine would become a beneficial treatment for acute myelocytic leukemia (AML) in adults.

* The double-helix structure of DNA, which revealed how DNA could be "unzipped" to be read or copied, would not be discovered by James Watson and Francis Crick until 1953.

While the new drugs were effective in treating cancer, however, they were still hard to tolerate.

Elion was determined to find a better drug. She continued searching for a less toxic compound, testing more than a hundred purines before finally discovering 6-Mercaptopurine (6-MP), which she created by minutely altering one of the compounds by replacing an oxygen atom on the purine ring with a sulfur atom. Testing on experimental animals showed 6-MP not only inhibited growth of tumors in mice but also caused a significant percentage to regress permanently. Treated mice also had survival times twice as long as those left untreated. At Sloan Kettering, Fred Philips tested it in dogs, which react to drugs much the same way humans do, and he determined the maximum dose, mode of delivery, and toxicities. 6-MP looked like a winner, and Burchenal rapidly proceeded to clinical trial.

Hitchings and Elion stayed in close contact with Rhoads and Burchenal and looked forward to having another advanced therapeutic option soon. The experience was "an emotional rollercoaster" for researchers, doctors, and patients alike, Elion recalled. "We would learn about patients who would have a remission, and then ultimately they would relapse and die. At that time, we thought we were very close to having the answer for the treatment of leukemia."

WITHIN A YEAR, BURCHENAL BEGAN a clinical trial of 6-MP and was obtaining remissions. The results, published in 1953, showed that the drug secured good remissions in fifteen of forty-five children with acute lymphoblastic leukemia. Another ten patients showed partial remissions and good clinical improvement. Importantly, it was also shown that 6-MP was effective in children whose disease failed to respond to the folic acid antagonists. 6-MP was the first lead doctors had with respect to the way additional chemical compounds could be used to solve the problem of drug resistance. It was the biggest success they had achieved with a new drug since Sidney Farber's trial of methotrexate. Although most of the patients eventually relapsed, Burchenal and his colleagues were learning how to extend lives—first month by month, then year by year. A more extensive study of 269 patients confirmed that 6-MP produced remissions in both adults and children with acute leukemia.

As the results from the study rolled in, Rhoads was so encouraged he persuaded Kettering to underwrite the Hitchings research program at Burroughs Wellcome. The donation came just in time: The pharmaceutical firm had decided to scale back the biochemistry department and had already issued pink slips to some of the laboratory staff. "We were rescued in the eleventh hour," said Hitchings of his saviors. Rhoads, unable to contain his excitement, talked up the great discovery of 6-MP to reporters. Walter Winchell, the famous newspaper columnist and radio commentator, announced the new treatment for leukemia on his influential Sunday night broadcast. When news of the clinical success broke, Hitchings was inundated with more than six hundred phone calls from doctors and patients.

The FDA broke a speed record by rushing through its approval of 6-MP before the end of 1953, only months after the results of the clinical trial were made available. "Supplies of 6-MP were extremely limited," recalled Dr. John Laszlo, the longtime national vice president of research for the American Cancer Society. "The company went full steam ahead to increase the synthesis of the drug, even though it had no idea of what the manufacturing cost would be, how it would distribute the drugs, or how it would respond to the many pathetic appeals it was receiving from dying patients." Hitchings, Elion, and their colleagues spent the Christmas holidays making as much of the drug as they could to meet the demand.

The following year, Burchenal gave Debbie Brown, a nine-year-old leukemia patient, two of the new anticancer drugs, 6-MP and methotrexate, and a slim chance at beating the odds against her. When first diagnosed, she was too sick to attend the third grade and had to be homeschooled. She was so weak she could scarcely crawl up the stairs to her family's second-floor apartment, and she bruised at the slightest contact. In the beginning, she went to see Burchenal three times a week for treatment. He never mentioned the word *cure*, but she slowly improved over time, and her visits to Sloan Kettering became less and less frequent. Debbie Brown would go on to become one of the first long-term survivors of acute lymphoblastic leukemia: She graduated from high school, married and had a child, and became a teacher in New Jersey.

Very quickly, 6-MP and methotrexate became the mainstays of the treatment of childhood leukemia. "Chemotherapy of cancer," Burchenal wrote, "was shown to be a not-impossible dream." These developments again raised expectations that cancer researchers were on the verge of a cure. And once again, the press was full of euphoric predictions of "wonder-drug remedies." A 1953 article in *Look* magazine offered the exalted prophecy that the disease would soon be conquered. *Newsweek* anticipated a vaccine against cancer.

Vigorously lobbying for increased federal funding for cancer research, and aware he needed the public on his side, Rhoads fueled the media speculation with his authoritative pronouncements. "I am convinced that in the next decade or maybe more, we will have chemicals as effective against cancer as the sulfa drugs are today against bacterial infections," he told the House Commerce Committee, which was holding hearings to appraise whether chemotherapy was scientifically promising enough to warrant government support. Rhoads and Farber were pushing for the National Cancer Institute (NCI) to take over the burden of drug testing from Sloan Kettering and to expand drug development to handle the mass screening of tens of thousands of new natural and synthetic compounds. More than ten thousand pure chemicals had been investigated, along with seven thousand crude extracts, "including everything from grape and apple pairings to mushrooms," Rhoads told the committee, insisting that they had barely begun to scratch the surface of nature's bounty.

Rhoads cited the case of Senator Robert Taft Sr., the late Republican majority leader whose cancer was diagnosed too late, as an example of what they were "fighting for." Taft, whose first symptom had been a pain in his left hip that he experienced during a round of golf with Eisenhower, had undergone a battery of tests at Walter Reed Hospital in late May of 1953, but they had failed to turn up anything. Feeling fatigued and limping badly, he traveled to a hospital in his hometown of Cincinnati, Ohio, where physicians found the tumors. Determined to hide his illness—a common impulse at a time when cancer victims still risked pariah status—he continued to work at his senatorial duties, rejecting advice to get treatment at Memorial. By the time he underwent exploratory surgery at New York Hospital on July 8, it was impossible for Rhoads and his other doctors to determine the origin of the tumors, because the abdominal cavity was "full of cancer." They closed him up, knowing the ferocious, fast-moving disease had spread beyond the scope of the knife, and any therapy would be at best palliative. Taft died of a brain hemorrhage several weeks later, at age sixty-three. A postmortem later revealed the cancer probably had originated in the pancreas.

As a measure of his belief in the new drugs, Rhoads suggested that such untimely deaths should be preventable, and he made a rash claim he would never quite live down: "Inevitably, as I see it," he declared, "we can look forward to something like penicillin for cancer." He later qualified the statement, explaining that they were not just looking for a single miracle drug, but rather "a variety of new drugs of similar effectiveness" that could wipe out the plague once and for all. But it was too late to pull it back, and his boast made headlines. TAFT'S DOCTOR SEES CANCER CURE NEAR, proclaimed the *Washington Post*.

Rhoads's rosy prognosis immediately drew fire from some of his colleagues, who argued that talk of a "penicillin for cancer" was premature. Some privately denounced him for raising unrealistic expectations in public. The following day, Dr. John C. Bugher, director of the division of biology and medicine of the United States Atomic Energy Commission, acknowledged the substantial strides that had been made in recent years, but he added tersely, "Most of the road lies ahead." A committee of the National Cancer Society assigned to assess the validity of the screening methods took the same view, deciding that the state of knowledge on chemotherapeutic drugs was too inconclusive to justify the design of a national "crash" program.

A noisy debate then ensued over the proper direction of cancer research. Academic investigators vigorously opposed the idea of a centralized national program, arguing it would have an adverse effect on the scientific community. They felt that an atmosphere of independence was required to foster advances. What they really wanted was to see money earmarked for research grants. In December, a compromise was reached, agreeing that there would be a program of voluntary cooperation among institutions engaged in cancer research. Agitating behind the scenes, Sidney Farber managed to enlist the support of the influential philanthropist and health activist Mary Lasker, who with her husband, Albert, had raised millions of dollars for the American Cancer Society, and he impressed her with his data on childhood leukemia. Lasker, whom the press dubbed "the fairy godmother of medical research," had first met Rhoads in 1944 and been struck by his "smoldering determination to conquer cancer," and what he and his "key Army associates" had accomplished at the Chemical Warfare Service and then at Memorial. At Lasker's urging, the Senate Appropriations Committee, frustrated by the intramural bickering and lack of progress, provided $5 million to the NCI, with a mandate to establish the new screening system.

Rhoads and Farber got their way. In 1955, the NCI set up the Cancer Chemotherapy National Service Center to investigate all manner of compounds with potential anticancer activity submitted by companies, institutions, and research scientists. The chemotherapy program quickly ballooned, and soon it was screening thirty thousand samples a year, ten times the output at Sloan Kettering. It changed the face of cancer research forever and ultimately spawned the multibillion-dollar cancer pharmaceutical industry. No sooner than it was established, the huge, costly, inefficient screening enterprise gave rise to a backlash against the focus on drug discovery and chemotherapy itself, with its narrow therapeutic window and meager results. As the distinguished British cancer researcher Isaac Berenblum complained to a Rockefeller Institute colleague in 1955, "Rhoads is making an all-out drive for a cure, and that is not the right way."

Opponents of chemotherapy pointed to Rhoads's dogged pursuit of a newly discovered substance called properdin as a case in point. It had long been observed that some animals were more resistant to cancer than others, indicating they might have some kind of immunity against the disease. In human patients, cases of "spontaneous regression" had been documented in which a cancer retreated for no apparent reason. Sloan Kettering scientists believed the explanation might be properdin, a natural defense chemical in the blood, so they decided to test the theory by injecting cancer cells into the skin of the forearm of fourteen healthy volunteers from the Ohio State Penitentiary. In all fourteen cases, a large patch of inflammation appeared, showing the body was rejecting the cancer cells. Later, the cancer cells were surgically removed and the cancer did not reappear in a single prisoner. When they tried the same experiment on fifteen cancer victims, in thirteen cases the cancer continued to grow and flourish until it was removed some weeks later. In four cases, the cancer recurred. The Sloan Kettering scientists found that the level of properdin in the blood varied directly with the ability of the individual to fight off the invading cancer. Overeager for a result, Rhoads announced that the tests showed "there clearly does exist in well persons a defense mechanism against the growth of cancer cells."

The study suggested there might be a way to build up the body's natural resistance by vaccination. Further studies were ordered. "A dramatic breakthrough seemed imminent," *Reader's Digest* later reported. "Hopelessly ill children were injected with the new substance. It was useless. Two years and tens of thousands of dollars had gone into one more crushing defeat. Dr. Rhoads must have been bitterly disappointed, but he never faltered. He simply kept testing—substance after substance." Immunotherapy—turning the body's natural defenses against cancer—was ahead of its time. Much work still needed to be done to understand natural immunity, and properdin would be revived as a treatment in years to come.

Chemotherapy had racked up a long list of controversies, and an increasingly vocal group of critics began to question whether the entire strategy for the control of cancer was wrong. "Skepticism surrounded the clinical usefulness of chemotherapy for cancer in the 1950s," noted Drs. Vincent DeVita Jr. and Edward Chu in their history of the experimental treatment. "A great deal of resources were being invested in a controversial effort to develop drugs, yet there was no evidence that drugs could cure or, for that matter, even help cancer patients in any stage despite some impressive antitumor responses."

The old defeatism and fatalism about cancer had returned, only this time it was an "aggressive skepticism," recalled DeVita, then a young doctor at the NCI. "They had seen chemotherapy and they *knew* it was going to fail." The esteemed hematologist William Dameshek of the New England Medical Center was the leader of the disaffected. He had tried prescribing huge doses of nitrogen mustards, and when the patients all died at his hands, it was too much for him to bear. Not only was he finished using chemotherapy, he became its most ardent foe. At the spring meeting of the American Society for Clinical Investigation, which was held annually in Atlantic City, he set up an informal group called the "Blood Club" with a number of like-minded physicians. The group would invite chemotherapists to come speak about their work, but it was just an excuse to excoriate them in front of their peers. "I had never seen anything like it before," said DeVita. "They would rip them to pieces for daring to try to cure leukemia."

Even within Memorial, a similar schism had developed. A "cabal" of senior surgeons, long the dominant faction in the hospital, was protesting the trends in modern cancer treatment and demanding their abolition. Cancer chemotherapy was cutting into their margins, according to Rhoads, and the surgeons were calling for what he caustically described as a "return to the good old days and sterling virtues" that brought distinction to the institution and filled their lucrative private practices. The simmering resentments and interdepartmental strife finally led to Rhoads being replaced as head of the hospital in 1953 and being given the honorific title of Scientific Director. He remained head of SKI, but thereafter Memorial was a house divided. Rhoads's enemies rejoiced. As *Time* later observed, a "willful band of little men in the New York County Medical Society" had been waiting for an excuse to oust Rhoads. "Jealous, they threatened him (always unofficially) with expulsion," and when that did not succeed, "harassed him for a decade."

Stung by the betrayal, Rhoads was deeply hurt and angry. He began talking of moving on. All the battles had begun to wear him down. "The history of medical advance is one of a struggle between those who gain by preserving the status quo and those who derive equal satisfaction by contributing to scientific progress, even at some financial loss," he wrote in a scathing memorandum to Memorial's President Laurance S. Rockefeller in July 1954. "For years we have struggled at Memorial to achieve by unified guidance, mutual understanding and tolerance between those two different points of view. The advances in medical science have been steadily brought into the Memorial organization in order to maintain progress and leadership. Until recently, the presence of new things and new people has been tolerated, if not welcomed."

Even though he had alienated the old guard with his relentless grandstanding, Rhoads had almost singlehandedly raised millions of dollars for Sloan Kettering's coffers. "So much of the support which SKI has received has been a direct result of his personal efforts and the success of the program which he has directed that it is an illusion to suppose that this money has been raised by any other person, things or agency," Warren Weaver, a trustee and member of SKI's Executive Committee, privately advised Rockefeller in December 1957, warning him to "consider most carefully any move that is likely to disturb him further."

But as before, Rhoads played a part in his own downfall. Once again, his arrogance and entrenched opinions got the better of him. His refusal to acknowledge the very real problem of drug resistance and toxicity, and to be more open-minded about the evolving possibilities in cancer treatment rather than concentrating all of his resources on the endless empirical search for new chemical entities, earned him the antipathy of those disappointed with chemotherapy's cure rates. Cancer researchers desperate for funds for innovative approaches and ideas, and cancer patients desperate for alternatives, decried his blinkered vision.

Rhoads remained adamant that he had drawn up the right lines of attack, and that drug development would pay dividends for both doctors and patients. Chemotherapists already had at least twenty agents that prolonged life in cancer victims, and the prospects of adding to the list were bright. His philosophy was that the new agents were not only ends in themselves but also served as tools for unlocking and probing nature's mysteries—the true nature of cancer itself and the code governing its development that had eluded scientists for centuries. "The essential fact is that we seem to be coming closer to the great secret," he preached. "The mass attack mounted by science, and backed by the public's dollars, is beginning to have its effect."

Meanwhile, Rhoads continued to hold the spotlight as "Mr. Cancer Research." Inspired by his example, dozens of institutions around the world plunged into the war on cancer, which has become the most concentrated medical effort in history. A tireless evangelist for the cause, he told *Collier's,* "It is no longer a question of *if* cancer will be controlled, but *when* and *how.*"

WHAT CHEMOTHERAPISTS NEEDED was proof of an actual cure, and that proof was shortly forthcoming. In 1956, Dr. Min Chui Li, a Sloan Kettering doctor who had recently moved to NCI, used methotrexate as an emergency treatment for a twenty-four-year-old woman with terminal choriocarcinoma, a rare tumor of the placenta that occurs during pregnancy, and achieved the first example of a drug-induced cure for cancer. The woman's cancer had metastasized to her lungs, and a lesion had ruptured, flooding the chest cavity with blood and air and leaving her near death. The doctors managed to stabilize her, and Li, who had observed that methotrexate inhibited the chorionic cells in mice while at Sloan Kettering, decided to try a large dose of methotrexate. To his surprise, the patient survived the night. The following day, he gave her another very large dose, and she steadily improved over the next several days. He then designed a regimen of high doses, and, after four months, the tumor masses completely disappeared. The woman went home from the hospital fully recovered from her disease. "As a sign of the times," wrote DeVita and Chu, even after an additional two women went into remission, "no one was prepared to believe the results were significant."

Already an outsider, Li, a political refugee from China, was regarded within NCI as something of a renegade. Now he had crossed the line and was trying a controversial approach to cancer treatment. He was employing the antifolate drug over an unusually protracted period— long after there were any signs of tumor and despite his patients' suffering from serious complications brought on by the excessive toxicity. To some of his colleagues, it appeared Li was poisoning his patients with dose after dose of the powerful drugs. Li was advised that if he continued his radical treatment, he would lose his position.

However, Li had observed that the women's tumor marker hormone, or "hcg level," was elevated, and he hypothesized that there was a correlation between the degree of elevation and the extent of malignancy. He carried on treating his patients with intermittent doses of methotrexate, convinced that microscopic collections of cancer cells, or micrometastases, shed from the original tumor lingered in the blood. He believed the patients required intensive systemic therapy until the hormone levels went down to zero and all the cancer cells were fully eradicated, even though there was no longer any clinical evidence of the disease. Li achieved the first cure of a solid tumor in a human being using chemotherapy alone. "It was a fantastic breakthrough," recalled his NCI colleague Dr. Emil J. Freireich. "That all went on right under my eyes. We talked to him every day, saw those ladies in the clinic." They were hopeful that when the usual five-year waiting period elapsed, the "cured" women would still show no evidence of the disease.

The Institutional Board at NCI did not see it that way. They felt Li had gone rogue, and his perseverance was rewarded with dismissal. "Li was accused of experimenting on people," said Freireich, a trailblazing cancer researcher in his own right, who maintained that all chemotherapists were essentially experimenting during that time. "To not experiment would mean to follow the old rules—to do absolutely nothing. So Li was fired for acting on his convictions, for doing something."

Li returned to Sloan Kettering, was later proved right, and would develop a similar cure for testicular cancer. But chemotherapy had a long way to go before it won acceptance at most medical centers. In the 1950s and 1960s, those tasked with administering the highly toxic agents continued to be regarded with scorn. Many doctors and nurses felt it was unethical to treat cancer patients—especially children—with the primitive, blunt-edged drugs. The term in general use by hospital staff for the new anticancer agents was still *poison*. Dr. DeVita, the former director of the NCI, recalled that, even in his own Clinical Center, the well-known hematologist Dr. George Brecher, who reviewed all the cancer patients' bone-marrow slides, routinely referred to the Leukemia Service as the "butcher shop" on rounds, "even while, quite literally, seeing the evidence of recovery magnified before his eyes."

Novice chemotherapists were the "Young Turks" of academic medicine, their methods questioned and assailed at every turn. "No one can ever cure a cancer. . . ," muttered Freireich, repeating the tired refrain that was thrown in his face every time he and his fellow clinicians proposed a new method of treatment. "So that's what we did. We made the leap from choriocarcinoma to curing childhood leukemia." Everybody was convinced that if surgery and radiation failed to control the local disease—that once it was systemic—it was hopeless. But Freireich and his NCI colleagues were the first people in the world who had seen that a systemic cancer could be cured with a chemical. They knew it could be done, and they were anxious to prove that it could be done again in the case of acute lymphoblastic leukemia in children.

Howard Skipper, the soft-spoken Southern "mouse doctor," as he called himself, made it possible by working out the kinetics of leukemia. His research showed that it was necessary to kill every last leukemia cell, because back extrapolations after treatment revealed that just one surviving cell was sufficient to kill a mouse. He came up with the "cell kill" paradigm, which stated that a given dose of a drug killed a constant fraction of tumor cells, not a constant number, therefore success would depend on the number of cells present at the beginning of each treatment. He suggested that the amount of residual cells could be measured, because even though it was impossible to count all the cells, an estimate could be made based on the time it took for the cancer to come back.

Skipper also found that by using drugs sequentially, he could increase the cell-kill ratio. Delivering drugs in combination could have a "synergistic" effect that could overcome the problem of resistance. When he found drugs that worked, he tried to determine the most effective schedule so that all of the agents attacked tumors, but each had different side effects, which reduced system toxicity. This meant that the drug's therapeutic effects were potentiated and the side effects were diffused. Until then, doctors had delivered a single drug on a daily or weekly basis to the point of toxicity, and then they waited for the patient to recover from the side effects before resuming the medication. Skipper's work changed the existing approach to dosing in favor of longer, more aggressive chemotherapy. The goal was to not just delay the disease's return but to permanently prevent its recurrence.

Following this new line of approach at Sloan Kettering, Burchenal began experimenting with the increasing number of drugs being shown to have activity against leukemia. Exploring the role of steroids in mice, he discovered that sometimes resistance to methotrexate could be overcome after a course of steroids. This generated a new group of steroid alkylating agents, which are still being used against several types of cancer. In another set of experiments, he found that a single large dose of cortisone could temporarily reduce the high leukocyte count in advanced cancers. When he tried using three anticancer agents—folic acid antagonist (methotrexate or aminopterin), cortisone, and 6-MP—in a sequential treatment program, the three-drug combo had a knockout effect. Sequential or combination therapy became the standard model of cancer chemotherapy, often as an adjunct to either or both surgery and radiation.

Clinicians realized that the mistake they had made was thinking that a single drug was the way to treat cancer, when it turned out that a combination of drugs was far more effective. Ironically, the idea of pumping patients full of multiple drugs was anathema to most doctors, regarded as sloppy and unsound practice. As usual, chemotherapists had to buck convention. At NCI, which offered free treatment to patients willing to participate in experimental cancer research programs, Freireich and his similarly named colleague, Dr. Emil "Tom" Frei III, saw what Burchenal was doing at Sloan Kettering and decided to try their own combination chemotherapy on children with leukemia who had relapsed following the best available treatment. Taking advantage of the newly discovered drug vincristine, they designed a four-drug chemo regimen known as VAMP (vincristine, amethopterin, 6-MP, and prednisone). Vincristine, a vinca alloid extracted from the Vinca rosea, or periwinkle, had been tested by the Eli Lilly Company and shown to have anticancer properties, as well as a peculiar toxicity that did not affect normal blood cells in the same way as other drugs in use. Freireich and Frei reasoned that because each of the drugs had a different method of killing cancer cells, and none overlapped, maximum doses could be administered without upping the toxicity.

When they first proposed running a trial of the VAMP protocol on children with leukemia, it was greeted with laughter, then outrage. A "verbal bloodbath" was the way one doctor described the reaction in the large solarium where NCI chemotherapists would present their latest work to their peers. The pair was already in trouble for giving their young patients platelet and white blood cell transfusions to reduce the bleeding caused by leukemia, a procedure so difficult and risky no one else even attempted it. VAMP horrified everyone. "At first I opposed it," recalled Dr. Gerald Bodey, a specialist in antibiotic therapy in children who worked with them. "Giving these kids four drugs all at once! As a Christian, I thought it was immoral because if they relapsed we would

have no fallback. I thought Freireich was crazy." After a lot of harangu-
ing, they were given permission to go ahead. The initial findings turned
the skeptics into true believers. Children who had been in a deep coma
woke up. Dying children went into remission. The results were spectacular. Bodey was stunned: "We had sixteen patients, and eleven were
cured. It was astonishing."

The VAMP study was a courageous leap forward, but it proved too
far to go at a single bound. After several rewarding months of watching
sick children return to normal and go home, some children suddenly
started relapsing. One after another returned to NCI complaining of
headache and numbness. The leukemia had returned, invading the central nervous system and lodging in the brain. The burden of responsibility borne by the young doctors was tremendous. Bodey was so upset
he sought counsel from his minister about the experiments they were
doing on the children. Of seventeen patients treated with VAMP, three
stayed in long-term remission and lived to old age. In the tumultuous
months that followed, the clinicians scrambled to surmount the defi-
ciencies of the original treatment program. When they modified the
dosage and interval of the treatment to make it more effective, there
was a steady increase in remission rates and duration.

Influenced by their clinical success, DeVita, Dr. Jack Moxley, and
another talented team at NCI cobbled together four chemotherapy
drugs—mechlorethamine (nitrogen mustard), Oncovin (the brand
name of the vinca alloid), methotrexate, and prednisone (MOMP)—and
reported the first cures of advanced Hodgkin's lymphoma. The intensive combination chemotherapy was designed to destroy the leukemia
cells lingering in the bone marrow and circulating in the bloodstream,
while the intervals between courses allowed time for the normal cells
to recover. According to DeVita, the MOMP and then the MOPP protocols (which substituted procarbazine for methotrexate) also met with
"fierce resistance" for being too big a departure from the norm. There

was not enough evidence to try the drugs against Hodgkin's, which started out as a solid tumor in the lymph nodes and then spread to the bloodstream. His superior argued: "It would be too dangerous." DeVita insisted it had to be worth a try. After careful deliberation, they agreed on an unheard-of ten-week duration for the therapy. "The results were startling," he recalled. "Remission rates went from near zero to 80 percent." Not a single patient died. MOPP did not disappoint: Sixty percent of the patients who attained complete remissions in the original study never relapsed, even with long-term follow-up exceeding forty years.

The epochal development revolutionized the treatment of advanced Hodgkin's: By 1965, 80 percent of all patients were going into complete remission and enjoying long-lasting, disease-free survival. With improved drugs and techniques, Hodgkin's lymphoma is now curable in 90 percent of cases.

By the end of the 1960s—the so-called Golden Age of Chemotherapy—it was firmly established that chemicals could eradicate some forms of cancer. The success of MOMP and MOPP represented a huge step forward and set the stage for even more effective combination therapies. The reports of the curability of choriocarcinoma, lymphomas, and acute leukemia with combination chemotherapy inspired Congress, spurred on by Mary Lasker, to pass the National Cancer Act of 1971, and launch another, even more lavishly funded and controversial "War on Cancer." In his State of the Union address that January, President Richard M. Nixon advocated a total commitment to finding a cure in language that harkened back to the inauguration of Sloan Kettering, calling for "the same kind of concentrated effort that split the atom and took man to the moon."

In the fall of 1972, Joe Burchenal, Vincent DeVita, Emil Frei, Emil Freireich, and Min Chui Li, along with a handful of others, received Albert Lasker Clinical Medical Research Awards for the development of curative chemotherapy for cancer. "It was heady validation," DeVita acknowledged. The following year, oncology was established as an official subspecialty of medicine, with chemotherapy as the principal tools of its trade. As part of its mandate, the National Cancer Act was to create new cancer centers to improve access to specialized care and advanced therapies. Regarded as a role model for what the new research hospitals should aim to be, the Memorial Sloan Kettering Institute was designated a national cancer center, and its name was changed once again to Memorial Sloan Kettering Cancer Center.

In the decades that followed, the cycles of hope and disappointment, praise and detraction, would continue to play out as doctors practiced the art of chemotherapy. The great gains in cancer treatment that came out of the wartime research inevitably stalled, and progress was slow. Learning how to optimize the potential of the chemicals was an even slower process. Drug succeeded drug as clinicians struggled to combat different forms of cancer while keeping the side effects at a manageable level. Numerous mustard derivatives were synthesized along the way, producing many new drugs with anticancer activity, including busulfan, thiotepa, myleran, chlorambucil, and melphalan. Using these compounds was like "walking a tightrope between toxic and therapeutic effect," recalled Irving Krakoff, who served for two decades as head of the chemotherapy program at Sloan Kettering. Over time, physicians improved the multidrug regimens, fine-tuned dose intensity and delivery, and introduced staging and prolonged treatment, achieving truly durable remissions. Last but not least, the development of supportive therapies has allowed doctors to safely deliver more intensive drug protocols, prevent the nausea and vomiting, and enable patients to endure the rigors of treatment that in the past would have been prohibitive.

While these chemicals were not panaceas, and all had their limitations, some contained the kernels of fresh insights that led to the creation of new medicines. 6-MP proved especially fruitful. George Hitchings and Gertrude Elion found that 6-MP also interfered with the immune system, and they went on to discover drugs that combated infectious diseases such as malaria, meningitis, and septicemia by targeting bacterial and viral DNA. Elion's discovery of azathioprine made it possible for people with compromised immune systems to receive organ transplants without concern about rejection. The drug Imuran remains in use for kidney transplants today. Antimetabolites were also used to create a treatment for gout, reducing the body's buildup of uric acid, which can cause painful arthritis. Her work on the antiviral activity of purines led to the synthesis of a compound that could interfere with the replication of the herpes virus, and it culminated in her colleagues' development of the AIDS drug azidothymidine (AZT). For their discovery of important principles of drug treatment, Hitchings and Elion were awarded a Nobel Prize in 1988.

In her Nobel speech, Elion proudly noted that in the 1940s, the life expectancy of children with acute lymphoblastic leukemia was only three to four months. "With the addition of 6-MP to the antileukemia armamentarium," she said, "the median survival time increased to 12 months in these children, and a few remained in remission for years with 6-MP and steroids . . . 6-MP remains one of the dozen or more drugs found useful in the treatment of acute leukemia. With the use of combination chemotherapy with three or four drugs to produce and consolidate remission, plus several years of maintenance therapy with 6-MP and methotrexate, almost 80 percent of children with acute leukemia can now be cured." Today, more than 90 percent of children survive the disease.

Over the course of his long career, DeVita has served as director of the NCI's Division of Cancer, physician-in-chief at Memorial Sloan Kettering and then at the Yale Cancer Center, and in each hospital where he worked he says he has watched cancer mortality rates drop, thanks to chemotherapy. The use of "adjuvant" chemotherapy—pairing cancer drugs with surgery and/or radiation—has led to a decline in mortality for common killers such as breast cancer, down 25 percent; colon cancer, down 45 percent; and prostate cancer, down 68 percent. Targeted therapy—drugs aimed at specific genes or proteins found in certain cancer cells—is making inroads against lung cancer and melanoma, tumors previously highly resistant to treatment. More recently, chemotherapy, together with refined surgery, radiotherapy, and immunotherapy, has made progress in patients with advanced melanoma, and very advanced leukemias and lymphomas. "All these things are chemotherapy," explains DeVita. "Chemotherapy was developed as the first systemic therapy for cancer. Anything that goes in the vein is a systemic therapy."

"We *are* winning the war on cancer," he asserts, good-humoredly batting away the habitual negativism that still pervades his profession. He is optimistic we have the ability to cure many more forms of cancer in the near future, and he is not afraid to use the word *cure*, even though it is not fashionable to talk in Rhoads-style absolutes. New, efficacious drugs have been developed, and he is impatient for the FDA to approve them so they can be put to use saving lives. "A lot of the things wrong in medicine are not because we don't have the right tools, but because the field is very slow to change."

Fortunately for cancer patients, the frontal assault on cancer launched in 1945 changed the culture for the better. "Cancer is a disease that's out in the open, so much so that people wear the colors of the cause," observes DeVita in his book *The Death of Cancer,* pointing to the pink ribbons, pink hats, and assorted pink accessories that emerge every October as symbols of cancer awareness. "People who have cancer are now seen as warriors—people who are fighting back and, what's more, people with a shot at winning—not victims."

Dusty Rhoads did not live to see the first real chemical cures of cancer. His sudden death on August 13, 1959, at age sixty-one, from a massive coronary occlusion, cut short his quest. "His death is a loss to humanity as well as to science," the *New York Times* wrote of the man who did more than anyone to shape the modern era of chemotherapy. "In laboratories and hospitals throughout the nation tens of thousands of workers are engaged in slow, painstaking research. Many of these workers are brilliant scientists. Some have international reputations. But the number of scientific giants among them is few. Friday morning our greatest killer—heart disease—took from us one of those scientific giants in the battle against cancer."

In a statement to Rhoads's shocked staff, Warren Weaver, SKI's vice president, said simply, "It is quite literally true he worked himself to death. But this occurred in a great cause; and however tragic the immediate incident, this is a noble way to die."

At his memorial service a month later, in a nod to the attacks Rhoads repeatedly endured during his pioneering leadership, one of his loyal colleagues, Dr. Chester Stock, stated that there could be no more fitting epitaph than the words of Theodore Roosevelt:

It is not the critic who counts, not the man who points out how the strong man stumbled, or where the doer of deeds could have done them better. The credit belongs to the man who is actually in the arena, whose face is marred by dust and sweat and blood; who strives valiantly; who errs and comes short again and again . . . who, at the best, knows in the end the triumph of high achievement; and who, at the worst, if he fails, at least fails while daring greatly, so that his place will never be with the cold and timid souls who know neither victory nor defeat.

Stock had come upon the book containing the speech, and the marked passage, in Rhoads's office.

• • •

THE STORY OF THE Memorial Sloan Kettering Cancer Center and the evolution of chemotherapy is a long one, too long to recount here. While the hospital and laboratory continue to be a living memorial to Rhoads's inspired vision, the institutional memory of nitrogen mustard's progress from battlefield to frontline cancer treatment died with him. His successors dropped the references to the wartime discoveries, perhaps not wanting to remind their patients of chemotherapy's sinister origins, deeming it incompatible with the hospital's healing message. Today, there is little to remind people of the uneasy alliance between the military and medical establishments that gave rise to the war on cancer. Nowhere in Memorial Sloan Kettering's pastel-hued lobbies and soothing waiting rooms is there a plaque honoring the young Army doctor who identified the killer of a cure, or the thousands who died so millions could live.

Rhoads believed that whatever treatments for cancer might be discovered in the future, it should forever remain part of the medical canon that chemotherapy owed a debt to the dead at Bari. He concluded his famous 1946 Mount Sinai Hospital lecture by paying homage to Stewart Alexander and the many doctors and research scientists who followed the instruction of Isaiah to "beat their swords into ploughshares" and forged the links in the long chain of discoveries that produced something of unparalleled value for civilization:

> The Bari incident has long been forgotten by most, and World War II is history. Chemical warfare, awaited with so much anxiety, has become, with the development of atomic energy, an obsolete weapon. All the fears and the precautions, the desperate efforts and anxious hours, proved to be of only prophylactic value. Despite this fact, perhaps from the studies of the mode of action of toxic chemicals, rather more salvage for human good has been made than is the case for most of the other military arms.

Belated Justice

The secrecy surrounding chemical weapons in World War II continued long after the need for secrecy ended. "There is something particularly ugly and unthinkable about poison gas that makes people want to turn away and relegate it to the periphery of history," observed Dr. Jules Hirsch, the former physician-in-chief of Rockefeller University Hospital, referring to the American and British governments' "persistent need to remain distanced from the Bari incident that has been referred to as a deliberate 'cover up.'" The official secrecy resulted in lost records, misinformation, and considerable confusion about how the toxic chemical came to be tamed for medical use. It also meant that the chronic effects of mustard gas exposure on the surviving sailors, naval personnel, and civilians were denied by the military, resulting in years of suffering, controversy, and lawsuits for compensation in America and Britain. "Apparently, secrecy during the war often leads to inaccuracies in reporting or erroneous memories," reflected Hirsch, "particularly for matters relating to poison gas."

In his eagerly anticipated memoir of the war years, published in the fall of 1948, Dwight Eisenhower could barely bring himself to write about the Bari bombing and the regrettable loss of Allied vessels and valuable cargo. Aware that some stories about the chemical-weapons accident had already leaked, he observed almost as an aside that "one of the ships was loaded with a quantity of mustard gas," calling the spillage "an unfortunate affair" and minimizing the episode in an attempt to control the narrative and prevent any more information from coming out. "Fortunately the wind was offshore and the escaping gas caused no casualties," he wrote. "Had the wind been in the opposite direction, however, great disaster could well have resulted. It would have been indeed difficult to explain, even though we manufactured and carried this material only for reprisal purposes."

Ironically, Eisenhower's deflection of the "disaster" to the realm of the theoretical, and his allusion to the difficulty he would surely have encountered in trying to explain the "most unfortunate repercussions," almost seems like a subconscious plea for understanding of the wartime pressures and calculations that led to the cover-up in the first place. An even more sanitized account had appeared a year earlier in *Battle Report,* a quasi-official history of the Allied naval campaigns written by Commander Walter Karig of the US Navy and two other officers. The authors omitted any mention of poison gas but made no apology for not telling the whole story, asserting in the foreword to their volume that there were "still some few details" that needed to remain secret: "As such, they are not deletions from the story of the Atlantic, but from the whole history of the war."

Lt. Col. Alphonsus d'Abreu, the officer in charge of the surgical division of the 98th British General Hospital in Bari, did not approve of the deletions or the whitewashing of history. "I hope you will forgive me when I deny the accuracy of your statement that the escaping gas caused no casualties," he wrote Eisenhower, his former commanding officer in Italy, on January 26, 1949. "I was stationed there at the time and was responsible for the management of some 1,280 casualties of all nationalities," he continued, adding that he still had his notes, "and

I am afraid the death toll was very high." Most of the casualties were caused by the mixture of mustard gas and oil in the harbor and "were in fact very severely contaminated and many of them died later of the well known lung complications of this fearful chemical." D'Abreu gave the general credit for telling at least part of the truth: "Your reference to a ship loaded with mustard gas is the first official reference I have seen in the accounts of the disaster." He ended his note by saying, "Please do not think, Sir, that this is in the slightest way intended as a criticism, but I thought that you yourself would like an accurate account of the affair."

Eisenhower acknowledged d'Abreu's "thoughtfulness" in writing to him about the extent of the toxic release and resulting casualties. "As a matter of fact," he replied, "it was only this week that an article in *Blackwood's Magazine* [a small highbrow British monthly] for June 1947 supporting your account was called to my attention."

The article, "Big Bang at Bari," was a straight-from-the-horse's-mouth account of the air raid by Scott Jeavons, the injured British first lieutenant in charge of the port who happened to be recuperating at the 98th General Hospital when the bombs began to fall. Once Jeavons returned to headquarters at Navy House, he "picked up the missing details of the disaster, later amplified by this and that official report. It did not make good hearing, but it had to be faced." His piece was riddled with errors and rife with conjecture, including the rumor that "every Liberty ship" in the harbor had been carrying a secret shipment of gas bombs loaded with a lethal chemical that was "one hundred percent American," most likely "lewisite." But Jeavons had also gleaned that the secrecy about the cargo had exacerbated the catastrophe: "So secure had the bills of lading of the convoys been kept that many precious hours were thus granted to the poison to work through the skins of those patients, poor devils." A review of the Bari losses listed "over a thousand Allied casualties, let alone local inhabitants, of whom some three or four hundred were killed outright or died later." As a consequence, he noted, the Allies made sure the accident received "little publicity," as it was "hardly palatable news outside of Germany."

Eisenhower, who was already mulling a run for the presidency, must have wondered how Jeavons managed to sneak his article past the military censors, and what headaches it would create. "While I have not yet had an opportunity to check back through the official records, I shall do so," he assured d'Abreu, "and a correction will be made in future printings." No correction was ever made.

In the fifth installment of his voluminous memoirs of World War II, *Closing the Ring*, published in 1951, Churchill continued to cling obstinately to his position that there was no mustard gas in Bari. Even though he makes frequent reference to Eisenhower's *Crusade in Europe* in his own book, Churchill chose to ignore Ike's account of the toxic release, conceding only that a "chance hit" by the German Luftwaffe blew up an ammunition ship and did a great deal of damage in the crowded harbor, causing "the sinking of sixteen other ships and the loss of 30,000 tons of cargo."

The controversy remained dormant for another two decades until an enterprising US Navy officer, Captain D. M. Saunders, decided to look into exactly why the twenty-minute German air raid was so "spectacularly successful," noting that "not since Pearl Harbor had so many Allied ships been lost at one time." He unearthed Stewart Alexander's June 20, 1944, "Final Report of the Bari Mustard Casualties," which the US Army had classified as Secret. "Although regraded to Unclassified in 1959," Saunders observed, "it does not appear that the story has ever been told, at least within Navy circles." This struck him as odd, since, as "one of the very few times that U.S. military personnel had ever been exposed to the effects of toxic warfare agents, there may be lessons to be learned from this tragic affair." Saunders's cogent analysis of the chemical-weapons accident appeared in the September 1967 issue of the US Naval Institute *Proceedings,* along with his recommendations for how to avoid a repetition of the same costly mistakes. Like Jeavons, he concluded that a key factor contributing to the disaster was "the tendency (which continues to this day) to cloak all matters pertaining to BW/CW agents in a mantle of secrecy and safety precautions. Had the knowledge of the SS *John Harvey*'s cargo been more widely held, someone would have remembered, and appropriate measures could have been taken."

The long-buried incident, which was known to a limited degree in medical and military circles, was slowly emerging, like the haunting remains of an old wreck. It was not until Glenn B. Infield, a former pilot in the US Air Force, heard about it from the doctor taking care of his mother, who mentioned that a World War II accident had led to the development of nitrogen mustard as the recommended treatment for her Hodgkin's disease, that the Bari incident finally found a writer with the skill and determination to get to the bottom of the story. While his mother underwent chemotherapy, which would prolong her life for another year, Infield, his "curiosity aroused," set out to discover everything he could about the fateful accident. As he soon learned, "even in the late 1950's, the military were extremely reluctant to release any details about the poison-gas episode at Bari in 1943." He was rebuffed at the National Archives, the repository of the incident's official reports and memoranda, which he was told remained classified. His inquiries at Edgewood Arsenal also brought no success. A letter to the newly elected President Eisenhower produced "a polite note from his military aide, but no more information."

Infield resorted to old-fashioned shoe-leather reporting. He spent years collecting the personal accounts of men and women who had been at Bari the night of the air raid. He traveled to Italy, where he spoke to locals who remembered when the *John Harvey* exploded, and to Germany, where he questioned some of the former Luftwaffe pilots who bombed the harbor. He located Otto Heitmann, captain of the doomed *John Bascom*. He eventually tracked down Stewart Alexander, who had never spoken to anyone about the classified incident and declined to be interviewed. Infield refused to take no for an answer. He argued that he already knew the true story, it was too important a historical event to ignore, and it was in everyone's interest that his account be as accurate as possible. Alexander, who by this time had been a family physician and cardiologist in New Jersey for more than thirty years and had not given the Bari episode so much as a second thought, phoned the War Department. After ascertaining that his final report on the mustard gas casualties, which had been published in *The Military Surgeon*, was a matter of public record, Alexander sent Infield a copy. He cautiously agreed to help him with the medical aspects of the accident, but only on background.

Alexander was fiercely loyal to Eisenhower—they remained friends after the war—and would not hear a critical word about him. As he saw it, Eisenhower had believed his diagnosis that the Bari deaths were due to mustard gas, so he allowed him to write his report despite Churchill's objections. He defended Ike's decision to omit the mustard gas casualties from *Crusade in Europe*, as it was published just after the war and the magnitude of the disaster had not yet been made public. In the intervening years, Alexander and his wife had become very close to Eisenhower and his wife, Mamie, and often visited the White House. When Ike announced he was running for office, he offered Bunny a job on his campaign staff, which she turned down because she had two young daughters. Finally, she agreed to serve as national vice-chairwoman of Citizens for Eisenhower and cochair of New Jersey Citizens for Eisenhower, and she worked to get out the vote in forty-six states, often accompanying the general on his campaign train. On election night, November 3, 1952, the Alexanders sat with Ike and Mamie as they waited for the returns to come in. Ike was so nervous that all he wanted to do was "talk of the war."

While Infield managed to get hold of a number of other derestricted documents, there were huge gaps in his knowledge. He never saw the *John Harvey*'s ordnance breakdown, so he incorrectly recounts the way the ship was carefully loaded with mustard bombs in Baltimore, Maryland, and imagines the concerns expressed by both captain and crew prior to sailing, when in fact the toxic munitions were already in a chemical depot in Oran. Infield did not know that both American and British port officials were aware of the presence of gas in the harbor from the beginning, that chemical warfare experts confirmed it the next morning, or that the Italian doctors recognized it almost immediately, but their suspicions were either ignored or never reached the responsible hospital authorities. Most notably, he never learned of Eisenhower's Board of Inquiry, or Alexander's part in it, and never had access to the reams of witness testimony and final investigation reports. Unfortunately, Infield filled the holes in his manuscript with pages of re-created scenes and dialogue—including the thoughts and remarks of men who died in the disaster—which make for an entertaining read but render his book, *Disaster at Bari,* a strange amalgam of fiction and nonfiction, and thus unreliable as history.

Nevertheless, Infield's book made a big splash when it was published in the fall of 1971. Alexander was embarrassed by all the attention. He was also a little uncomfortable with some of the liberties the author took with the story. The climactic scene in which a dock officer phones with the report that the bomb fragments recovered from the harbor floor were German, supposedly providing stunning evidence the Nazis might be to blame, never happened, and, as he instructed a subsequent author, were "not correct." The idea that he "had not considered that the mustard might have been used by the Luftwaffe" was also absurd— it was the very contingency that prompted Eisenhower to request a chemical-weapons expert be assigned to AFHQ. Moreover, the bomb casings were clearly marked with American serial numbers. Once found by Allied divers, there was never the slightest doubt about their origin. Alexander attributed the inventions to the author's desire to enhance the drama, putting it down to "literary license."

Italians for the most part embraced Infield's exposé of the poison gas accident, which shed some light on the price they paid as a result of the Allied occupation. At the same time, some Italian experts found the description of the deadly vapor rolling into town exaggerated, and they disputed his estimate of more than "one thousand deaths among civilians," a figure that has been cited in virtually every subsequent article and book about the disaster. World War II historians Vito Antonio Leuzzi and Pasquale Trizio, who have spent decades researching the accident and subsequent cleanup efforts, maintain the true number of Italian fatalities is closer to three to four hundred. They believe it is probable that Infield confused two events, and his inflated figure includes the death toll from a second massive explosion in Bari Harbor that took place a month before the end of the war. On the morning of April 9, 1945, another American Liberty ship, the SS *Charles Henderson,* exploded while its cargo of bombs and ammunition was being unloaded, killing all fifty-six members of the crew and 317 Italian dockworkers and wounding another six hundred Italian naval personnel and civilians. That midday massacre, which in an instant robbed the town of all its young men, was a far greater tragedy for Bari, and it remains an indelible memory in the minds of its citizens today.

The air raid that rocked Bari on December 2, 1943, is still remembered in the region not so much for the loss of life—the majority of those killed had been American and British servicemen, not Italian— but for the poison gas shells littering the harbor floor. All kinds of rusting munitions, from German mines to unexploded mustard and phosphorous bombs, lay on the seabed at depths of 50 to 700 feet all along the Puglia coastline in a wide arc from Bari to Molfetta and Manfredonia, posing a hazard to ships, ferries, and fishermen. In the first few years after the war, dozens of cases of mustard gas poisoning were reported after fishing nets accidentally dislodged gas canisters and resulted in contamination—the men's red, blistered arms and racing pulses telling local doctors all they needed to know. Young boys who dove in dangerous waters to salvage scrap iron for pocket money were also affected.

The reports were mostly anecdotal until the cleanup operation of Bari Harbor began in earnest in the spring of 1947. In the course of surveying the twenty-two submerged wrecks still cluttering the port, Italian Navy divers found stores of unexploded mustard shells in the cargo hold of the *John Harvey*, "a time bomb at the bottom of Bari harbor," as Professor Trizio put it. The alarming discovery necessitated a far more rigorous salvage operation, undertaken by the Puglia Demining Nucleus, and required a working team composed of a senior naval officer, four experienced divers, along with a medic, nurse, paymaster, and weapons technician. The cleanup operation took seven years, and some two thousand mustard gas canisters were reportedly recovered from the *John Harvey* alone. They were carefully transferred to a barge, which was towed out to sea and sunk. Not everything could be recovered. A stray canister still occasionally emerges from the mud and causes injuries.

In the spring of 1944, the British Army moved their dead servicemen from the municipal cemetery in Bari to a new military cemetery five miles away, in a secluded spot outside the tiny village of Triggiano. Many of the American servicemen killed in the disaster were buried at sea, but those who were put in makeshift graves were later reinterred at the Sicily–Rome American Cemetery in Nettuno, including twenty-four of the seventy-eight lost crew members of the *John Harvey*. In this breathtaking seventy-seven-acre burial ground are the remains of nearly 7,900 American men and women who lost their lives in the liberation of Sicily, the landings in Salerno and Anzio, and in the heavy fighting northward.

By breaking the story of "one of the best kept secrets of World War II," Glenn Infield succeeded in lifting the official veil on the chemical-weapons accident and bringing it far-reaching publicity in the form of book reviews, related articles, and a lengthy excerpt in the October 1971 issue of *American Heritage* magazine. Feature stories inspired by his account of the devastating air raid continued to appear in various publications for years afterward. There can be no imagining the surprise and dismay of the survivors of the disaster—not to mention all the servicemen, doctors, and nurses present that night—who stumbled on the news items and learned for the first time about the poison gas that leached into the harbor, and its terrible lingering effects.

The young British nurse Gwladys Rees, who after the war married a Canadian Army doctor named Robert Aikens and settled in Halifax, Nova Scotia, had always wanted confirmation of what the young sailors on her ward had been contaminated with, but her request to the British War Office had "produced no information." Then one day, out of the blue, she received a clipping about the incident from an acquaintance at the Maritime Museum of the Atlantic in Halifax. The article was entitled, MUSTARD GAS HORROR AT BARI. She had felt so betrayed by the deception the authorities had perpetrated in 1943, when they ordered the hospital staff to mislead the patients and alter their medical charts. Yet, looking back on it, she thought that Churchill might have been right to suppress the truth about the incident in order to prevent Germany from retaliating and initiating a chemical war. "Had the mustard gas incident been made public, the consequences could have been far worse," she reflected in her memoir, *Nurses in Battledress*. "Who knew in those days what Hitler was prepared to do?"

Not everyone was prepared to forgive and forget, especially when the secrecy came at the expense of the Bari survivors' welfare. In July 1976, George Southern, a gunlayer on HMS *Zetland*, organized a reunion of some fifty former officers and men at the aptly named Zetland Arms, a charming Victorian corner pub in South Kensington, London. One of his shipmates had read Infield's book and told him there had been poison gas in Bari Harbor on the night of the bombing, and it was probable they had all been exposed in the aftermath of the explosions. "It came as a tremendous shock as until then we members of the ship's crew had known nothing about mustard gas," explained Southern, aged ninety-eight, old and deaf, but still sharp as a tack.

Strict censorship had applied for more than thirty years, but even so, he and his friends asked themselves how one of the worst incidents of the war could have been covered up so completely. Southern, who was awarded the British Empire Medal for his heroic actions during the air raid, was convinced it was an orchestrated "cover-up." Given the dreadful memories of poison gas from World War I, he felt certain that news of the chemical weapons accident would have inspired protests at home and abroad and turned world opinion against them. The cover-up, he argued, was ordered to avoid the political fallout: "It was purely for the purpose of keeping the populations of the UK and USA from knowing both countries were stockpiling and transporting mustard gas to the front."

Furious, Southern decided that the official silence about the Bari incident had gone on long enough. He immediately began work on a firsthand account of his harrowing ordeal that night in 1943, when he and four others fought fires to keep the *Lyman Abbott* from being consumed and pulled sailors out of what they now realized was a "deadly cocktail of mustard and oil." He had been in the middle of the harbor from the time the first bomb dropped to almost dawn the next morning, all the while breathing in the fumes and getting repeatedly soaked by the filthy contaminated water. When he tried to obtain Ministry of Defence documents to corroborate his account, he was told there was no official record of the catastrophe. He received the same reply from the Royal Army Medical Corps: "We have no knowledge of this incident." Frustrated by his inability to access the Bari archives, Southern placed a series of advertisements in the local papers, appealing for more information from sailors who were present during the December 2 air raid. He knew that not everyone exposed to the mustard had died— good luck, a quick shower, change of clothes, and prompt treatment had allowed many to return home safely. Until then, Southern had always been "content to be in one piece." The blisters and burns on his arms and hands had healed, and although he was left with a hacking cough that he was never quite able to shake, his wounds had been comparatively minor. As one survivor after another answered his ads, however, he soon learned that hundreds of men had not been so lucky.

The British government's refusal to acknowledge what had happened in Bari meant that many sailors who still bore the scars never got the help they needed. "The cover-up meant some victims' claims of mustard gas exposure were not believed and not treated seriously by medical authorities," he said. Others unknowingly suffered myriad health problems from inhaling the fumes, manifested as debilitating lung, throat, and eye disorders, as well as a variety of respiratory cancers, which reduced them to invalids. Then there were the psychological problems, particularly depression and post-traumatic stress syndrome. Proving their ailments were due to a mustard gas accident that officially did not exist, and was not cited anywhere in their medical records, was an almost impossible task. "It made me all the more determined to tell the true story," said Southern, his anger still raw. "The British government had censored and was continuing to censor the details of the Bari raid."

A deeply personal work, *Poisonous Inferno* is based on dozens of interviews with fellow survivors. It throbs with outrage at the Allied authorities who authorized the cover-up of the mustard gas and condemned hundreds of servicemen who did their patriotic duty to a lifetime of suffering. A case in point was Able Seaman Bertram Stevens, who was aboard the *Vulcan* when it was engulfed in the explosions.

After being drenched by a huge wave of seawater and oil, he and the rest of the crew spent days living and sleeping in their sodden uniforms before they reached Brindisi, where they were treated by the medics. Stevens was transferred from the hospital in Italy to his home base at the Royal Naval Barracks in Portsmouth, England, but he was never examined by a doctor or provided with any follow-up care for his blurry eyes and bad headaches. When he completed his military service in January 1948, he was given a cursory checkup and discharged from the Royal Navy as A1, the designation for "fit for further service." Within four years, Stevens's health began to deteriorate: He became impotent and suffered from bouts of gastritis, bronchitis, and conjunctivitis. His eyes were painful and watered uncontrollably, forcing him to wear dark glasses all the time. Walking was difficult due to the large blisters that had formed on the soles of his feet. By 1968, his breathing became labored, and he was ill so often that he could no longer continue working as a longshoreman.

In 1982, Stevens was admitted to London's Whitechapel Hospital for a series of tests and diagnosed with cancer of the lip, which quickly spread to his neck. Quite by chance, after Stevens underwent an operation to remove the tumor, his wife, Betty, overheard the doctor discussing his case. It was the first time she had ever heard the words *mustard gas*. With a sudden, awful recognition, she understood the cause of her husband's long-drawn-out illness.

In a strange twist, it turned out that the Whitechapel doctor had been part of a fact-finding team sent to Bari six years after the war to investigate why some local citizens were suddenly dying. When Stevens stated that he thought his chronic health problems dated back to the injuries he sustained during the 1943 air raid, the doctor listened intently. He questioned Stevens about the events of that night, his hospitalization, and the symptoms that had appeared in the hours and days that followed. "Did at any time anyone tell you the cause of your irritations?" he asked, scribbling notes. Stevens replied, "No." The doctor explained that his interest in the case stemmed from his visit to Bari, but for reasons of "security," he said he could not elaborate. He promised Stevens he would be able to tell him more at a later date. He never did. Even so, many years after the fact, the doctor still felt constrained from telling his patient the truth about his condition. "He never volunteered one word about mustard gas," recounted Southern. "Bert had encountered the British establishment's obsession with secrecy."

Betty Stevens led the fight for justice for her husband and the other British survivors contaminated at Bari. Believing that they were deliberately misinformed and denied disability benefits, she spent three years battling the War Pensions Board, which initially rejected Stevens's claim for compensation. The Ministry of Defence also refused to release his medical records, making it more difficult to prove their case. Betty Stevens did not give up. She continued to lobby Parliament for change, and she enlisted the media's assistance in drawing attention to the heartless and unfair treatment of the ailing veterans. Finally, in December 1985, Bert Stevens's application was granted, and he became the first survivor to be officially recognized as a Bari mustard gas victim and awarded a pension. Because he was never informed about the contamination, the authorities grudgingly agreed his pension should be backdated to when his symptoms first began to appear. After ten more years of struggling to breathe, an oxygen cylinder and mask always by his side, Stevens passed away at the age of seventy-three.

In 1986, as a direct result of the onslaught of victims' claims that followed in the wake of the news coverage of Bert Stevens's petition, the Department of Health and Social Security in England undertook what it called a "special exercise" to trace the remainder of the British casualties involved in the Bari incident to see whether similar compensation was appropriate. According to their figures, of the 693 casualties stemming from the Bari Harbor incident, 141 died or were declared missing.

No information was available on how many of their widows received war pensions. As of 1991, another 185 claims for war pensions had been submitted, of which 106 were successful. By then, of course, many of the aging, infirm Bari veterans had passed away. A bitter and disgusted George Southern believes that number is a drop in the bucket compared to the hundreds of affected servicemen who were never told they had been exposed to gas. They were treated by ship's surgeons, sick-berth attendants, and first-aid personnel at the scene who were either ignorant of the danger or sworn to secrecy. "As it has turned out—a lifetime's secrecy," he wrote. "How many more people suffered like Bert Stevens, and his family, totally unaware of the real reason, we shall never know."

The censorship of the Bari episode also impeded American veterans from acquiring the information and assistance needed to cope with their own health problems. In 1961, the National Academy of Sciences attempted to conduct a study of the physical conditions of the American victims of mustard gas contamination, but the follow-up agency appointed by the Division of Medical Sciences to examine the personnel records found its efforts blocked by both American and British military red tape. Officials fell back on the well-worn excuses that documents could not be found or were not available. Stewart Alexander offered to help in any way he could, but he was eventually informed that the project could not go forward because of the difficulty of tracing victims. "All the records said 'burns due to enemy action,'" he recalled. "They couldn't tell who had [thermal] burns and who had mustard burns." Even if the victims could be located, the agency's director was unsure whether the men should be informed of the chemical exposure at such a late date. "Should we frame our approach in terms of the Bari disaster or conceal our underlying interest in a general study?" he asked Alexander, still hesitant to violate military security.

In response to the long-delayed official admission that American servicemen had been exposed to mustard gas and other chemical warfare agents during World War II, the US Department of Veterans Affairs in 1991 requested that a committee of the Institute of Medicine (IOM) of the National Academy of Sciences look into the matter. In January 1993, the results of a comprehensive study were made available to the public in the IOM document *Veterans at Risk: The Health Effects of Mustard Gas and Lewisite*. The report castigated the armed forces for taking nearly fifty years to acknowledge that US servicemen had been used as human experimental subjects in mustard gas testing programs. The Department of Defense had failed to provide follow-up medical care and to anticipate the long-term health consequences of exposure to the toxic agents. Finally, the report noted that the continued secrecy maintained by the military about chemical-weapons research created a barrier to proper medical assessments. The American survivors of the Bari incident—the only US mustard gas combat casualties of the war—made up only a tiny percentage of the approximately sixty thousand affected servicemen, at least four thousand of whom suffered the kind of serious mustard exposure likely to cause chronic health problems. "There can be no question," the IOM committee stated, "that some veterans, who served our country with honor and at great personal cost, were mistreated twice"—first by the secrecy and second by the official denials that lasted for decades.

In the January 1993 press conference, the Veterans Administration announced plans to relax the standard of proof for gas victims and ease the way for compensation claims. It also promised to heed the committee's advice to seek out an additional ninety thousand military and civilian munitions workers—many of them women—who may have been exposed to toxic concentrations of mustard gas at sites such as Edgewood Arsenal, where the air reportedly was thick with mustard throughout the war years. The VA had great difficulty locating the personnel records and had to file requests repeatedly under the Freedom of Information Act to obtain the necessary data from the Department of Defense. By the fall of

1994, the VA had managed to identify another eight thousand individuals who may have faced gas exposure in military exercises of accidents, rather than as research subjects, though not all of these were confirmed cases. Approximately five hundred of those names were from the Bari disaster. Warren Brandenstein, the young gunner aboard the *John Bascom* who was blinded for two weeks by mustard gas following the raid, was contacted by the IOM about his experience to supplement the scanty medical knowledge about the Bari survivors' health status: "[We] have heard from only a few veterans who were present," Constance Pechura, the IOM study director, wrote Brandenstein. "It would be helpful to our committee if you could provide a little bit more information on your immediate health problems and injuries at the time."

Another part of the IOM committee's task was to try to understand the historical context of the Chemical Warfare Service's preparations, including the "extraordinary" experiments with lethal gases. In June 1942, six months after Pearl Harbor, when fears that Germany or Japan might initiate a gas attack were at their peak, the War Department authorized the use of human "volunteers" for chemical warfare research in order to obtain better data than the animal models could provide. The so-called volunteers were US servicemen who were recruited with offers of extra privileges, additional leave, or a change of scene, but official reports revealed that the men were not told of the true nature of the tests until it was too late to back out. Many were later threatened with prison if they violated the terms of secrecy. The highly classified experiments, which were designed to test defensive and offensive equipment and techniques, were carried out under the auspices of the Chemical Warfare Service and the Naval Research Laboratory and were part of a larger Allied program involving Britain, Australia, Canada, and India.

The mustard gas experiments were of three basic types: the "patch tests," in which drops of the chemical were painted on a small area of skin and the potency of the agent was assessed; "chamber tests," in which thousands of US Navy personnel at the Great Lakes Training Center in Illinois were repeatedly exposed to varying concentrations of mustard gas to determine the effectiveness of protective clothing; and field tests, in which men outfitted in different kinds of protective gear were subjected to mustard gas attacks, marched across contaminated ground, or entered contaminated areas to collect data, in order to see how well the equipment stood up and how sailors and soldiers could function at different levels of impairment. The chamber and field tests were also called "man-break tests," with the level of exposure extending from mild skin burns to severe tissue injury that took more than a month to heal. The Army conducted field experiments at a number of sites, including Edgewood Arsenal; Camp Sibert, Alabama; Bushnell, Florida; Dugway Proving Ground in Utah; and San José Island, Panama.

By studying the toxic effects on the men's bodies, CWS researchers were able to improve equipment, and medical scientists learned more about the action of mustard agents. Howard Skipper, who worked under Rhoads at the CWS, spent two years on Australia's Great Barrier Reef assisting a British–Australian–American team studying how effective mustard gas might be against Japanese forces defending an island, and whether it could be used to minimize Allied casualties in an offensive. The scientists staged mock "bombings" of the deserted Barrier islands, and Skipper and his team, dressed in protective gear, would go in and collect samples of the poisonous vapor and perform tests on Navy "volunteers." Early on, he observed that mustard damaged bone marrow, and he endeavored to reverse the inhibitory effects, but he never found an antidote. Skipper later said he was very relieved that mustard gas was never used, because it was "a terrible weapon." He was glad that after the war he was able to use what he learned firsthand about its toxicity to make significant contributions to the scourge of cancer. But as one US Navy veteran put it bluntly, he "was injured, not by the enemy, but by his own countrymen."

In late 1943, the CWS selected San José Island, off the coast of Panama, as the site for a test project to ascertain how chemical weapons could be used in a land invasion of Japan and its occupied islands. United States military scientists believed poison gas would be more lethal in the Pacific because enemy soldiers in the hot, steamy environment exposed more skin than their counterparts in Europe. Rhoads was assigned to establish the Chemical Warfare Service's medical program in Panama. The San José Project, run by Brigadier General Egbert F. Bullene, bombed more than seven hundred acres on the island with a variety of chemical agents—from mustard gas and phosgene to hydrogen cyanide, butane, and napalm—to investigate how the toxins acted in jungle conditions and to measure their effects on rabbits and goats. Because skin reactions vary greatly from species to species, and sulfur mustard penetrates human skin faster at higher ambient temperatures, it was considered necessary to use soldiers as test subjects.

One series of mustard gas experiments compared the blistering on Puerto Rican and American "white" mainland soldiers to determine whether there was a difference in skin sensitivity. It was theorized that the thickness of skin might affect susceptibility, and that black skin might react differently to antigens than white skin. In the course of the tests, some of the men were hospitalized with severe burns and irritated eyes. None of the experimental data supported the concept that there was a difference in the rate of sulfur mustard penetration between black and white skin. The race studies in Panama, another blemish on the US Army's record, were just a small part of extensive wartime testing on the dermatological effects of mustard gas.

At the time, no formal set of rules existed governing the clinical conduct of tests on human subjects, whether healthy volunteers or sick patients. The Nuremberg Code, a set of ten ethical guidelines—including the essential requirement of voluntary consent—regarding the proper use and treatment of human subjects in medical research was established in 1947 as a reaction to Nazi human experimentation. (Since military and intelligence agency testing using human subjects continued well into the 1960s, there is no evidence the Army felt bound by the codes.) In their book *Veterans at Risk*, Constance Pechura and David Rall closely examined the World War II chemical warfare experiments and the testimony of 250 participants in order to attempt to portray the atmosphere in which the tests were conducted and to describe the attitudes of the military researchers who carried them out. The IOM committee affirmed that the individual investigators involved in the testing programs, spurred by the fury of the conflict in Europe and Japan, "were convinced of the likelihood of great numbers of gas casualties and that they believed their work to be necessary to save lives."

Yet they also found that the full body of knowledge available to the scientists as to the harmful effects of the toxic agents was not applied to their conduct of the human experiments, and this resulted in excessive exposure levels, injuries, and enduring health problems. "It was a war," concluded Pechura and Rall. "A worldwide emergency that understandably required certain goals to take precedence over others, possibly to the detriment of sound medical research practices concerning individual well-being."

Rhoads and his wartime cohort of scientists successfully bridged the worlds of military and civilian medical research, but their legacy remains controversial. "The laboratory and the battlefield marked two paths through which scientific investigators in the early 1940s learned about mustard gas and nitrogen mustards and then tested their ideas on sick people," observed the historian Susan Smith in her book *Toxic Exposures*. While doctors at the time drew a distinction between the experimental use of nitrogen mustard on military volunteers and its therapeutic use on terminal patients, in many ways the lines became blurred. In his eagerness to translate what he had learned from the laboratory and the battlefield to the clinic, and to transform chemical weapons into a new type of cancer treatment, Rhoads moved with a speed and lack of due caution that many of his colleagues found troubling. His critics felt that because of his easy equivalence of research and therapy goals, Rhoads tended to lose sight of the fact that he was using patients as experimental proxies in cancer trials, and that enrolling them in the studies was not entirely for their benefit, with the result that sometimes the individual patient's welfare could be compromised. The path through this ethical thicket is no easier now than it was for Rhoads and other early chemotherapists, but today the progression to clinical trial would be much slower and more deliberate, with each step debated in planning conferences and in peer review committees.

Rhoads's legacy as a pioneering cancer researcher is further complicated by his notorious letter joking about killing Puerto Ricans, which inflicted a wound on the island's soul that continued to fester. In November 1950, the controversy flared again when Rhoads's letter made news as the apparent motivation behind the attempt of two Puerto Rican nationalists to invade Blair House in Washington, DC, and assassinate President Harry Truman. One assailant was shot dead after killing a policeman, and the other, Oscar Collazo, was wounded before being arrested. He later confessed he had dedicated his life to the Puerto Rican Nationalist Party after hearing its leader, Pedro Albizu Campos, talk about the abuses of American imperialism as symbolized by Rhoads's plot to exterminate Puerto Ricans. Collazo was convicted and sentenced to death, but in 1952 Truman commuted his sentence. In 1979, President Jimmy Carter reduced his sentence to time served, and the elderly Collazo was released. He received a hero's welcome on his return to Puerto Rico.

The Rhoads letter was publicized again in the fall of 2002 by biology professor Edwin Vázquez, who came across it while preparing a lecture for his students at the University of Puerto Rico. Deeply offended by the letter, on October 5 Vázquez wrote to the American Association for Cancer Research (AACR) and demanded that the organization remove Rhoads's name from its coveted award for achievement in cancer research that was established in his honor. "I find it morally unacceptable that you confer an award named after a person whose work was inhuman and unethical," he wrote. After Vázquez brought the allegations to the attention of the AACR, the renewed media attention inspired fresh outrage in Puerto Rican academic, medical, and social communities. It also brought fresh calls for "belated justice" from Pedro Aponte-Vázquez (no relation), a professor of history at the University of Puerto Rico, who had been researching and writing about Rhoads for more than two decades. In the last of a series of books on the subject, *The Unsolved Case of Dr. Cornelius P. Rhoads: An Indictment*, he argued that Rhoads's letter should be regarded as "a written confession of the multiple murders he committed in Puerto Rico and the ones he tried to commit."

Most historians and medical ethicists do not agree that the case is that clear-cut. "Few people seriously believe that Rhoads injected patients with cancer cells," opined Douglas Starr in *Science* magazine, noting that "what shocks some observers is not only the contents of the letter but the collegial treatment Rhoads received after they became public." Susan Lederer, author of a scholarly essay exploring the murky ethical landscape of the Rhoads letter, took the position that it was a private joke for his own consumption, albeit one with an "incredibly racist element." Yet she does not believe that the many controversial groundbreaking figures in medicine should simply be stricken from history for their questionable actions. She noted that there were many prominent researchers like Rhoads who made major contributions to medical science but had a darker side to their pasts, adding, "If we are going to tar Rhoads, the net has to be cast a lot farther." What was needed in Rhoads's case, most scholars and ethicists agreed, was a perspective that did not condone what he wrote or thought but that gave him "due appropriate credit for his accomplishments as well as acknowledgment of his faults and sins."

Toward that end, the AACR commissioned an independent investigation into the seventy-year-old charges that Rhoads caused the death of eight Puerto Ricans by injecting them with cancer cells. The organization also suspended its annual $5,000 award in his name. In April of 2003, the investigation by Jay Katz, an emeritus professor of law, medicine, and psychiatry at Yale Law School and a specialist in medical ethics, concluded that although there was no evidence that Rhoads killed patients or transplanted cancer cells, or participated in any medical misconduct, the letter itself was sufficiently reprehensible to warrant removing his name from the prize.

Now, Rhoads's name has been reduced to a footnote at the cancer institute he was instrumental in founding. The imposing oil portrait of him in his white lab coat that once hung in the lobby has been taken down, but if you look closely enough, there is a glimpse of him in a small group photo in the historical mural in Memorial's main building. In its "About Us" brochure, part of its public relations package, Memorial Sloan Kettering Cancer Center states of its first director: "Dr. Rhoads' ties to the military and charges of unethical human experimentation would later sully his reputation as a pioneer of chemotherapy."

As THE YEARS PASSED, Stewart Alexander followed the developments in cancer treatments based on nitrogen mustard, the mystery compound he had tested in his Edgewood laboratory in 1942. A modest, affable, and unassuming man, he never boasted of his wartime exploits to his colleagues but became more open about discussing his work with the Chemical Warfare Service after the publication of the Infield book. He took quiet pride in the fact that it was recognized in most medical texts that "the modern age of chemotherapy for malignant diseases dates from the Bari Harbor episode." It did not matter to him that he was never mentioned by name. He was already respected and beloved as Park Ridge's premiere physician and cardiologist, who had continued a private practice that had existed since 1865 and had looked after some area families for more than a hundred years. He was director of medicine at Bergen Pines County Hospital for eighteen years, was affiliated with Pascack Valley Hospital among several others, and taught part time at both Columbia and New York University Medical Schools. As public-spirited as his father, he served on numerous community boards and medical organizations and was a past president of the Bergen County Medical Society, Bergen County Heart Association, and New Jersey Academy of Medicine.

By the spring of 1987, the seventy-two-year-old Alexander had retired from private practice, and was recovering from a bout of surgery, when he received a phone call from Nicholas Spark, a precocious seventeen-year-old high school junior in Tucson, Arizona. Spark had spotted an excerpt from Infield's book in a hardbound collection of *American Heritage* magazines bought at a yard sale, and he was enthralled by the story of the young World War II doctor's desperate search for answers to the medical mystery at Bari. He showed the article to his father, Ronald Spark, a pathologist, who was also intrigued and helped dig up Alexander's final report and other medical papers on the origins of chemotherapy. Young Spark was sure he had found the "perfect topic" for his school essay for "National History Day." If not for Alexander's determination, it was possible mustard gas might never have been identified as the culprit in the catastrophe—or a cure in disguise.

After reading Infield's book, however, Spark worried that it was too much of a "historical novel," and that he would never be able to figure out how to "sort out fact from fiction." He thought that if he could just talk to Dr. Alexander and clarify some of the key points, he could submit a well-researched paper that had a chance of advancing in the essay contest. However, when he learned that a 1973 fire at the National Personnel Records Center in St. Louis, Missouri, had destroyed hundreds of veterans' files, he doubted he would ever be able to find the doctor before his deadline.

The theme of that year's history essay was personal liberty, and Spark wanted to show how the young chemical warfare doctor had put his career on the line, and very possibly his liberty, by challenging Churchill: "The idea that somehow a person like Dr. Alexander had managed to save so many lives, risked so much, and altered the course of medical history, and yet was deprived of even a letter of commendation really did bother my conscience," he recalled. He was spurred on by his youthful indignation over the way Alexander had been treated by the British authorities, and his naive belief that he could do something about it and perhaps right a wrong. Spark was also inspired by an example closer to home. His father was actively battling the big tobacco companies in Tucson at the time—and eventually succeeded in getting cigarette vending machines banned citywide—so he understood something of what it meant to try to "speak truth to power."

Against all odds, the VA located Alexander's damaged personnel file and forwarded the Tucson University High School student's letter to his New Jersey address. When Spark's mother shouted from the kitchen in late March that "a Dr. Alexander is on the phone for you," Nick could hardly believe it. After that, he was able to interview Alexander several times about his medical sleuthing and his clash with British officials. The conversations were necessarily brief—long-distance calls were expensive in those days—and he taped their fifteen-minute exchanges on a small telephone-recording device he had bought at Radio Shack with money saved from his allowance. Alexander was very cordial and answered all his questions, though Spark sensed that he did not quite approve of his efforts to spotlight his work at Bari. But Alexander went along with it, "not believing for a second that it would amount to anything." Spark's sixteen-page paper, "For the Benefit of My Patients," took him all the way to the state finals, where it won first place. Alexander wrote to congratulate the youngster and wished him good luck in the National History Day competition.

In the weeks that followed, Spark could not rid himself of the idea that it was unfair that he should win an award, while Dr. Alexander had never been decorated for his actions. "With his name removed from all official records," Spark wrote in his essay, "the true hero of Bari became an invisible man." Spark did not win the national competition in Washington DC, but he garnered a special award from the Naval Historical Foundation and a $250 prize. He later received a $7,000 college scholarship from the Flynn Foundation. At an event at the Hart Senate Office Building, when the contestants lined up to shake hands and pose for photos with their state representatives, Spark approached Arizona Senator Dennis DeConcini about Alexander's case, making as strong an argument as he could muster that the government should acknowledge the doctor's courageous actions at Bari. Much to Spark's surprise, after hearing him out, DeConcini said it sounded like something he would like to look into further.

DeConcini's office took up the issue with the Army. A detailed review of Alexander's personnel records—water-stained from the fire, but still legible—showed that he had been awarded a half-dozen military honors, including the Bronze Star for meritorious service in support of combat operations in Italy and France in 1944, the American Defense Medal with Foreign Service Clasp, an EAME medal with seven battle stars, D-Day Arrowhead, and Victory Medal, among others. No documentation could be found to show the Army had attempted to decorate him at Bari but had not done so because of British objections and the potential embarrassment. Suffice it to say that, after dozens of letters to former officers at AFHQ in North Africa, inquiries to the American and British military authorities, and extensive research by

DeConcini's staff, as well as that of New Jersey Congressman Robert Torricelli, the US Army Awards Division finally agreed to make a rare exception and review the case. On October 9, 1987, the *American Medical News* reported, "Thus, 44 years after Bari, and 22 years since Churchill's death, the division is delving into musty, old, never released records and into the role of Stewart Alexander, MD, then a brash young lieutenant colonel and chemical warfare expert, who made what was one of the most politically sensitive diagnoses ever made."

The "persistent" inquiries from Torricelli's staff eventually provoked a testy response from Whitehall: "Dr. Alexander was quite correct in thinking Churchill was skeptical about the suggestion that casualties were (partly) suffering from Mustard gas poisoning," Stephen Dunn of the Ministry of Defence informed officials in the British Embassy in Washington. "After all, the ship was US in origin and it was some time before US authorities could confirm Dr. Alexander's diagnosis." He disputed the suggestion that Churchill attempted to "'cover up' the exact cause of injuries," explaining that, "in the absence of a confirmed diagnosis, he [Churchill] preferred to call the injuries 'chemical burns,' etc." However, advised that two influential senators, Bill Bradley of New Jersey and Dennis DeConcini of Arizona, had taken a personal interest, and might well decide to pursue the matter further, his office was willing to concede that it was not Churchill's finest hour: "You can say that with the benefit of hindsight things might have been handled better. It must be considered that this was one incident amongst many which were exercising Allied commanders at the time."

In the end, US Army historians confirmed the story to their satisfaction. On Friday, May 20, 1988, at a small ceremony in the Capitol, a white-haired Alexander, with Bunny by his side, received the long-overdue military honor. Senator DeConcini made a short speech praising Alexander's heroism and Spark's pursuit of the truth. Also officiating at the ceremony was Senator Bradley, who said he was pleased Alexander's

Belated Justice + 319

medical detective work was being recognized, because his efforts had an impact that reached far beyond his patients and became "a catalyst for developing chemotherapy." While a beaming Spark looked on, they presented Alexander with a Certificate of Appreciation signed by the Army surgeon general. "Without his early diagnosis and rapid initiation of appropriate and aggressive treatment, many more lives would have been lost and the severity of injuries would have been much greater," the commendation read. "His service to the military and civilians injured during this catastrophe reflects the finest measure of a soldier and physician."

At the end of the ceremony, Spark apologized to Alexander for taking more than eight months to get him the recognition he deserved, but the two senators, both visibly wincing, said nearly in unison that, "for Washington, getting something done in only eight months is pretty amazing." Alexander thanked Spark for his efforts in bringing his story to the public's attention. Then, in a solemn act of remembrance, he paused to commemorate all those who had perished at Bari and gave their tomorrows to the country's defense and to medical science.

In the press conference afterward, Captain Mark Yow, assistant executive officer to the surgeon general, explained that the US Army could not have honored Alexander until recently, when the British declassified the documents relating to the incident. (The British are the masters of the slow reveal: The bulk of the Bari incident files were declassified in 1971, a group of Air Ministry papers a decade later, but some were not opened until 2008. Still others will not be released until 2044.) It was noted that the British government had no plans for any official UK honor for the doctor's work at Bari. Looking somewhat abashed at the scrum of reporters and cameras, Alexander said simply, "This [award] is not something I ever sought. I did what I saw as my duty at the time, as I always have all my life."

When asked by a journalist who reached him at home whether he felt vindicated, Alexander said, "I'm very gratified, it's not a question of vindication at all." He added that he had great admiration for the former prime minister, whom he called one of his political heroes, and he understood the need to put victory before transparency in 1943. "I think Churchill was right," he said of the decision to deny the mustard gas accident, if not his diagnosis of toxic exposure. "But I think he was unduly harsh in his management of it."

The next day, the papers could not resist the political angle, and the headline in the *Arizona Daily Star* read, TUCSON TEENAGER RIGHTS INJUSTICE BY WINSTON CHURCHILL.

That fall, the story of Alexander's investigation at Bari, along with the Army Surgeon General's award, were read into the *Congressional Record*. Representative Margaret "Marge" Roukema of New Jersey saluted Alexander and offered the tardy but well-deserved recognition of the fact that he might fittingly be called "The Father of Chemotherapy."

Three years later, Alexander was packing for a Thanksgiving vacation in the Caribbean with his daughter and grandchildren when a call came from London that the British government would belatedly like to honor him for his work at Bari. He replied that, after so many years, it would have to wait a little longer. He was leaving on holiday and would be happy to discuss the matter on his return. It was a bittersweet moment. Alexander was terminally ill, and he knew he would not live to see that day. He died on the island of Mustique two weeks later, on December 11, 1991, at the age of seventy-seven. The cause was a malignant melanoma—skin cancer—that he had diagnosed himself.

His obituary in the *New York Times* made no reference to the Bari incident or chemotherapy.

In September 2006, the year marking the sixtieth anniversary of the first report of a trial of cancer chemotherapy, Dr. Jules Hirsch paid tribute to Dr. Stewart Alexander in the *Journal of the American Medical Association*, reminding readers of the Bari disaster and the inquisitive physician investigator "who sifted through the horrors and extracted a gem—something potentially useful for the abatement of human disease."

Acknowledgments

Quite simply, this book would not have been possible were it not for the extraordinary generosity of Stewart F. Alexander's two daughters, Diane and Judith. They enthusiastically embraced the idea of a book about their father's classified mission in Bari, Italy, and provided a wealth of wartime letters, reports, documents, recorded memoirs, and photos. Their hospitality at the family retreat on Block Island was more than any author could ask for, and I am most grateful for their kindness. Nick Spark was similarly generous with his time and teenage recollections, and he deserves my thanks. By some miracle, he—and his proud mother—preserved all of his taped conversations with Dr. Alexander, as well as a thick file of correspondence with the office of Arizona Senator Dennis DeConcini, and dozens of local newspaper articles. What a treasure trove! I was especially fortunate in being able to interview George Southern, a survivor of the Bari disaster and a gifted storyteller in his own right. With the assistance of his son, Paul, a fellow historian, he was able to answer all my prodding questions. Sadly, George passed away on November 17, 2019, before this book went to press. I am forever grateful to the Southern family.

I also want to thank Sabina Castelfranco, my Rome asset, for all her help with research, reporting, and translation in Italy. The trip to Bari would not have been nearly as productive—or fun—without her. The author Francesco Morra was also a great help, and he provided invaluable information about the impact of the disaster on his hometown of Bari. I have Roberto Dall'Angelo of SD Cinematografica to thank for the rare morning-after images of the catastrophe.

This book involved hundreds of hours spent ransacking the National Archives in both the US and the UK. I am hugely indebted to my talented and resourceful research assistant, Ruth Tenenbaum, whose terrierlike instincts unearthed many buried treasures. She alone managed to track down Alexander's original classified 1942 report on the captured sample of German nitrogen mustard gas, Compound 1130, which Edgewood Arsenal informed us was lost. She spent more days than either of us care to count helping me go through the documents, catching things I missed or might never have noticed. This was our sixth book together, and at this point she knows what I am looking for before I do. I cannot thank her enough.

I also received tremendous assistance at The National Archives UK from Simon Fowler, who helped decipher the intricacies of the censorship process, and fielded dozens of requests to dig deeper. Also at the National Archives at College Park, Tim Nenninger, and in NARA St. Louis, George Fuller, who ventured into the "burn bay" to look through sealed refrigerated units containing personnel records damaged in the 1973 fire. Holly Reed and Michael Bloomfield helped to find the still photographs. Steve Greene of Historicity is responsible for the fine reproductions of faded World War II images. Thank you to Duane Miller at the U.S. Army War College Library, Valoise Armstrong and Mary Burtzloff at the Dwight D. Eisenhower Presidential Library and Museum, and to the entire staff of the Library of Congress. A very special thank you to Susan D. Weil of Memorial Sloan Kettering Cancer Center and her compliance office for making every effort to secure the copyrights and permissions for the photographs provided to me from their collection.

I am also indebted to numerous doctors and experts who helped elucidate the complex medical material, especially Dr. Vincent T. DeVita Jr., a pioneering figure in the history of chemotherapy, whose writings helped inform this book. Also the brilliant Dr. Charles Sawyers, who took the time to read the work-in-progress, made insightful suggestions, and saved me from some embarrassing errors. Those that remain are my own. I am most appreciative of his assistance. Dr. Michael Nevins contributed important background information about his colleague and friend Dr. Stewart F. Alexander, guided me to other doctors and nurses who knew him, and sent me related medical books and articles.

I am lucky to be surrounded by a wonderful team. Kris Dahl, my longtime agent, has been a constant source of support and encouragement. I must record my immense gratitude to my editor, John Glusman, for having faith in this book from the very beginning. I am deeply indebted to him and his Norton team, particularly Helen Thomaides, for their care and attention to the manuscript, and Kathleen Brandes for her meticulous copyediting. Morgan Entrekin of Grove Atlantic was typically generous with his advice, and I am fortunate to have him as my British publisher.

Last but not least, I must thank Cavelle Sukhai for keeping the world at bay while I disappeared everyday into my foxhole. For cheering me on through thick and thin, my heartfelt thanks to James Jacoby and Tav Holmes. My mother was a lively interlocutor and her unfailing enthusiasm for the project week in and week out helped me see it to completion.

Above all, I wish to thank my husband, Steve, and son, John, my bag man and companion in Bari, for being my champions. After listening to so many war stories for so many years, they insisted I tell this one. Now that I come to the end, there are no words to express my gratitude. I dedicate this book to them.

Jennet Conant, Sag Harbor, 2019

Notes

Prologue: "Little Pearl Harbor"

ix **When the two:** The movements and observations of Will Lang and George Rodger come from Will Lang, Will Lang notebooks, 1943–1945, notebook #9, "Bari Raid," USMA Special Collections, West Point.

x   **"Knocked out":** Vincent Orange, *Coningham: A Biography of Air Marshal Sir Arthur Coningham* (Washington DC: Center for Air Force History, 1992), 175; Dwight D. Eisenhower, *Crusade in Europe* (London: William Heinemann, 1948), p. 226.

xi **The invasion of Sicily:** Details are drawn from Lang, notebooks; Rick Atkinson, *The Day of the Battle: The War in Sicily and Italy, 1943–1944* (New York: Henry Holt, 2007); Samuel Eliot Morison, *Sicily–Salerno–Anzio* (Boston: Little, Brown, 1962); Richard Lamb, *War in Italy 1943–1945: A Brutal Story* (New York: Da Capo Press, 1993).

xiii **"snail's progress":** "Snail's Progress," *Time*, Dec. 27, 1943.

xiii **"misery march":** Dispatches from *Time* Magazine Correspondents: First Series, 1925–1955, Will Lang (MS Am 2090 112), Houghton Library, Harvard University.

xiii **"There are no":** Jon B. Mikolashek, *General Mark Clark: Commander of U.S. Fifth Army and Liberator of Rome* (Philadelphia: Casemate, 2013), p. 66.

xiii **"They don't seem to have":** Lang, notebooks.

xiv **"*Madonna, Madonna mia*":** Lang, notebooks; "Disaster at Bari," *Time*, Dec. 27, 1943.

xv **"There goes Monty's":** Dispatches from Time Magazine Correspondents: First

Series, 1925–1955, Will Lang (MS Am 2090 112), Houghton Library, Harvard University.

xv   **"Let's get out"**: Ibid.

xv   **"Fiery panorama"**: Ibid.

xvi   **"Help, help!"**: Ibid.

xvi   **"There are a lot"**: Ibid.

xvi   **"damage was done"**: "Bari Facts," *Time,* Dec. 27, 1943; *New York Times*, Dec. 16, 1943.

xvi   **"sneak attack"**: *Washington Post,* Dec. 16, 1943.

xvii **"napping"**: Ibid.

xvii **"No! I will not comment"**: "Bari Facts," *Time,* Dec. 27, 1943.

xvii **"Belated and patently embarrassed"**: Ibid.

xvii **Rocket-driven glide bomb**: *New York Times,* Dec. 6, 1943; *Los Angeles Times*, Dec. 17, 1943.

xvii **"Bari had all the makings"**: Robert J. Casey, *This Is Where I Came In* (New York: Bobbs-Merrill, 1945), p. 78.

xviii **"little Pearl Harbor"**: "Little Pearl Harbor," *Newsweek,* Dec. 27, 1943.

xviii **"You're going to hear"**: "Bari Facts," *Time,* Dec. 27, 1943.

Chapter One: "A Regiment of Wizards"

1–2   **"Red light"**: Stewart F. Alexander, "Bari Harbor and the Origins of Chemotherapy," Lecture delivered at Englewood Hospital on Nov. 11, 1987, unpublished, SFAP; Stewart F. Alexander, "Bari Harbor—and the Origins of Chemotherapy for Cancer," *CML Army Chemical Review* (July 1990): pp. 21–26; Nicholas Spark interviews with S. F. Alexander, March 31 and April 4, 1987, NSP; Glenn B. Infield, *Disaster at Bari* (New York: Macmillan, 1971), p. 179.

2   **"Expert advice"**: Ibid.; Stewart F. Alexander, "Final Report of the Bari Mustard Casualties," June 20, 1944, Appendix #1, "Memorandum by O i/c Surgical Division, 98th General Hospital, Dec. 5, 1943," SFAP and AFHQ, Office of the Surgeon, RG492, 704, box 1757, NARA.

3   **Overstretched hospitals**: Ibid.; WWII US Medical Research Center, "26th General Hospital," https://www.med-dept.com/unit-histories/26th-general, accessed June 2019.

3–6   **Alexander family background**: Stewart F. Alexander, *SFA: An Autobiography by Stewart F. Alexander,* ed. Judy Connelly, Unpublished, 1992, SFAP, pp. 1–7. Stewart F. Alexander, "Samuel Alexander, M.D., and the Uniform Medical Practice Act," *Journal of the Medical Society of New Jersey,* vol. 81, no. 9 (Sept. 1984): pp. 759–62.

6   **"Available any time"**: Alexander, *SFA*, p. 8.

6 **"We must do":** Ibid.

7 **"Well below":** Ibid.

8 **Patented gas-mask design:** Ibid.; *Bergen* [NJ] *Evening Record*, Nov. 23, 1943.

8 **"I really think":** Ibid., p. 18.

8–9 **"harden," "Won't I get into trouble":** Alexander, *SFA*, pp. 13–14.

9 **"Exciting":** Ibid., p. 33.

9 **"investigation, development, manufacture":** Al Mauroni, "The U.S. Army Chemical Corps: Past, Present and Future," Army Historical Foundation, Jan. 28, 2015; the history of the Chemical Warfare Service (CWS) was drawn from Leo P. Brophy and George J. B. Fisher, *United States Army in World War II: The Technical Services. The Chemical Warfare Service: Organizing for War* (Washington, DC: Center of Military History, 1989), pp. 18–23.

9 **"Let Us Rule":** Mauroni, "The U.S. Army Chemical Corps: Past, Present and Future."

9 **"defensive necessities":** Brophy and Fisher, *Organizing for War,* p. 22.

10 **"every living soul":** *New York Times*, Jan. 3, 1943.

10 **king of battle gases:** Robert Harris and Jeremy Paxman. *A Higher Form of Killing: The Secret Story of Chemical and Biological Warfare* (New York: Hill and Wang, 1982), p. 42.

10 **He learned to identify:** Alexander, *SFA*, pp. 26–27.

11 **Chart of Chemical Warfare Agents:** Chemical Warfare Service, 1942, SFAP.

11 **Medical Research Laboratory:** Alexander, *SFA*, pp. 26–29; Edgewood Arsenal Medical Research Division bulletins, memoranda, and reports 1941–1942, SFAP; Brooks E. Kleber, and Dale Birdsell. *The Chemical Warfare Service: Chemicals in Combat. USAWWII* (Washington DC: United States Army, 1966), pp. 90–93.

12 **"It's the natural fear":** *New York Times,* Jan. 3, 1943.

13 **CWS budget soared:** Harris and Paxman, pp. 116–17; Jonathan B. Tucker, *War of Nerves: Chemical Warfare from World War I to Al-Qaeda* (New York: Anchor Books, 2006), p. 89.

14 **"The Supreme Court":** *New York Times,* Jan. 3, 1943.

14 **"Smoke saves blood":** Ibid.

15 **"It will look better":** Alexander, *SFA*, p. 27.

15 **"a very heady time":** Ibid., p. 28.

15 **"defensive preparedness":** Kleber and Birdsell, *Chemicals in Combat,* p. 48.

16 **1925 Geneva Protocol and details of German gas production:** Harris and Paxman, *A Higher Form of Killing*, pp. 44–45, 51.

16 **gas at Yichang:** *Time,* Feb. 1, 1943. Barton J. Bernstein, "Why We Didn't Use Poison Gas in World War II," *American Heritage*, vol. 35, issue 5 (Aug./Sept. 1985).

16 **"authenticated reports":** *New York Times*, Jan. 3, 1943.

17 **"horror propaganda":** Ibid.

17 **"The best defense":** Ibid.

17 **"perverted science":** Winston S. Churchill, *Churchill: The Power of Words*, ed. Martin Gilbert (New York: Da Capo Press, 2013), p. 394.

17 **"the attitude of the British government":** Ibid.

17 **"I wish now to make plain":** "World Battlefronts: Gas," *Time*, May 18, 1942; Brophy and Fisher, *Organizing for War*, p. 63; Edward M. Spiers, *Chemical Warfare* (New York: Palgrave Macmillan, 1986), p. 73.

18 **"drew on everything":** Eisenhower, *Crusade in Europe*, p. 69.

18 **"To preserve the image":** Harris and Paxman, *A Higher Form of Killing*, p. 115.

18 **Axis powers were unlikely to conduct gas warfare:** Kleber and Birdsell, *Chemicals in Combat*, p. 75.

19 **Eisenhower's cable:** Alexander, *SFA*, pp. 33–34.

20 **"evolve as needed":** Ibid., p. 35.

20 **"a regiment of wizards":** Kleber and Birdsell, *Chemicals in Combat*, p. 91.

20 **Western Task Force:** Alexander, *SFA*, p. 35.

21 **"Well, I'll fix you":** Ibid., p. 38.

21 **"Yes, Sir, I have very little knowledge":** Ibid.

21 **naval battle at Casablanca:** William Manchester and Paul Reid, *The Last Lion: Winston Spencer Churchill, Defender of the Realm (1940–1965)* (New York: Little, Brown, 2012), pp. 585–87; Charles M. Wiltse, *The United States Army in the Second World War, Technical Services, The Medical Department in the Mediterranean Theater and Minor Theaters* (Washington, DC: Office of the Chief of Military History, 1965), pp. 116–20; Rick Atkinson, *An Army at Dawn: The War in North Africa, 1942–1943* (New York: Henry Holt, 2002), pp. 130–40.

22 **"very haphazard":** Alexander, *SFA*, p. 39.

22 **Casablanca Conference:** Ibid., p. 40–43; Meredith Hindley, *Destination Casablanca: Exile, Espionage and the Battle for North Africa in World War II* (New York: Public Affairs, 2017), pp. 351–55.

22 **"potential hazards":** Alexander, *SFA*, p. 40.

23 **Anfa Hotel:** Hindley, *Destination Casablanca*, p. 352.

25 **"shot in the arm":** Alexander, *SFA*, p. 42.

25 **"unconditional surrender":** Atkinson, *An Army at Dawn*, p. 294.

25 **"small potato," "I don't know":** Stewart F. Alexander to his parents, Feb. 2, 1943, SFAP and Rauner Special Collections Library, Dartmouth College, Hanover, NH.

25 **"splendid manner":** Letter of Commendation from Roosevelt to Eisenhower, Jan. 27, 1943, and copy sent by Brigadier General T. J. Davis to Alexander, SFAP.

26 **"bulldog meeting a tomcat":** Eisenhower, *Crusade in Europe*, p. 85.

26 **"unity of purpose":** Ibid.; Alexander, *SFA*, pp. 44–45.

26   **"I'm rather glad":** Alexander, *SFA*, p. 45.1.

28   **"all at loose ends":** Edward D. Churchill, *Surgeon to Soldiers: Diary and Records of the Surgical Consultant, Allied Force Headquarters, World War II* (Philadelphia: J. B. Lippincott, 1972), p. 82.

28   **"steal":** Alexander, *SFA*, p. 47.

29   **Air evacuation:** Ibid., pp. 45–46. Details of air transport in the Tunisia campaign were also drawn from Wiltse, *Medical Department in the Mediterranean*, p. 204.

29   **Defeat at Kasserine Pass:** Details of the Kasserine battle are drawn from Eisenhower, *Crusade in Europe*, pp. 163–64, 172.

29   **"Pack and run":** Albert E. Cowdrey, *Fighting for Life: American Military Medicine in World War II* (New York: Free Press, 1994), p. 118.

30   **"bleak, difficult place":** Alexander, *SFA*, p. 54.

30   **"The sooner they give":** Stewart F. Alexander to his parents, Feb. 2, 1943, SFAP and RSC.

30   **fears of chemical warfare heightened:** Spiers, *Chemical Warfare*, pp. 76–77; Stephen L. McFarland, "Preparing for What Never Came: Chemical and Biological Warfare in World War II," *Defense Analysis,* vol. 2, no. 2, 1986, pp. 107–8.

30   **"capable of initiating":** AFHQ, Secret Operation Memorandum, Chemical Warfare Policy, April 23, 1943, Records of the Chemical Warfare Service, RG 175 1917–1994, 175.2, NARA.

31   **"though less remote than hitherto," "Hitler, faced," "British resources":** Spiers, *Chemical Warfare*, p. 77; *New York Times*, April 23, 1943.

31   **"increasing unease," "military sources":** UPI, April 22, 1943.

31   **"likely to employ," "pulling down the pillars":** *New York Times*, April 22, 1943.

31   **"making significant preparations," "shall under no":** Harris and Paxman, *A Higher Form of Killing*, p. 118.

32   **"made the most minute preparations":** Spiers, *Chemical Warfare*, p. 77.

32   **"threatened that if Italy":** Prime Minister to Gen. Ismay for Chiefs of Staff, TNA: PREM 3/88/3; Atkinson, *Day of the Battle*, p. 272.

32   **"gas reprisals":** Spiers, *Chemical Warfare*, p. 77.

32   **"call forth immediate":** Spiers, *Chemical Warfare*, p. 77.

33   **"Adolf will turn":** Spiers, *Chemical Warfare*, pp. 76–77; Atkinson, *Day of the Battle*, p. 272.

33   **Enigma decrypt:** Ibid.

33   ***Tentative Lessons Bulletins:*** Lina Grip and John Hart, "The Use of Chemical Weapons in the 1935–36 Italo-Ethiopian War," SIPRI Arms Control and Non-Proliferation Programme, October 2009, p. 4.

33   **Seronio chemical factory:** Spiers, *Chemical Warfare*, pp. 76–77.

33   **"It is probably":** Stewart F. Alexander letter to Col. William D. Fleming, Office of the Chief Surgeon, European Theater of Operations, Sept. 15, 1943, SFAP.

34   **Wehrmacht policy:** Spiers, *Chemical Warfare*, pp. 77–78; Comm. Walter Karig, Lt. Earl Burton, and Lt. Stephen L. Freeland, *Battle Report: The Atlantic War* (New York: Farrar & Rinehart, 1946), p. 272; Author interview with Dr. Vito Antonio Leuzzi, Bari, Italy, Oct. 2018.

34–35 **"The development," "among the first":** Alexander, *SFA*, pp. 27–28.

35   **AFHQ October 13, 1943 minute** is also cited as the chemical-weapons policy "for the maintenance of Italy," in "Report on the Circumstances in Which Gas Casualties Were Incurred at Bari on December 2/3, 1943," March 14, 1944, RG 492, MTO, Chemical Warfare Section, 350.01 (entry 166, box 1747, loc 290/54/16/6), NARA; "Implementation of Theater Plans for Gas Warfare," August 18, 1943, War Department, and related Chemical Warfare Service operations memoranda dated April 23, Aug. 30, and Sept. 7, 1943, RG 492, MTO, Chemical Warfare Section, 381, box 1706, NARA; TNA: WO 204/5452.

35   **"We were always":** Eisenhower, *Crusade in Europe*, p. 226.

Chapter Two: "The Die Is Cast"

36   **"Their agitation":** Alexander, "Bari Harbor," lecture.

37   ***"Acqua, acqua":*** George Southern, *Poisonous Inferno: World War II Tragedy at Bari Harbour* (Shrewsbury, UK: Airlife Publishing, 2002), p. 70. Details of the bomb damage and aftermath in Bari are also drawn from Amy Louise Outterside, "Occupying Puglia: The Italians and the Allies, 1943–1946" (PhD diss., University of Newcastle upon Tyne, 2015), pp. 52–58; Author interview with Dr. Vito Antonio Leuzzi, and Dr. Pasquale Trizio, Bari, Italy, Oct. 2018.

37   **98th British General Hospital:** Gwladys M. Rees Aikens, *Nurses in Battledress: The World War II Story of a Member of the Q.A. Reserves* (Halifax: Nimbus Publishing, 1998), pp. 83–85.

38   **"With every fresh":** Cocks, E. M. Somers, *Kia-Kaha: Life at 3 New Zealand General Hospital 1940–1946* (Christchurch, NZ: Caxton Press, 1958), pp. 242–45.

38   **nightmarish scene:** Ibid.; Aikens, *Nurses in Battledress*, pp. 89–90; Scott Jeavons, "Big Bang at Bari," *Blackwood's Magazine*, vol. 261, June 1947, p. 462; Stanley Scislowski, *Not All of Us Were Brave* (Toronto: Dundurn Press, 1997), p. 93; Infield, *Disaster at Bari*, pp. 127–28.

39   **"death ward":** Southern, *Poisonous Inferno*, p. 89.

40   **"considerably puzzled," "immersion" cases:** Alexander, "Final Report," Appendix no. 1.

40   **"smarting eyes":** Ibid.

40 **"such a nuisance":** Southern, *Poisonous Inferno*, p. 93.

40 **"cot case":** Jeavons, "Big Bang at Bari," p. 462.

40 **"We worked":** Aikens, *Nurses in Battledress*, p. 90.

40 **"unusual":** Stewart F. Alexander, "Toxic Gas Burns Sustained in the Bari Harbor Catastrophe," Dec. 27, 1943, cited hereafter as "Preliminary Report," included in Alexander, "Final Report."

41 **"rather well":** Ibid.

41 **"No treatment":** Stewart F. Alexander to William D. Fleming, Dec. 26, 1943, RG 112, MTO surgeon general, 390/17/8/2–3. 319.1, box 6, NARA.

41–42 **"odd," "as big as balloons":** Aikens, *Nurses in Battledress*, p. 91.

42 **"We began to realize":** Ibid.

42 **"gritty, as though":** Alexander, "Preliminary Report."

42 **"Force them to open":** Ibid.; Alexander, "Final Report," Appendix #3, "Report of Ophthalmologist, 98th General Hospital."

42 **"eye teams":** Ibid.

43 **"as rumors were heard":** Ibid.

43 **"Dermatitis N.Y.D.":** "Report on Circumstances," NARA.

43 **"Among the battle casualties":** Cocks, *Kia-Kaha*, p. 243.

44 **"good condition":** Alexander, "Preliminary Report."

44 **"much mental anguish":** Alexander, "Final Report."

44 **"With what little knowledge":** Aikens, *Nurses in Battledress*, p. 91.

45 **"We did everything":** Ibid.

45 **"That's when the rumors":** Warren Brandenstein, *2 Dicembre 1943: Hell over Bari*, documentary, directed by Fabio Toncelli, script by Fabio Toncelli and Francesco Morra, Rome: SD Cinematografica, 2014.

45 **"Their eyes asked":** Aikens, *Nurses in Battledress*, p. 91.

46 **"early death," "as dramatic":** Alexander, "Preliminary Report."

46 **"Individuals that appeared":** Ibid.

46 **"cyanosed and respirations":** Alexander, "Final Report," Appendix #4 "Representative Case Records."

46 **"abruptly died":** Alexander, "Preliminary Report."

46 **"no prognostic signs":** "Report on Circumstances," NARA.

47 **"no or only very minimal":** Alexander, "Preliminary Report."

47 **"not conform," "official manual":** Alexander, "Final Report," Appendix #1.

47 **"At the moment":** Ibid.

48 **"considerable anxiety":** D.D.M.S. 2 DIST., Col. J. H. Bayley, War Diary, Dec. 1–31, 1943, UK National Archives UK NA: WO 177/133.

48 **"strange deaths":** Alexander, "Bari Harbor," lecture.

49 **"certain patterns":** Alexander, "Preliminary Report."

50 **The three most common blister agents:** Description of poison gases taken from

"Medical Bulletin No. 17," Office of the Chief Surgeon, European Theatre of Operations, March 15, 1944, SFAP; Rudolph Hecht, "The Dermatologic Aspects of Chemical Warfare," Office of the Chief Surgeon, European Theater of Operations, A.P.O. 871, SFAP; Harris and Paxman, *A Higher Form of Killing*, pp. 24–27.

51   **"textbook":** Alexander, "Final Report."

51   **"twelve to fourteen hours":** Alexander, "Preliminary Report."

51   **"rather dilute":** Ibid.

51   **"strikingly brawny":** Ibid.

53   **"unfortunate souls":** Alexander, "Bari Harbor," lecture.

53   **"almost absolute correlation":** Alexander, "Final Report."

53   **"What is that odor?":** Infield, p. 181; Alexander, "Bari Harbor," lecture; Rosemary Lunardini, "The Birth of a Notion," *Dartmouth Medical School Alumni Magazine,* Fall 1988, pp. 17–21; Interview with Alexander by Nicholas Spark, March 31, 1987, NSP.

53   **"Traces of an odor":** Alexander, "Bari Harbor—and the Origins of Chemotherapy."

54   **"I feel these men," "None":** Infield, p. 182.

54   **"Have you checked," "I have":** Ibid.

55   **"highest degree":** Interview with Alexander by Nicholas Spark, March 31, 1987, NSP.

55   **"careful and complete":** Alexander, "Bari Harbor—and the Origins of Chemotherapy," p. 23.

55   **"great protest," "Did he not know":** Alexander, "Bari Harbor," lecture.

56   **"Certain of the scientific":** Alexander, "Final Report."

56   **"remarkable that no":** Alexander, "Preliminary Report."

56–57 **"Some of the survivors," "In the hustle":** Ibid.

57   **"rumor," "A rumor had been heard":** Ibid.

57   **"obtain no verification":** Alexander, "Final Report."

58   **"No attempt was made," "It must be,":** Alexander, "Preliminary Report."

58   **"The speed with which":** Memorandum to All Medical Officers, Task Force "A," October 10, 1942; and many similar CWS bulletins and memoranda, SFAP.

58   **"The die is cast":** *Post Review,* May 26, 1988.

59   **"absolutely denied":** Alexander, "Bari Harbor," lecture.

59   **"Something funny":** Interview with Alexander by Nicholas Spark, March 31, 1987, NSP.

59   **"gut feeling," "mustard gas poisoning":** Alexander, "Bari Harbor," lecture.

Chapter Three: "Angels in Long Underwear"

60   **"significant grief":** Alexander, "Bari Harbor," lecture, SFAP.

60   **responsible for 4,500 nurses:** *The Record* (Bergen County, NJ), Nov. 30, 2005.

61 **"carefully take down," "strong-willed":** Alexander, *SFA*, p. 49.

61 **"an obstructionist," "fought over the phone":** Ibid., p. 51.

61–62 **Red Cross–Harvard Field Hospital Unit, "Typhoid Mary":** Pete Martin, "Angels in Long Underwear," *Saturday Evening Post*, July 31, 1943; Gertrude Madley, *Bulletin of the American Association of Nurse Anesthetists,* May 1994; "My Assignment as a Red Cross Nurse," *The Record* (Bergen County, NJ), Nov. 30, 2005.

62 **North Africa invasion:** *New York Times*, May 21, 1943; Martin, "Angels in Long Underwear."

63 **"night and day," "The biggest":** *New York Times,* Oct. 28, 1943.

63 **"hid his clothes," "Boston Nurse":** *Daily Boston Globe*, April 27, 1943; Martin, "Angels in Long Underwear."

63 **"in an awful hurry":** *Daily Boston Globe,* April 27, 1943.

63 **Round-trip ticket:** "On Leave from Africa," *The American Journal of Nursing*, vol. 43, no. 6 (June 1943): p. 559.

64 **promotion and impromptu ceremony:** Martin, "Angels in Long Underwear."

64 **"so that others":** *Harrisburg* [PA] *Telegraph,* June 4, 1943.

64 **"I'd tell her":** Martin, "Angels in Long Underwear."

64–65 **"facing the horrors," "her girls":** Ibid.

65 **"Wilburnice":** Transcript of dedication speech at opening of the nurses' villa, SFAP.

65 **"Let's pray together":** Alexander, *SFA*, pp. 56–57; Eisenhower, *Crusade in Europe*, pp. 198–201.

65 **"General, I guess":** Eisenhower, *Crusade in Europe*, p. 198.

65 **"nervous":** Atkinson, *An Army at Dawn*, pp. 147–48.

65–66 **"You coward," "gutless bastards":** Ibid.

66 **"I can't help it":** Ibid.

66 **"slapping incidents":** Eisenhower, *Crusade in Europe*, p. 198.

67 **"I must so seriously":** Martin Blumenson, *The Patton Papers: 1940–1945* (New York: Houghton Mifflin, 1974), pp. 328–30.

67 **"Tell me why," "I didn't do anything":** Alexander, *SFA*, p. 57.

67 **"shirking":** Eisenhower, *Crusade in Europe*, p. 199.

67 **exhaustion:** Cowdrey, *Fighting for Life*, p. 142.

68 **"Old Blood & Guts":** Edward Churchill, *Surgeon to Soldiers*, p. 478.

68 **"If you have two":** Cowdrey, *Fighting for Life*, p. 132.

68 **"a maniac driving":** Ibid.

68 **"The problem," "Of course":** Alexander, *SFA*, p. 58.

69 **"It is impossible":** Edward Churchill, *Surgeon to Soldiers,* p. 8.

69 **"frantic but somewhat fruitless," "hush-hush":** Ibid.

69 **blast injuries:** Ibid.

69–70 **"great gaps," "disaster management":** Ibid., pp. 18, 20.

70   **Cocoanut Grove fire:** Edward Churchill, "Management of the Cocoanut Grove Burns at the Massachusetts General Hospital," Office of the Surgeon General, May 24, 1943; Jeffrey R. Saffle, "The 1942 Fire at Boston's Cocoanut Grove Night Club," *The American Journal of Surgery*, vol. 166 (Dec. 1993); Oliver Cope, MD, "Care of the Victims of the Cocoanut Grove Fire at the Massachusetts General Hospital," *New England Journal of Medicine* (July 22, 1943): pp. 138–47.

73   **"miracle drug":** Lesch, John E., *The First Miracle Drugs: How the Sulfa Drugs Transformed Medicine* (Oxford: Oxford University Press, 2007), p. 3; "Champ Lyons: Brief Life of an Innovative Surgeon: 1907–1965," *Harvard Magazine*, May–June 2016.

73   **"rescue something":** Edward Churchill, *Surgeon to Soldiers*, p. 24.

73   **"essential to preserve an open mind":** Ibid.

73   **"When external violence":** Ibid.

Chapter Four: "Journey into the Nightmare"

74   **Description of bombed harbor and cleanup effort:** Jeavons, "Big Bang at Bari"; Capt. D. M. Saunders, "The Bari Incident," US Naval Institute *Proceedings*, vol. 93, no. 9 (Sept. 1967): pp. 35–39.

74   **"the ugly ducklings":** Peter Elphick, *Liberty: The Ships That Won the War* (Annapolis, MD: Naval Institute Press), pp. 18–19.

76   **Hitler might wage gas warfare:** Alexander, "Bari Harbor," lecture, SFAP; Interviews with Alexander by Nicholas Spark, March 31 and April 4, 1987, NSP; Circular Letter No. 5, "Nitrogen Mustards," Office of the Chief Surgeon, European Theater of Operations APO 871, April 13, 1943, SFAP; Mark D. Arvidson, "A Mustard Agent Tragedy—the air raid on Bari," *CML Army Chemical Review* (July 1994).

76   **"The Germans are now known":** Most Secret, "Memorandum on a New German Odourless Gas," 1943, pp. 8–10, SFAP.

76   **"The principal danger":** Ibid.

76–77 **Substance "S," "Winterlost":** CWS Memorandum, undated, SFAP; Joel A. Vilensky, *Dew of Death: The Story of Lewisite, America's World War I Weapon of Mass Destruction* (Bloomington: Indiana University Press, 2005), p. 102; Constance M. Pechura and David P. Rall, eds., *Veterans at Risk: The Health Effects of Mustard Gas and Lewisite* (Washington, DC: National Academy Press, 1993), p. 22.

77   **"spray attack":** Hecht, "The Dermatologic Aspects of Chemical Warfare, Office of the Chief Surgeon, European Theater of Operations, A. P. O. 871, SFAP;

77   **"Zahlost":** Alexander to Col. E. P. Rhoads, Office of the Chief of the Chemical Warfare Service, Sept. 14, 1943, SFAP.

77 **"thickened mustard preparations"**: Alexander to Col. E. P. Rhoads, Office of the Chief of the Chemical Warfare Service, Sept. 14, 1943, SFAP.

78 **Germans possessed bombs:** Alexander to Col. Charles S. Shadle, Chief Chemical Officer, AFHQ, December 2, 1943, SFAP; Hecht, "The Dermatologic Aspects of Chemical Warfare, Office of the Chief Surgeon, European Theater of Operations, A. P. O. 871, SFAP.

78 **"full blast"**: Alexander to Col. Rhoads, Sept. 14, 1943, SFAP.

79 **"nursemaid squad"**: "Bari Air Raid," Dec. 1943, UK NA: 17 ADM 199/739.

80 **No Smoking!:** *2 Dicembre 1943: Hell over Bari,* doc., Toncelli.

80 **"Mustard?" "That's impossible":** Interviews with Alexander by Nicholas Spark, March 31 and April 4, 1987, NSP.

81 **"state categorically":** Alexander, "Bari Harbor—and the Origins of Chemotherapy," p. 23.

81 **"unity of purpose":** Eisenhower, *Crusade in Europe,* p. 85.

81 **"It is imperative":** Alexander, "Final Report."

81 **Of the 534 men:** D.D.M.S. 2 DIST., Col. J. H. Bayley, War Diary, Dec. 1–31, 1943, UK NA: WO 177/133; Alexander, "Preliminary Report."

81 **"it could only":** Alexander, "Bari Harbor—and the Origins of Chemotherapy," p. 23.

82 **diver sent down:** Ibid.; Alexander, "Bari Harbor," lecture; Lunardini, "The Birth of a Notion"; Karel Margry, "Mustard Disaster at Bari," *After the Battle,* no. 79, 1993.

83 **"no trace of mustard":** "Report on Circumstances," NARA.

83–84 **"To understand," "pattern had been made clear":** Alexander, "Final Report."

84 **"Reading the reports":** Alexander in *2 Dicembre 1943: Hell over Bari,* doc., Toncelli.

84 **preliminary postmortem results:** Alexander, "Final Report," Appendix #4.

85 **Seaman Stone, "early deaths," "A generalized," "curious black":** Ibid.

86 **Seaman McLaughlin chart, "living tissue":** Ibid.

87 **"It would appear":** Alexander, "Final Report."

88 **"Blast Deaths," "grave derangement":** Alexander, "Preliminary Report."

89 **"a German airborne delivery":** Alexander, "Bari Harbor—and the Origins of Chemotherapy," p. 23.

89 **"Everyone, including the Post Commander":** Ibid.

89–90 **American M47A2 bombs:** Alexander, "Bari Harbor—and the Origins of Chemotherapy," p. 23; Margry, "Mustard Disaster at Bari"; USS *John Harvey*'s bill of lading in "Report on Circumstances," NARA; TNA: 17 ADM 199/739.

90 **many problems associated with the M47A1 bombs:** Thomas Spoehr, *CML Army Chemical Review* (January 1990): p. 33.

91 **Advised hospital staffs on proper treatment:** Alexander, "Bari Harbor—and

the Origins of Chemotherapy," p. 23; Alexander, "Bari Harbor," lecture; Margry, "Mustard Disaster at Bari"; "Report on Circumstances," NARA.

91   **"Sufficiently superior":** Alexander, "Preliminary Report."

91   **running list of treatments:** Ibid.

92–93 **great majority of patients, "treatment of choice," "a bit more poorly":** Ibid.

93–94 **"A casualty with burns," "a minimum of success," "relatively little effect":** Ibid.

94   **"most discouraging":** Alexander, "Final Report."

94   **"Allies' own supply":** Alexander, "Bari Harbor," lecture.

94   **"frightful international import," "If they were going to accuse":** Lunardini, "The Birth of a Notion."

95   **"Grave political implications":** Alexander, "Bari Harbor," lecture.

95   **"fullest possible retaliation":** Alexander, "Bari Harbor—and the Origins of Chemotherapy," p. 24.

95   **"The political significance":** Ibid.

95   **Death toll spiked:** Alexander, "Preliminary Report."

96   **"The burns in the hospitals":** Alexander to DDMS AFHQ, December 11, 1943, in Alexander, "Final Report," Appendix #1.

97   **"Please keep me":** Alexander, "Bari Harbor," lecture; Alexander, "Bari Harbor—and the Origins of Chemotherapy," p. 24; Nadine Epstein, "MD Remembers Role in Treating WII's Bari Victims," *American Medical News*, Oct. 9, 1987; Margry, "Mustard Disaster at Bari"; Infield, *Disaster at Bari*, pp. 203–4.

97   **"your man in the field":** Interview with Alexander by Nicholas Spark, March 31, 1987, NSP.

97   **"proof," "we not acknowledge," "scientist on the ground":** Epstein, "MD Remembers Role in Treating WII's Bari Victims."

98   **"beyond any doubt":** Alexander, "Bari Harbor," lecture.

98   **"the symptoms," "The doctor should reexamine":** Alexander, "Bari Harbor—and the Origins of Chemotherapy," p. 24; Lunardini, "The Birth of a Notion," p. 19.

98   **"strange exchange," "lowly, lonely American":** Alexander, "Bari Harbor," lecture; Margry, "Mustard Disaster at Bari."

Chapter Five: "A Special Affinity"

99   **most important question:** Alexander, "Bari Harbor—and the Origins of Chemotherapy," p. 25.

99–100 **World War I fatality rate, "minimally present":** Ibid.

100   **"In this group of cases":** Alexander, "Preliminary Report."

100   **"The effect upon the white blood cells":** Alexander, "Final Report."

101 **"It all added up":** Barbara T. Musso, "Medical Detective Work: Chemotherapy Owes Debt to Dr. Stewart Alexander," *Pascack Valley* [NJ] *Community Life*, July 16, 1980.

101 **"If mustard could":** Ibid.

102 **Classified samples tested:** Alexander, *SFA*, p. 31; Alexander, "Bari Harbor," lecture; Alexander, "Bari Harbor—and the Origins of Chemotherapy," p. 21.

102 **Structure of nitrogen mustard compounds:** Ibid.

103 **Experiments on compound 1130:** T. W. Kethley and C. B. Marquand, MD (EA) Memorandum Report 59, *Preliminary Report on Hematological Changes in the Rabbit Following Exposure to Lethal Doses of 1130* (June 30, 1942), National Library of Medicine.

103 **"normalcy," "The changes":** Ibid.

104 **"bad batch of rabbits":** Alexander, *SFA*, p. 31.

104 **"shrunken little shells":** Ibid.

105 **Twenty-one copies distributed:** T. W. Kethley and C. B. Marquand, MD (EA) Memorandum Report 59; Alexander, "Bari Harbor—and the Origins of Chemotherapy," p. 22.

106 **History of poison as a cure:** M. Weatherall, *In Search of a Cure: A History of Pharmaceutical Discovery* (Oxford: Oxford University Press, 1990), pp. 3–45; Guy B. Faguet, *The War on Cancer: An Anatomy of a Failure, A Blueprint for the Future* (Dordrecht: Springer, 2005), pp. 28–35.

106–7 **"antitoxins," "chemotherapies":** Weatherall, *In Search of a Cure*, pp. 55–64; Morton A. Meyers, *Happy Accidents: Serendipity in Major Medical Breakthroughs in the Twentieth Century* (New York: Arcade, 2007), pp. 39–47.

107 **"special affinity," "magic bullet":** Ibid.

107 **poison gas as useful medicine:** "Medicine: Gas Therapy," *Time*, May 12, 1923; Thomas Faith, " 'As Is Proper in Republican Form of Government': Selling Chemical Warfare to Americans in the 1920s," *Federal History online*, 2010, p. 34.

108 **"all of the depression":** Ibid., p. 35.

108 **Vedder's defense of gas:** Ibid.; Vilensky, *Dew of Death*, p. 70.

109 **Winternitz background and character:** Dan A. Oren, *Joining the Club: A History of Jews and Yale* (New Haven, CT: Yale University Press, 1985), pp. 136–45.

109 **"Winter," "Napoleonic in outlook":** Averell A. Liebow and Levin L. Waters, "Milton Charles Winternitz, February 19, 1885–October 3, 1959," *Yale Journal of Biology and Medicine,* vol. 32 (December 1959): pp. 143, 145.

110 **"bizarre blood findings," "We found that the agent":** Alexander, "Bari Harbor—and the Origins of Chemotherapy," p. 22.

110 **"unreliable," "if this did happen":** Alexander, *SFA*, pp. 32–33.

111 **"If such a thing," "a little bit":** Ibid.; Alexander, "Bari Harbor—and the Origins of Chemotherapy," p. 22.

111 **"mustard gas did, in truth"**: Ibid., p. 25.

112 **yelling for more blood tests**: Interview with Alexander by Nicholas Spark, March 31, 1987.

112 **First Seaman Theodore M. Fronko chart**: Alexander, "Final Report," Appendix #4.

113–14 **Ensign K. Vesole chart**: Ibid.

115 **"The striking features"**: Alexander, "Preliminary Report."

115 **Preparing samples for Edgewood**: Ibid.; Alexander, "Bari Harbor—and the Origins of Chemotherapy," pp. 24–25; Alexander, "Bari Harbor," lecture.

116 **"It was just rumors"**: Bob Wills, *2 Dicembre 1943: Hell over Bari,* doc., Toncelli.

116 **"warm, pleasant sensation"**: Ibid.; Southern, *Poisonous Inferno*, p. 54.

117 **"There were dead servicemen"**: Bob Wills, *2 Dicembre 1943: Hell over Bari,* doc., Toncelli.

117 **"Cover that man's face"**: Southern, *Poisonous Inferno*, p. 89.

117 **"He looked ever so young"**: Bob Wills, *2 Dicembre 1943: Hell over Bari,* doc., Toncelli.

117–18 **"proper coffins," "We had to take"**: Ibid.

118 **"We were most surprised," "Some of the guys"**: Ibid.

119 **"We were sworn"**: Ibid.

119 **"We were at a loss," "Most of those dear boys," "We felt so betrayed"**: Aikens, *Nurses in Battledress,* p. 92.

119 **Italian doctors recognized gas, sailors spread rumors**: Author interviews with Drs. Vito Antonio Leuzzi and Pasquale Trizio, Bari, Italy, Oct. 2018; Naval Command Bari, Prot. N. 771, "Deposizione del Comandante della R.N.A. Barletta Cap. Corv. Corrao Salvatore Rigaurdante il Sinistro Occorso la Sera del 1/12/43," Ufficio Storico Marina Militare (Archival Office of the Italian Navy), Rome.

119 **"stab-in the-back"**: Author interviews with Drs. Vito Antonio Leuzzi and Pasquale Trizio, Bari, Italy, Oct. 2018.

120 **"There were thousands," "no explanation"**: Interview with Francis James Vail by Eileen M. Hurst, Sept. 4, 2004, Veterans History Project, Library of Congress.

120 **"security issue," "very few casualties," "strong offshore wind"**: Nicholas Spark interview with Alexander, March 31, 1987.

121 **"Sharing an underground"**: Southern, *Poisonous Inferno*, p. 102.

121 **Italian response to bombing**: Author interviews with Drs. Vito Antonio Leuzzi and Pasquale Trizio, Bari, Italy, Oct. 2018; Author interview with Francesco Morra, Rome, Oct. 2018; also, Outterside, "Occupying Puglia," pp. 17–20, 57–58.

122 **"USE OF TOXIC GAS"**: Telegram from COMINCH and CN to CINCLANT, CINCPAC, COMNAVEU, etc., Dec. 15, 1943, Map Room Papers, Box 103, MR 302, Sec. 1–Chemical Warfare 1942–1945, NARA.

122–23 **"would be effective," "initiating use of gas":** Ibid., Naval message from CINCLANT to COMINCH, Dec. 18, 1943.

123 **Nazi SS heard rumors:** Glenn B. Infield, *Secrets of the SS* (New York: Military Heritage Press, 1981), pp. 91–93.

123 **"The Allies could begin":** Atkinson, *The Day of the Battle*, p. 278.

123 **"I see you boys":** Ibid.; Infield, *Disaster at Bari*, p. 207; Nicholas Spark interview with Alexander, April 4, 1987.

124 **"Axis Sally was right":** Lunardini, "The Birth of a Notion."

Chapter Six: "Recommendation to Secrecy"

126 **"mental picture":** Alexander, "Bari Harbor—and the Origins of Chemotherapy," p. 24.

126 **Port defenses weak and phone line out of order:** Air Ministry and Ministry of Defence, Royal Air Force Overseas Commands, reports and correspondence, 242 GROUP, Air Attacks on Italy, 1943, TNA: AIR 23/1481.

126 **"on a plate":** TNA: AIR 23/1481.

127 **Mooring positions:** Drawn from "Bari Berthing Plan" on the night of Dec. 2, 1943, TNA: ADM 1/24248.

128 **Sketch of "Ship Positions 2 Dec. 1943":** Alexander, "Final Report," SFAP, NARA; also in "Report on Circumstances," NARA.

128 **"war supplies" and other cargo descriptions:** "Summary Statements by Survivors of the SS *John Bascom*," Office of the Chief of Naval Operations, Memorandum for File, 28 February 1944, TNA: AIR 23/1481; Infield, *Disaster at Bari*, p. 275; Southern, *Poisonous Inferno*, pp. 7–8.

129 **"walked," order in which the ships were bombed:** Margry, "Mustard Disaster at Bari"; Arthur R. Moore, *A Careless Word . . . A Needless Sinking* (Kings Point, NY: American Merchant Marine Museum at the US Merchant Marine Academy, 1983), p. 155; Saunders, "The Bari Incident," pp. 36–39.

129 **Sinking of *John Bascom*:** Ibid.; Karig, Burton, and Freeland, *Battle Report*, pp. 276–78.

130 **"This must be":** Southern, *Poisonous Inferno*, p. 69.

130 **heroic actions of Ensign "Kay" Vesole:** Karig, Burton, and Freeland, *Battle Report*, pp. 276–78; *Commendatory Conduct of Armed Guard Unit Assigned to SS Samuel J. Tilden, U.S. Cargo Ship* (Wash DC: Navy Dept., Office of Chief of Naval Operations, 18 January 1944).

131 **"huge Roman candle":** Jeavons, "Big Bang at Bari," p. 46.

131 **" 'Gas!' Many of the crew":** Alexander, "Preliminary Report," SFAP, NARA.

132 ***Bascom* crew rescued, Vesole taken to 98th General Hospital:** Margry, "Mus-

tard Disaster at Bari;" Karig, Burton, and Freeland, *Battle Report*, pp. 277–78; *The Daily Times,* Davenport, IA, March 12, 1944.

132 **"mysterious death":** Alexander, "Bari Harbor—and the Origins of Chemotherapy for Cancer," p. 21.

133 **"no longer existed":** Ibid., p. 23.

133 **casualty distribution chart:** Alexander, "Final Report," SFAP, NARA.

134 **breakdown of mustard deaths:** Ibid.; Lunardini, "The Birth of a Notion," p. 18.

134 **concern for mustard casualties diverted to other ports:** Nicholas Spark interview with Alexander, April 4, 1987, NSP.

135 **No information about Italians except for ten cases:** Alexander, "Final Report," SFAP, NARA.

135 **"held it up to their nose":** Nicholas Spark interview with Alexander, March 31, 1987, NSP.

136 **one hundred tons of mustard gas:** Alexander, "Bari Harbor—and the Origins of Chemotherapy for Cancer," p. 24; Margry, "Mustard Disaster at Bari"; Paxman and Harris, *A Higher Form of Killing*, p. 121.

136 **"acknowledged the mustard gas":** Alexander, "Bari Harbor," lecture; Alexander, "Bari Harbor—and the Origins of Chemotherapy," p. 24.

136 **"to deny the presence":** Ibid.

136 *John Harvey* **loaded with mustard at Oran, and official orders and invoice:** "Report on Circumstances," NARA.

136–37 **Official paper trail, shipping wire and manifest sent via air courier:** Ibid.

137 **"cargo of mustard gas":** Ibid.

137 **"U and E boat activities":** Ibid.

137 **"low priority," "in as safe a place":** Ibid.

137 **Wilkinson at wheel of his jeep and actions during raid:** Southern, *Poisonous Inferno*, p. 48.

138 **"dangerous," "scuttle":** "Report on Circumstances," NARA.

138 **"order every," "horror," "If you can't":** Marcus Sieff, *Don't Ask the Price: The Memoirs of the President of Marks & Spencer* (London: George Weidenfeld & Nicholson, 1987), pp. 124–25.

138 **Four messages:** "Report on Circumstances," NARA.

139 **"It picked me up":** Southern, *Poisonous Inferno*, p. 48.

139 **"a brilliant white light":** Ibid., p. 49.

139 **"a direct hit":** Sieff, *Don't Ask the Price*, p. 124.

139 **thirty broken casings, "tidal wave":** "Report on Circumstances," NARA.

139–40 **"just had time," "but with a thick":** Southern, *Poisonous Inferno*, p. 50.

140 **"gas in the dock area":** "Report on Circumstances," NARA.

140 **"definite," "general warning":** Ibid.

140 **2:15 p.m. meeting at harbormaster's office and decisions taken:** Ibid.

141 **"unanimous in their opinion," "in order to maintain":** Ibid.

141 **"Recommendation to secrecy":** Ibid.

142 **"No direct information":** Alexander, "Final Report," SFAP, NARA.

142 **"Mustard problem":** Nicholas Spark interview with Alexander, March 1987, NSP.

142 **"The cover-up," "It was the same factor":** *Mojave Daily Miner,* May 20, 1988.

143 **First inspection failed to detect toxic site:** "Report on Circumstances," NARA.

143 **"at least 2,000–3,000 pounds of mustard":** Alexander, "Preliminary Report," SFAP, NARA.

143 **"not of major degree":** Ibid.

144 **"It was the mixture," "The burns sustained":** Ibid.

145 **"young and foolhardy":** Alexander, "Bari Harbor," lecture, SFAP.

145 **"professional integrity":** Lunardini, "The Birth of a Notion," p. 21.

145 **"Gas has very few":** Tim Cook, *No Place to Run: The Canadian Corps and Gas Warfare in the First World War* (Canada: UBC Press, 2001), p. 4.

146 **"as if they were something":** Southern, *Poisonous Inferno*, p. xiv.

146 **full support of his superiors:** Epstein, "MD Remembers Role in Treating WII's Bari Victims," p. 54.

146 **"complicated the clinical":** Alexander, "Final Report," SFAP, NARA.

146 **"reexamined all the data," "If the Prime Minister":** Alexander, "Bari Harbor," lecture, SFAP; Alexander, "Bari Harbor—and the Origins of Chemotherapy," p. 24; Lunardini, "The Birth of a Notion," p. 19.

147 **Col. Bayley memo to Surgeon WFTD MED FLAMBO:** UK National Archives UK NA: WO 177/133.

147 **"burns due to enemy action":** Alexander, "Bari Harbor," lecture, SFAP; Alexander, "Bari Harbor—and the Origins of Chemotherapy," p. 24; Lunardini, "The Birth of a Notion," p. 19; Nicholas Spark interview with Alexander, April 4, 1987, NSP.

147–48 **"It was a high secret":** "Wartime Nursing in North Africa and Italy," Jessie Park Smith's experiences, accessed Sept. 16, 2019, http://www.bbc.co.uk/history/ww2peopleswar/stories/92/a2090792.shtml.

148 **"court martialed":** Alexander, "Bari Harbor," lecture, SFAP; Alexander, "Bari Harbor—and the Origins of Chemotherapy," p. 24; Lunardini, "The Birth of a Notion," p. 19; Nicholas Spark interview with Alexander, March 31, 1987, NSP.

148 **"safety and wellbeing":** Alexander, "Bari Harbor," lecture.

Chapter Seven: "Magnum Opus"

149 **"the closer you get":** Ernie Pyle, *Brave Men* (Lincoln, NE: Bison Books, 2001), p. 44.

149 **discovered a whole new group:** Alexander, "Bari Harbor," lecture, SFAP; Alexander, "Final Report," Appendix #2.

150 *Bicester* **crew contaminated, "odor of garlic":** Ibid.; Comm. Guinness's Comprehensive Report of Bari Air Raid, Reports from Commanding Officers of the *Bicester, Zetland* and *Vulcan*, TNA: AIR 23/1481.

151 **Medical report on Alfred H. Bergman, "due to leaking":** Jay M. Salzman, Captain, M.C., Ward Surgeon to Chief of Surgical Services, 7th Station Hospital, APO 774, U.S. Army, 4 Jan. 1944, SFAP.

151 *Bicester* **admissions:** TNA: PIN 15/5071 and 15/5217/3, and TNA: AIR 23/1481.

152 *Vienna,* **"necessary precautions":** "Report on Circumstances," NARA.

152 *Vulcan,* **"owing to temporary blindness":** TNA: AIR 23/1481; TNA: WO 169/13885.

153 **"the lucky ones":** Southern, *Poisonous Inferno,* p. 98.

153 **"covered in blisters":** Judith Perera and Andy Thomas, "Britain's Victims of Mustard-gas Disaster," *New Scientist,* Jan. 30, 1986.

153 **"the size of an old penny":** Southern, *Poisonous Inferno,* p. 98.

154 **"eye-only" casualties chart:** Alexander, "Final Report."

154 **"universal," "their fear," "instructions as to the exact":** Medical Officer's Journal, HMS *Bicester,* Dec. 23, 1943, TNA: PIN 15/5071.

155 **"representative cases," "at least twelve":** Alexander, "Preliminary Report."

155 **"a plea for":** Alexander, "Final Report."

155 **"a bit of a heavy heart," "But I did have":** Alexander, "Bari Harbor," lecture, SFAP.

157 **"short report," "certain cases," "A request":** Alexander, "Final Report," Appendix #2; "Report on Circumstances," NARA.

157 **"observations of Casualties" memorandum:** TNA: WO 204/7613.

159 **"Superior to what?":** Ibid.

159 **"a gigantic attack":** Franklin D. Roosevelt, Dec. 24, 1943: Fireside Chat 27: On the Tehran and Cairo Conferences, https:///www.docs.fdrlibrary.marist.edu.

160 **"Toxic Gas Burns":** Alexander, "Preliminary Report."

160 **"The facts are related":** Ibid.

160 **"due to mustard," "The point":** Ibid.

161 **"not likely to," "severe systemic effects," "far greater significance":** Ibid.

161–62 **"The lack of warning," "the pattern":** Churchill, *Surgeon to Soldiers,* p. 305.

162 **"calls particular attention":** Col. Standlee cover letter to Col. Shadle, Dec. 26. 1943 (TNA): WO 204/1105.

162 **"I have really been":** Alexander to Col. W. D. Fleming, Dec. 24, 1943, Report of Bari Harbor Blast 1943, Office of the Surgeon General, RG 112, Box 6, NARA.

163 **"Dear Colonel Wood":** Alexander to John R. Wood, Dec. 27, 1943, SFAP; Infield, *Disaster at Bari,* pp. 202–3.

164 **"magnum opus":** Lunardini, "The Birth of a Notion," p. 19.

164 "offending the Prime Minister": Alexander, "Bari Harbor," lecture, SFAP.

164 "Dear Colonel Alexander": Rhoads to Alexander, Jan. 15, 1944, SFAP; Infield, *Poisonous Inferno,* p. 284.

165 "worth bearing in mind": Alexander to Capt. George M. Lyon, Dec. 27, 1943, SFAP; Infield, *Disaster at Bari,* pp. 201–2.

165 "Col. Shadle was most": Lyon to Alexander, March 28, 1944, SFAP.

165 "quite bursting," "Such solutions": Col. W. D. Fleming to Alexander, Jan. 6, 1944, SFAP.

165–66 "at the earliest," "Chemical intelligence": Fleming, Circular Letter to Port Commanders, Jan. 11, 1944, enclosed in letter to Alexander, SFAP.

166 "Your report," "Relations with the CWS": Fleming to Alexander, Jan 11, 1944, SFAP.

166 "should be left": TNA: CAB 79/68/18.

167 "The Royal Navy": Maj. Gen. Lowell Rooks to G-1, AFHQ, Dec. 22, 1943, TNA: WO 204/1105.

167 "no secret," "report these casualties," "We should state": Ibid.

167 "the straight facts," "without concealment": Ibid., Rooks telegram.

167–68 "Enemy action," "bronchitis, etc.," "these terms": Ibid., Eisenhower, "Most Secret and Immediate" telegram, Jan. 2, 1944; also in TNA: AIR 2/13585.

168 "Allied policy is not": Ibid.; also "Report on Circumstances," NARA.

168 "injuries to eyes": Ibid., Air Ministry to AFHQ, Jan. 5, 12, 1944; also in AIR 2/13585.

168 "Breaking": Ibid., Chiefs of Staff Committee Meeting, note of draft telegram.

168 "a large party," "repercussions": TNA: AIR 2/13585, Air Marshal Richard Peck, Jan. 9, 1944.

168 "I agree": Ibid., Peck, Jan. 14, 1944.

168 "kept on ice": Ibid.

169 "strongly recommended," "It is believed": TNA: WO 204/1105, "Important and Most Secret" telegram from Gen. Wilson, Jan. 11, 1944; also in AIR 2/13585.

169 "unjust distribution," "Even had the defenses": Ibid., Air Chief Marshal Tedder to AFHQ, "Report on Adequacies of Protective Measures at Bari," Dec. 23, 1943.

170 "The Prime Minister": TNA: PREM 3/88/3.

170 "thank you letter": *New York Times,* Dec. 30, 1943.

170 "unknown destination," "A few weeks": Ibid.

170 "at the end": Winston S. Churchill, *The Second World War, Volume V: Closing the Ring* (Boston: Houghton Mifflin, 1951), p. 373.

171 "so tired out": *New York Times,* Dec. 30, 1943.

171 "absolutely vile": Churchill, *Closing the Ring,* p. 372.

171 **"White House":** Eisenhower, *Crusade in Europe*, p. 214.

171 **"Am stranded amid":** Churchill, *Closing the Ring*, p. 374.

171 **"I am distressed":** Ibid.

171 **"soft underbelly":** Eisenhower, *Crusade in Europe*, p. 213.

172 **"risky affair":** Ibid., p. 233.

172 **"could be more dangerous":** Churchill, *Closing the Ring*, p. 387.

173 **"at an alarming pace":** J. A. Vale and J. W. Scadding, "In Carthage Ruins: The Illness of Sir Winston Churchill at Carthage, December 1943," *Journal of the Royal College of Physicians of Edinburgh*, vol. 47, issue 3 (Sept. 2017): p. 290.

173 **"I judge he is":** Ibid., p. 292.

173 **"I have not at any time":** *New York Times*, Dec. 30, 1943.

Chapter Eight: "Forgotten Front"

174 **"serious blow":** Eisenhower, *Crusade in Europe*, p. 22.

174 **"end-run":** Manchester and Reid, *The Last Lion*, p. 784.

175 **"specific answers," Eisenhower's questions:** "Report on Circumstances," Brig. Gen. E. J. Davis to the Board of Officers, Jan. 2, 1944, NARA.

176 **"Some of the details":** Ibid.

177 **"We considered that no":** Ibid., Brig. Chichester-Constable's summary report.

177 **"had the impression":** "Report on Circumstances," NOIC Comm. E. J. Guinness's Bari Comprehensive Report, Feb. 22, 1944, Section VII, "The Report of the Gas," NARA; also in TNA: ADM 199/739.

178 **"whether the alleged":** "Report on Circumstances," Brig. Chichester-Constable's report, NARA.

178 **"reticence of authorities," "The outstanding fact":** Ibid.

179 **"special notification," "mixed cargo," "If there is reason":** Ibid.

179–80 **"very much concerned," "In checking," "most evident":** "Report on Circumstances," Col. Shadle to Gen. Adcock, "Inspection of the Port of Bari, Italy," Dec. 20, 1943; also in TNA: WO 204/1105.

180 **"at least some," "red":** Ibid.

181 **"There appears to be," "recommendation":** "Report on Circumstances," Brig. Chichester-Constable's report, NARA.

181 **"the relationship," "Normally, the principle":** Ibid.

182 **List of specific answers:** "Report on Circumstances," NARA.

183 **"It was an unlucky raid":** J. F. M. Whiteley to J. N. Kennedy, Dec. 21, 1943, TNA: WO 204/307.

184 **"Had the ship concerned exploded":** "Report on Circumstances," NOIC Comm. E. J. Guinness's Bari Comprehensive Report, Feb. 22, 1944, NARA; also in TNA: ADM 199/739.

184   **"Bloody River"**: Todd DePastino, *Bill Mauldin: A Life Up Front* (New York: W. W. Norton, 2008), p. 145.

184   **"It added to"**: Harry C. Butcher, *My Three Years with Eisenhower: The Personal Diary of Captain Harry C. Butcher, USNR, Naval Aide to General Eisenhower, 1942 to 1945* (New York: Simon & Schuster, 1946), pp. 511–12.

185   **"gung-ho" marines**: DePastino, *Bill Mauldin*, p. 139.

185   **"While planning"**: Tucker, *War of Nerves*, pp. 64–65.

186   **"biological warfare," "two principal types," "Due to his steady"**: Memorandum for the Adjutant General, Subject: Biological Warfare, The Secretary of War Directs, Feb. 9, 1944, SFAP; War Dept. memorandum, Subject: BW, to Comm. Gen., NATOUSA, Feb. 19, 1944, SFAP; Interim Report on Bacteriological Warfare, AFHQ, Feb. 21, 1944, SFAP; McFarland, "Preparing for What Never Came," pp. 111–15.

186   **"highest evaluation," "definite report," "The Germans"**: Alexander to John P. Marquand, Jan. 7, 1944, SFAP.

187   **"neutralize any such," "This is to let"**: Ibid.

187   **D-day planners**: Kleber and Birdsell, *Chemicals in Combat*, pp. 156, 167; McFarland, "Preparing for What Never Came," pp. 111–15; Spiers, *Chemical Warfare*, pp. 78–79.

188   **"It is recommended"**: Alexander to Chief Surgeon, NATOUSA, Jan. 16, 1944, SFAP.

188   **"I see Comp'ny E"**: Kleber and Birdsell, *Chemicals in Combat*, p. 176.

189   **"tremendous"**: Alexander, "Bari Harbor," Lecture, SFAP.

189   **"Your cooperation in furnishing"**: Rhoads to Alexander, April 15, 1944.

189   **"It is most," "scanty"**: Alexander to Rhoads, April 17, 1944, "Report on Circumstances."

190   **"The systemic effects"**: Ibid.

190   **"Inadequacy of the material," "In general"**: Arnold Rich and Arthur M. Ginzler, MRL (EA) Report no. 20, "Pathological Changes in the Tissue of the Victims of the Bari Incident," May 18, 1944, Edgewood Arsenal, Army Medical Library, Washington, DC.

191   **"systemic mustard," "a study be made"**: Ibid.

191   **"silver leaf merger"**: *New York Herald Tribune*, May 5, 1944.

193   **"This officer"**: Transcript of Perrin Long's toast, SFAP.

193   **"forgotten front"**: DePastino, *Bill Mauldin*, p. 168.

Chapter Nine: "A Riddle Wrapped in a Mystery"

194   **"classic medical paper"**: Tom Mahoney, "What We Know Now About Cancer," *American Legion Magazine*, July 1959, p. 16; also Cornelius P. Rhoads, "The

Sword and the Ploughshare," *Journal of The Mount Sinai Hospital,* vol. 13, no. 6 (1946): p. 300.

194 **"Under military security":** C. P. Rhoads, MD, "Report on a Cooperative Study of Nitrogen Mustard (HN2) Therapy of Neoplastic Disease," *Transactions of the Association of American Physicians,* vol. 60, issue 1 (1947): p. 110.

195 **"Dusty":** "Frontal Attack," *Time,* June 27, 1949.

195 **"A riddle wrapped":** Mahoney, "What We Know Now About Cancer," p. 17.

195 **"Scientifically inaccessible":** Cornelius P. Rhoads, "Ewing: The Experimental Method and the Cancer Problem," *Bulletin of the N.Y. Academy of Medicine* (Oct. 1951): p. 607.

195–96 **Rhoads background, "Trudeau Group":** "Mr. Cancer Research," *Time,* Aug. 24, 1959; Obituary, "C. P. Rhoads, M.D., D.Sc.," *British Medical Journal* (Aug. 29, 1959).

196 **"melancholy statements":** Rhoads, "Ewing: The Experimental Method," p. 620.

197 **"What drugs will not," discovery of radium:** Faguet, *The War on Cancer,* p. 26.

198 **"cancer might be regarded":** Rhoads, "Ewing: The Experimental Method," p. 608.

198 **"Melted away":** Musso, "Medical Detective Work: Chemotherapy Owes Debt to Dr. Stewart Alexander," *Pascack Valley* [NJ] *Community Life,* July 16, 1980; Rhoads, "The Sword and the Ploughshare," p. 308.

198 **"Most promising substance":** Rhoads, "Report on a Cooperative Study of Nitrogen Mustard," p. 110.

198 **"Since mustard gas":** *Asheville* [NC] *Citizen Times,* Oct. 3, 1953.

198 **"disturbed bone-marrow," "direct toxic action":** E. B. Krumbhaar and Helen D. Krumbhaar, "The Blood and Bone Marrow in Yellow Cross (Mustard Gas) Poisoning: Changes Produced in Bone Marrow of Fatal Cases," *Journal of Medical Research,* vol. 40, no. 3 (July 10, 1919): pp. 497–508.

199 **"We fully recognize":** Frank E. Adair and Halsey J. Bagg, "Experimental and Clinical Studies on the Treatment of Cancer by Dichloroethylsulphide (mustard gas)," *Annals of Surgery,* vol. 93, no. 1 (January 1931): p. 193.

199 **"anti-carcinogenic action":** I. Berenblum, "Experimental Inhibition of Tumour Induction by Mustard Gas and Other Compounds," *Journal of Pathology,* vol. 40 (1935): pp. 549–58.

200 **"Penicillin for cancer":** *Asheville* [NC] *Citizen Times,* Oct. 3, 1953.

200 **"Tower of strength":** Alexander, "Bari Harbor—and the Origins of Chemotherapy," p. 25.

201 **"Dusty, as I knew him":** Alexander, "Bari Harbor," lecture, SFAP.

201 **Winternitz assigned study, "substance X":** Alfred Gilman Sr., "The Initial Clinical Trial of Nitrogen Mustard," *American Journal of Surgery,* vol. 105 (May 1963): p. 574.

201   **"enemy did not intend," "battery of syringes":** Ibid., p. 575.

202   **"Close contact," "The point":** Ibid., p. 574.

202–3 **"unique properties," "sensitivity," "The problem":** Ibid., pp. 574–75.

203   **"lone mouse":** Ibid.

203   **"Amazement":** Tom Urtz, "On the Trail of a Cancer Cure," *Yale–New Haven Magazine,* Yale–New Haven Hospital publication, Fall 1983, p. 8.

203   **"This was quite":** Gilman, "The Initial Clinical Trial of Nitrogen Mustard," p. 575.

203–4 **"prolongation of survival," "therefore came up":** Ibid., p. 576.

204   **"act of a charlatan":** Ibid., p. 577.

204   **"Without consulting anyone":** Gene Cooney, "Cancer Chemotherapy" from Battlefield . . . to the Laboratory . . . to the Bedside," *Yale–New Haven Magazine,* Winter 1992, p. 20, and Urtz, "On the Trail of a Cancer Cure," p. 11.

204   **"sufficiently encouraging":** Gilman, "The Initial Clinical Trial of Nitrogen Mustard," p. 576.

204   **"Any drug that gave":** Urtz, "On the Trail of a Cancer Cure," p. 9.

205   **"JD":** John E. Fenn and Robert Udelsman, "First Use of Intravenous Chemotherapy Cancer Treatment: Rectifying the Record," *Journal of the American College of Surgeons,* vol. 212, no. 13 (March 2011): pp. 413–17.

205   **"The patient's outlook":** Ibid., p. 415.

206   **"unwarranted confidence":** Gilman, "The Initial Clinical Trial of Nitrogen Mustard," p. 577.

206   **"softening," "all cervical," "For a short time":** Ibid.

207   **"serious error," "fortunate guess":** Ibid.

208   **"very narrow":** Louis S. Goodman, Maxwell M. Wintrobe, William Dameshek, Morton J. Goodman, Major Alfred Gilman, and Margaret T. McLennan, "Nitrogen Mustard Therapy: Use of Methyl –Bis (Beta-Chloroethyl) amine Hydrochloride and Tris (Beta-Chloroethyl) amine Hydrochloride for Hodgkin's Disease, Lymphosarcoma, Leukemia, and Certain Allied Disorders," *Journal of the American Medical Association* (henceforth *JAMA*), vol. 132, no. 3 (Sept. 21, 1946): pp. 126–32.

209   **"to obtain data":** Rhoads, "The Sword and the Ploughshare," p. 308; *New York Times,* Jan. 9, 1946.

210   **"enemy dared not," "same wartime system":** *The Gazette and Daily* (York, PA), Jan. 5, 1945.

211   **"He dreamed of an approach":** Joseph Burchenal, "Cornelius P. Rhoads, M.D., 1895–1959," *CA: A Cancer Journal for Clinicians,* vol. 28, no. 5 (Nov./Dec. 1959), http://onlinelibrary.wiley.com, accessed July 2019.

211   **"Bench-to-bedside research":** C. P. Rhoads, "Cancer University," *Kettering Digest,* Dayton, OH, National Cash Register Co. (1956): p. 84.

212 **"This may be the key":** Musso, "Medical Detective Work," *Pascack Valley Community Life*, July 16, 1980.

212 **"That the Bari Harbor contribution":** Alexander, "Bari Harbor," lecture, SFAP.

Chapter Ten: "Frontal Attack"

213 **"First atomic bomb," "harnessed," "a marvel":** *New York Times*, August 7, 1945.

214 **"organized science":** Ibid.

214 **"a fresh page":** Paul Boyer, *By the Bomb's Early Light: American Thought and Culture at the Dawn of the Atomic Age* (Chapel Hill: University of North Carolina Press, 1985), p. 134.

214 **"Dream team":** Stuart W. Leslie, *Boss Kettering: Wizard of General Motors* (New York: Columbia University Press, 1983), p. 122.

214 **"American industrial research," "the amazing":** *New York Times*, Aug. 8, 1945.

214 **"Very rapid progress," "apparently hopeless," "I cannot help":** Ibid.

215 **"direct":** C. P. Rhoads, "Cancer University," p. 83.

215 **"Help to conquer":** *New York Times*, Aug. 7, 1945.

216 **"There is something":** *New York Herald Tribune*, Aug. 9, 1945.

216 **"persuasive tongue":** "Frontal Attack," *Time*, June 27, 1949.

216 **"He's no Scrooge":** *New York Times*, Feb. 18, 1966.

217 **"Moral fraud":** David Farber, *Sloan Rules: Alfred P. Sloan and the Triumph of General Motors* (Chicago: University of Chicago Press, 2002), p. 209.

217 **"economic royalists":** Ibid., p. 185.

217 **"All are alike":** Ibid., p. 209.

217 **"eminently proper":** *New York Times*, Feb. 18, 1966.

217 **"Our attention":** Farber, *Sloan Rules*, p. 211.

218 **"frontal attack":** Rhoads, "Cancer University," p. 81; "Frontal Attack," *Time*, June 27, 1949.

218 **"skeleton plan," "[W]hether the whole":** Ibid., p. 80.

219 **"tomorrow," "screwdriver and pliers":** Ibid., pp. 32, 82.

219 **"well-defined," "too diffuse":** Ibid., p. 79.

219 **"the interminable labor":** Ibid., pp. 81–82.

220 **Standard Oil and GM business ties to Nazi Germany:** Henry Ashby Turner Jr., *General Motors and the Nazis: The Struggle for Control of Opel, Europe's Biggest Carmaker* (New Haven, CT: Yale University Press, 2005); "Corporations and Conscience," *New York Times*, Dec. 6, 1988; Michael Straight, "Standard Oil: Axis Ally," *New Republic*, April 6, 1942; Michael Dobbs, "Ford and GM

Scrutinized for Alleged Nazi Collaboration," *Washington Post,* Nov. 10, 1998; Charles Higham, *Trading with the Enemy: An Exposé of the Nazi-American Money Plot, 1933–1949* (New York: Dell, 1984); Edwin Black, "Nazis Rode to War on GM Wheels," *San Francisco Chronicle,* Jan. 7, 2007; Edwin Black, *Nazi Nexus: America's Corporate Connections to Hitler's Holocaust* (New York: Dialog Press, 2017).

221 **"arsenal of Democracy," "Arsenal of Fascism":** Dobbs, "Ford and GM Scrutinized"; GM Opel will dominate European market in *New York Times,* March 18, 1929, and March 18, 1932.

221 **"a strong virile nation":** Turner Jr., *General Motors and the Nazis,* p. 45.

222 **"Now I believe," "In other words":** Ibid., p. 27.

223 **"outclassed on mechanical":** Farber, *Sloan Rules,* p. 225.

223 **"Blitz truck":** Dobbs, "Ford and GM Scrutinized."

223 **"camouflage":** Black, "Nazis Rode to War on GM Wheels."

223 **"did not assist":** Dobbs, "Ford and GM Scrutinized" and "Automakers and the Nazis: GM Responds," *Washington Post,* Dec. 14, 1998.

224 **"a plan has been worked":** Turner, *General Motors and the Nazis,* p. 97.

224 **"a hostage":** Ibid., p. 151.

224 **"more than ten thousand":** Turner, *General Motors and the Nazis,* p. 98.

224–25 **"Distinguished services," "inspiration":** Dobbs, "Ford and GM Scrutinized."

225 **"League of Benedict Arnolds," "treasonable":** Turner, *General Motors and the Nazis,* p. 122.

225 **"wasting his time":** Ibid., p. 126.

225 **"outlaw," "anything but force":** Ibid.

225 **"a Nazi sympathizer":** Farber, *Sloan Rules,* p. 229.

226 **"there will be a blast":** Ibid., p. 231.

226 **Kettering "bug," "flying bug":** Leslie, *Boss Kettering,* pp. 297–99.

227 **"horsepower is war power," "super fuel":** Ibid., pp. 301–5.

227 **"He is so engrossed":** Ibid., p. 307.

228 **"If you are going":** Farber, *Sloan Rules,* p. 234.

228 **"Victory Is Our Business":** Ibid., p. 235.

228 **"approximately $22.7 million":** Black, "Nazis Rode to War on GM Wheels," *New York Times,* Nov. 2, 1948.

229 **"rendered GM guilty":** Turner, *General Motors and the Nazis,* p. 158.

229 **"War reparations":** Black, "Nazis Rode to War on GM Wheels."

229 **"unaware of any":** "Automakers and the Nazis: GM Responds," *Washington Post,* Dec. 14, 1998.

229 **"Corporate officials":** "Corporations and Conscience," *New York Times,* Dec. 6, 1988.

230 **"principal target":** *New York Times,* Aug. 27, 1944.

230   **"war on cancer":** *New York Times,* Jan. 20, 1942.

230   **"the greatest curse":** Farber, *Sloan Rules,* p. 241.

230   **"Kettering Will Direct," "scientific community":** Rhoads, "Cancer University," p. 83.

231   **"professional amateur":** Ibid.

231   **"As such it now ranks":** *Williamsport* [PA] *Sun-Gazette,* Jan. 10, 1946.

231   **"The Nazis were":** "Frontal Attack," *Time,* June 27, 1949.

232   **"All I can do":** Ibid.

232   **"There is a tendency":** Smith, *Toxic Exposures,* pp. 110–11.

232   **"in the war of science," "Coordinated research":** *New York Times,* Oct. 18, 1945.

233   **"important observation":** Rhoads, "The Sword and the Ploughshare," p. 3.

233   **"lead to a cure":** Alexander, "Bari Harbor," lecture, SFAP.

234   **"Stewart had many," "Perhaps more than any":** Author interview with Dr. Michael Nevins; Michael Nevins, testimonial speech (undated), included in Alexander, *SFA.*

234   **"volunteering," narrowly escaped injury:** *The Record* (Bergen County, NJ), Nov. 30, 2005.

235   **"army of children":** Author interview with Diane and Judith Alexander, July 2018.

235   **"I was young":** Lunardini, "The Birth of a Notion," p. 20.

Chapter Eleven: Trials and Tribulations

236   **"too much power":** "Frontal Attack," *Time,* June 27, 1949.

236   **"arbitrary and autocratic":** "Mr. Cancer Research," *Time,* Aug. 24, 1959.

236   **"publicity seeking":** Ibid.

236   **"wartime emergency":** "Frontal Attack," *Time,* June 27, 1949.

237   **"tower of hope":** Ibid.

237   **"human guinea pig":** Mary Woodward Lasker, "The Unforgettable Character of Dusty Rhoads," *Reader's Digest,* April 1965, p. 166.

237   **"Pure research," "no necessary," "purposeful":** Warren Weaver, Draft of remarks at Memorial Service for Dr. Rhoads, Sept. 22, 1959, Warren Weaver Papers, Box 7, 76–96, Rockefeller Archive Center, hereafter RAC.

237   **"Hawk-like eyes," "outspoken, frequently blunt," "stepped on":** *New York Times,* Oct. 10, 1956.

238   **John D. Rockefeller and medical research:** Frances R. Frankenburg, *Human Medical Experimentation: From Smallpox Vaccines to Secret Government Programs* (Santa Barbara, CA: Greenwood, 2017), pp. 341–43.

238   **"big ideas":** Dr. William Bosworth Castle, transcript of an oral history interview conducted 2008, ASH Oral History, "Legends in Hematology," American Society of Hematology Project, Columbia University, New York City, pp. 1–3.

239   **"scientific value" and Castle's report on patients:** General Statement of Dr. William Castle, director of The Anemia Commission of the Rockefeller Foundation (hereafter RF) on their work and Dr. Rhoads's case, typescript, March 7, 1932, pp. 1–4, RF, RG 1.1, 243 Anemia, box 1, folder 7: 2, RAC.

239   **"Exciting experiment," "We now have":** C. P. Rhoads to Simon Flexner, Sept. 19, 1931, RF, RG 1.1, 243 Anemia, box 1, folder 7, RAC.

240   **For various descriptions of events surrounding the Rhoads letter to Fred "Ferdie" Stewart:** Susan E. Lederer, " 'Porto Ricochet': Joking about Germs, Cancer and Race Extermination in the 1930s," *American Literary History* 14, no. 4 (Winter 2002): pp. 720–46; Laura Briggs, *Reproducing Empire: Race, Sex, Science and U.S. Imperialism in Puerto Rico* (Berkeley: University of California Press, 2002), pp. 60–62; Pedro Aponte-Vázquez, *The Unsolved Case of Dr. Cornelius P. Rhoads: An Indictment* (San Juan: Rene Publications, 2004), pp. 57–63.

240   **"very much surprised":** Interview with Dr. William Galbreath, Director of Presbyterian Hospital, in Quiñones file, Feb. 9, 1932, RF, RG 1.1, 243 Anemia, box 1, folder 5, RAC.

240–41   **"High regard," "all a joke":** Ibid.

241   **"Fear" and "distrust":** Sworn Statement of Luis Baldoni in Quiñones file, Jan. 2, 1932, RF, RG 1.1 243 Anemia, box 1, folder 5, RAC.

241   **"considered the matter":** H. H. Howard to George Payne, Jan. 30, 1932, RF, RG 1.1, 243 Anemia, box 1, folder 6, RAC.

241–242   **"it would be ideal" and text of Rhoads letter:** Page 2 of Special Attorney José Ramón Quiñones to Honorable Governor of Porto Rico, Feb. 11, 1932, RF, RG 1.1, 243 Anemia, box 1, folder 5, RAC.

242   **"inoculate," "tuberculosis and other":** Ibid.

242   **"Confession of murder" and "libel":** Gov. James R. Beverley to Col. F. F. Russell of RF, Jan. 30, 1932, RF, RG 1.1, 243 Anemia, box 1, folder 5, RAC.

243   **"poison Ivy," "spin doctor":** Pedro Aponte-Vázquez, *The Unsolved Case of Dr. Cornelius P. Rhoads*, p. 26; David Miller and William Dinan, *A Century of Spin: How Public Relations Became the Cutting Edge of Corporate Power* (London: Pluto Press, 2008).

243   **"Regret very much":** "Porto Ricochet," *Time*, Feb. 15, 1932.

243–44   **"It tells of eight," "friend," "parody":** *New York Times*, Jan. 30, 1932.

244   **Payne interview:** Payne interviewed by William A. Sawyer of RF, Feb. 9, 1932, RF, RG 1.1, 243 Anemia, box 1, folder 6, RAC.

244   **"safety valve":** Lederer, "Porto Ricochet: Joking about Germs, Cancer and Race Extermination," p. 735.

244   **"Only a few years":** Ibid., p. 734.

245   **"The incident casts," "news":** Telegram from Henry R. Luce to Ivy Lee, Feb. 9, 1932, RF, RG 1.1, 243 Anemia, box 1, folder 6, RAC.

245   **"He and Dr. Castle," "His parody":** "Porto Ricochet," *Time,* Feb. 15, 1932.

245–46   **"acting on my instructions," and observations about patient deaths and Rhoads:** General Statement of Dr. William Castle, typescript, March 7, 1932, pp. 1–4, RF, RG 1.1, 243 Anemia, box 1, folder 7: 2, RAC.

246   **"by direct or indirect," "untrue":** Quiñones to Hon. Gov. of Porto Rico, Feb. 11, 1932, RF, RG 1.1, 243 Anemia, box 1, folder 5, RAC.

246   **"Dr. Rhoads Cleared":** *New York Times,* Feb. 15, 1932.

246   **"very happy," "Incidentally":** Gov. James R. Beverley to W. A. Sawyer of RF, Feb. 17, 1932, RF, RG 1.1, 243 Anemia, box 1, folder 6, RAC.

247   **"I think we have":** Payne to Doctor H. H. Howard of RF, Feb. 25, 1932, RF, RG 1.1, 243 Anemia, box 1, folder 6, RAC.

247   **"To him," "genuine interest," "No patients":** Rafael Arroyo Zeppenfeldt to Editor of *La Correspondencia,* Jan. 29, 1932, RF, RG 1.1, 243 Anemia, box 1, folder 4: 2, RAC.

248   **"The work he began," "His work":** Dr. George Minot to Dr. Herbert S. Gasser, Cornell University Medical College, Sept. 25, 1935, RF, RG 1.1, box 25, folder 20, RAC.

248   **"and his skill":** George W. Corner, *A History of The Rockefeller Institute, 1901– 1953: Origins and Growth* (New York City: Rockefeller Press, 1964), p. 477.

248   **"Porto Rican episode":** Business manager of RF in response to Rhoads request, March 6, 1942, RF, RG 1.1, 243 Anemia, box 1, folder 7, RAC.

Chapter Twelve: "The Sword and the Ploughshare"

250   **"For a moment":** Rhoads, "The Sword and the Ploughshare," p. 299.

251   **"A medical officer":** Ibid.

252   **"to produce more," "striking proportions":** D. A. Karnofsky, "The Nitrogen Mustards and their Application in Neoplastic Diseases," *New York State Journal of Medicine,* vol. 47, issue 9 (May 1947): pp. 992–93.

252   **"chemical tool," "unique group":** Rhoads, "The Sword and the Ploughshare," p. 309.

252   **"It is quite true":** Ibid.

253   **"undreamed of only":** *Cincinnati Enquirer,* April 2, 1947.

253–54   **Goodman and Gilman landmark studies:** Goodman et al., "Use of Methyl-Bis (Beta-Chloroethyl)amine Hydrochloride and Tris (Beta-Chloroethyl)amine Hydrochloride for Hodgkin's Disease, Lymphosarcoma, Leukemia and Certain Allied Disorders," *JAMA,* vol. 132, no. 3 (Sept. 21, 1946): pp. 126–32; Alfred Gilman and Frederick S. Philips, "The Biological Actions and Therapeutic Applications of the B-Chloroethyl Amines and Sulfides," *Science,* vol. 103, no. 2675 (1946): pp. 409–15.

254 **"prompted," "the experience":** *New York Times,* April 21, 1946.

254 **"deadly artillery":** "Medicine: Mustard Against Cancer," *Time,* Oct. 21, 1946.

254–55 **"War Gases Tried," "fifteen or twenty years":** *New York Times,* Oct. 6, 1946.

255 **"Medicine: Mustard Against Cancer":** "Medicine: Mustard Against Cancer," *Time,* Oct. 21, 1946.

255 **"significant remissions," "had been kept":** Ibid.; Leon O. Jacobsen, Charles L. Spurr, E. S. Guzman Barron, Taylor R. Smith, Clarence Lushbaugh, and George Dick, "Nitrogen Mustard Therapy: Studies on the Effect of Methyl-Bis (B-Chloroethyl) Amine Hydrochloride on Neoplastic Disease and Allied Disorders of the Hemopoietic System," *JAMA,* vol. 132, no. 6 (Oct. 5, 1946): pp. 263–71.

255 **"potentially dangerous drug":** Smith, *Toxic Exposures,* p. 107.

256 **"Alfred, you belong":** Vincent DeVita Jr. and Edward Chu, "A History of Cancer Chemotherapy," *Cancer Research,* vol. 68, no. 21, American Association for Cancer Research (Nov. 2008): pp. 8643–53.

256 **"Those who have not":** Joseph Holland Burchenal, "The Historical Development of Cancer Chemotherapy," *Seminars in Oncology,* vol. 4, no. 2 (June 1977): p. 136.

257 **"neochemotherapists":** "Joseph H. Burchenal: In Memoriam (1912–2006)," *Cancer Research,* American Association for Cancer Research (Dec. 2006).

257 **"studies of a fundamental":** C. P. Rhoads, "Perspectives in Cancer Research," in New York Academy of Medicine, ed., *Perspectives in Medicine* (New York: Columbia University Press, 1948).

258 **"briefly interrupt":** David Karnofsky, Walter H. Abelmann, Lloyd F. Craver, and Joseph H. Burchenal, "The Use of Nitrogen Mustards in the Palliative Treatment of Carcinoma," *Cancer* (November 1958): p. 655.

258 **Karnofsky Performance Status Scale, "disabled":** Carsten Timmermann, " 'Just Give Me the Best Quality of Life Questionnaire': The Karnofsky Scale and the History of Quality of Life Measurements in Cancer Trials," in *Chronic Illness,* vol. 3 (Sept. 2013): pp. 179–90.

259 **"C-Day Landing":** *New York Times,* April 16, 1948.

260 **SKI colony of mice, "take":** *Lawton* [OK] *Constitution,* May 9, 1948.

260 **"In the fight":** Ibid.

260 **"Differential effect":** "Frontal Attack," *Time,* June 27, 1949.

261 **"It was a sad":** Rhoads, *Kettering Digest,* p. 84.

262 **"There is no place":** *Muscatine* [IA] *Journal and News-Tribune,* Feb. 22, 1949.

262 *Symphony of the Air:* Leslie, *Boss Kettering,* p. 310.

262 **"All research is 99.9 percent":** A. H. Alexander, "The World's Most Dissatisfied Man," *Philadelphia Inquirer,* July 13, 1957, p. 136.

263 **Farber folic-acid experiments:** Siddhartha Mukherjee, *The Emperor of All Mal-*

adies: A Biography of Cancer (New York: Scribner, 2010), pp. 27–36; Meyers, *Happy Accidents*, pp. 128–29.

263 **"Devastation rather than triumph":** Meyers, *Happy Accidents*, pp. 128–29.

264 **"Babe" Ruth, one of the first chemo patients:** Lawrence K. Altman, MD, "The Doctor's World: Ruth's Other Record: Cancer Pioneer," *New York Times*, Dec. 29, 1998.

265 **"pulmonary complications," "asked no questions":** Ibid.

265 **"famous national figure," "a cure":** *Wall Street Journal*, Sept. 11, 1947.

265 **"hot news":** *New York Times*, Aug. 22, 1948.

266 **"no special drug," "had been previously":** *New York Times*, Aug. 18, 1948.

266 **"bold" play, "complicated the struggle," "In spite of":** "Toward the Cancer Goal," *Newsweek*, Oct. 18, 1948.

267 **Farber's repeated remissions, Burchenal confirmed:** Angela Thomas, "Joe Burchenal and the Birth of Combination Chemotherapy," *British Journal of Hematology*, vol. 133, issue 5 (June 2006), pp. 493–503.

267 **"Anti-metabolic effect":** *New York Times*, Oct. 5, 1948.

268 **Howard Skipper background:** Alexander, *SFA*; Linda Simpson-Herren and Glynn P. Wheeler, "Howard Earle Skipper: In Memoriam (1915–2006)," *Cancer Research*, American Association for Cancer Research (Dec. 2006).

268 **"Cancer Fighter":** "Frontal Attack," *Time*, June 27, 1949.

269 **"We can help only," "no callous," "Some people ask":** Ibid.

270 **"rational" method, Gertrude Elion:** John Laszlo, MD, *The Cure of Childhood Leukemia: Into the Age of Miracles* (New Brunswick, NJ: Rutgers University Press, 1996), pp. 62–85.

270 **Burchenal "2,6" tests:** William Wells, with the assistance of Gertrude Elion and John Laszlo, "Curing Childhood Leukemia," *Beyond Discovery: The Path from Research to Human Benefit* (Washington, DC: National Academy of Sciences, 1997); Thomas, "Joe Burchenal and the Birth of Combination Chemotherapy"; Laszlo, *The Cure of Childhood Leukemia*, pp. 54–55.

271 **Burchenal trial of 6-MP:** Wells, "Curing Childhood Leukemia"; Thomas, "Joe Burchenal and the Birth of Combination Chemotherapy"; Laszlo, *The Cure of Childhood Leukemia*, pp. 56–57.

272 **"We were rescued":** Ibid., p. 70.

272 **"Supplies of 6-MP":** Ibid., p. 71.

272–73 **Debbie Brown, *"cure"*:** Wells, "Curing Childhood Leukemia."

273 **"Chemotherapy of cancer":** Burchenal, "The Historical Development of Cancer Chemotherapy," p. 136.

273 **"wonder-drug remedies":** *Asheville* [NC] *Citizen-Times*, Oct. 3, 1953; *Oneonta* [NY] *Star*, Oct. 5, 1953; *Burlington* [VT] *Free Press*, Nov. 5, 1953.

273–74 **"I am convinced," "including everything":** *Asbury Park* [NJ] *Press*, Oct. 3, 1953; also in C. P. Rhoads testimony, Health Inquiry (Heart Disease, Cancer) Hearing, Oct. 1–3, 1953, Committee on Interstate and Foreign Commerce, House Sudoc No. Y4.In8/4:H34/7/pt.1, CIS #83 H1420–5-A, Microfiche group 3, link: https://congressional.proquest/congressional/docview/t29/.d30.hrg-1953-fch-0012.

274 **"fighting for," "full of cancer":** *New York Times,* Oct. 3, 1953.

274 **"Inevitably, as I see it," "a variety":** Ibid.

274 **"Taft's Doctor":** *Washington Post,* Oct. 3, 1953.

275 **"Most of the road," "crash":** *New York Times,* Oct. 4, 1953.

275 **"fairy godmother":** James S. Olson, *Making Cancer History: Disease and Discovery at the University of Texas M. D. Anderson Cancer Center* (Baltimore, MD: Johns Hopkins University Press, 2009), p. 46.

275 **"smoldering determination":** Lasker, "The Unforgettable Character of Dusty Rhoads," p. 164.

276 **"Rhoads is making":** Warren Weaver Diary, 4 October 1955, p. 91, Rockefeller Foundation, RG 12 Officers' Diaries, RAC, retrieved from https://storage .rockarch.org/58721bae-3476–469f-875a-a9b4a726911b-rac_rfdiaries_12–2_weaver_1932–1959_040.pdf.

276 **"spontaneous regression":** Mahoney, "What We Know Now About Cancer," *American Legion Magazine,* p. 44.

277 **"there clearly does":** Claude Stanush, "Medicine's Greatest Hunt—For Chemicals to Starve Out Cancer," *Collier's* (Nov. 23, 1956), p. 31; Sidney Katz, "Is There a Drug to Cure Cancer?" *Maclean's Magazine* (April 12, 1958), pp. 78–79.

277 **"A dramatic breakthrough":** Lasker, "The Unforgettable Character of Dusty Rhoads," p. 170.

277 **"Skepticism surrounded":** DeVita and Chu, "A History of Cancer Chemotherapy."

277 **"aggressive skepticism," "They had seen":** Author interview with Dr. Vincent T. DeVita Jr., August 2019.

278 **"Blood Club," "I had never seen":** Ibid.; Vincent T. DeVita Jr. and Elizabeth DeVita–Raeburn, *The Death of Cancer: After Fifty Years on the Front Lines of Medicine, A Pioneering Oncologist Reveals Why the War on Cancer Is Winnable—And How We Can Get There* (New York: Farrar, Straus and Giroux, 2015), p. 83.

278 **"Cabal," "return to the good old days":** C. P. Rhoads to Reginald G. Coombe and Laurance Rockefeller, July 19, 1954, Warren Weaver Papers, Box 7, folders 76–96, RAC.

278 **"willful band," "Jealous":** "Mr. Cancer Research," *Time,* Aug. 24, 1959.

278 **"The history of medical":** C. P. Rhoads to Reginald G. Coombe and Laurance Rockefeller, July 19, 1954, Warren Weaver Papers, Box 7, folders 76–96, RAC.

279 **"So much of the support":** Warren Weaver to Frank A. Howard and Laurance Rockefeller, Dec. 16, 1957, accompanying "Memorandum Concerning Memorial Center—Hospital, SKI, ETC.," Warren Weaver Papers, Box 7, folders 76–96, RAC.

279 **"The essential fact":** *The News-Messenger* (Fremont, OH), Nov. 14, 1956.

280 **"Mr. Cancer Research":** "Mr. Cancer Research," *Time*, Aug. 24, 1959.

280 **"It is no longer":** Stanush, "Medicine's Greatest Hunt—For Chemicals to Starve Out Cancer," *Collier's* (Nov. 23, 1956), p. 31.

280–81 **Min Chui Li background, "As a sign," "hcg level":** DeVita Jr. and Edward Chu, "A History of Cancer Chemotherapy"; Emil J. Freireich, "Min Chui Li: A Perspective in Cancer Therapy," *Clinical Cancer Research,* vol. 8, issue 9 (Sept. 2002); Mukherjee, *The Emperor of All Maladies*, pp. 137–38.

281 **"It was a fantastic":** Emil J. Freireich, transcript of an oral history interview conducted by Gretchen A. Case at Dr. Freireich's offices at the University of Texas M. D. Anderson Cancer Center on June 19, 1997, National Cancer Institute Oral History Project, History Associates Inc., p. 76.

281 **"Li was accused":** Mukherjee, *The Emperor of All Maladies*, pp. 137–38.

282 ***"poison":*** DeVita Jr. and Chu, "A History of Cancer Chemotherapy."

282 **"butcher shop," "even while":** DeVita Jr. and DeVita–Raeburn, *The Death of Cancer,* p. 60.

282 **"Young Turks":** Laszlo, *The Cure of Childhood Leukemia*, p. 57.

282 **"No one can ever":** Freireich, transcript of an oral history interview, p. 77.

282–83 **"mouse doctor," "cell kill," "synergistic":** DeVita Jr. and Chu, "A History of Cancer Chemotherapy"; Mukherjee, *The Emperor of All Maladies*, pp. 193–42.

283 **Burchenal and combination therapy:** Thomas, "Joe Burchenal and the Birth of Combination Chemotherapy," pp. 498–501.

284 **At NCI, VAMP:** DeVita Jr. and DeVita–Raeburn, *The Death of Cancer,* pp. 49–63.

284 **"verbal bloodbath":** Ibid., p. 49.

284 **"At first I opposed it":** James S. Olson, 2nd Reading from "Making Cancer History— Frei and Freireich Combination Chemotherapy," University of Texas M. D. Anderson Cancer Center Project, video transcript, retrieved from https://www.mdanderson .org › transcripts › making-cancer-history-2, accessed July 2019.

285 **MOMP, "fierce resistance":** DeVita Jr. and Chu, "A History of Cancer Chemotherapy."

286 **"It would be too dangerous":** DeVita Jr. and DeVita–Raeburn, *The Death of Cancer,* p. 77.

286 **"The results were startling":** DeVita Jr. and Chu, "A History of Cancer Chemotherapy."

286 **Golden Age:** G. Bonadonna, "Does Chemotherapy Fulfill Its Expectations in Cancer Treatment?" *Annals of Oncology*, vol. 1, no. 1 (1990): p. 12.

286 **"War on Cancer":** DeVita Jr. and DeVita–Raeburn, *The Death of Cancer*, p. 244.

286 **"the same kind":** Richard A. Rettig, *Cancer Crusade: The Story of the National Cancer Act of 1971* (New York: Authors Choice Press, 1977), p. 77.

286 **"It was heady":** DeVita Jr. and DeVita–Raeburn, *The Death of Cancer*, p. 137.

287   **"walking a tightrope"**: Glenn Infield, "Out of Calamity: Chemotherapy," *Roche Image: Of Medicine and Research* (Nov. 1972): p. 30.

288   **Hitchings and Elion discover new drugs**: Wells, with the assistance of Gertrude Elion and John Laszlo, "Curing Childhood Leukemia," *Beyond Discovery: The Path from Research to Human Benefit* (Washington, DC: National Academy of Sciences, 1997); Laszlo, *The Cure of Childhood Leukemia*, pp. 54–55.

288   **"With the addition of 6-MP"**: Gertrude B. Elion, "The Purine Path to Chemotherapy," Nobel Prize Lecture, December 8, 1988, Wellcome Research Laboratories, Burroughs Wellcome, Research Triangle Park, retrieved from https://www.nobelprize.org/uploads/2018/06/elion-lecture.pd.

288–89   **"adjuvant," "All these things"**: Author interview with Dr. Vincent T. DeVita Jr., Aug. 2019; decline in mortality figures from DeVita Jr. and DeVita–Raeburn, *The Death of Cancer*, p. 245.

289   **"We *are* winning"**: Ibid., p. 245.

289   **"*cure*," "A lot of the things"**: Author interview with Dr. Vincent T. DeVita Jr., Aug. 2019.

289   **"Cancer is a disease"**: DeVita Jr. and DeVita–Raeburn, *The Death of Cancer*, p. 246.

289   **"His death is a loss"**: "Crusader Against Cancer," *New York Times*, editorial, Aug. 15, 1959.

290   **"It is quite literally"**: Warren Weaver, SKI Chairman of the Board, transcript of his Statement to the Staff of Memorial Center, Aug. 18, 1959, Warren Weaver Papers, Box 7, folders 76–96, RAC.

290   **"It is not the critic"**: Lasker, "The Unforgettable Character of Dusty Rhoads," p. 172.

291   **"Beat their swords"**: Isaiah 2:4, retrieved from https://biblehub.com › Isaiah.

291   **"The Bari incident"**: Rhoads, "The Sword and the Ploughshare," p. 309.

Epilogue: Belated Justice

292   **"There is something," "Apparently, secrecy"**: Jules Hirsch, "An Anniversary for Cancer Chemotherapy," *JAMA*, vol. 296, no. 12 (Sept. 27, 2006): pp. 1518–20.

293   **"one of the ships," "Fortunately"**: Eisenhower, *Crusade in Europe*, p. 226.

293   **"disaster," "most unfortunate"**: Ibid.

293   **"still some few details"**: Karig, Burton, and Freeland, *Battle Report*, p. v.

293   **"I hope you"**: Lt. Col. A. L. d'Abreu to Gen. Dwight D. Eisenhower, Jan. 26, 1949, Dwight D. Eisenhower Presidential Papers, Pre-Presidential 1916–1952, name series, Box 30, Dwight D. Eisenhower Presidential Library.

294   **"thoughtfulness," "As a matter"**: Gen. Dwight D. Eisenhower to Col. A. L. d'Abreu, Feb. 14, 1949, Ibid.

294 **"picked up the missing"**: Jeavons, "Big Bang at Bari," pp. 462–63.

295 **"While I have not yet"**: Gen. Dwight D. Eisenhower to Col. A. L. d'Abreu, Feb. 14, 1949, Dwight D. Eisenhower Presidential Papers, Pre-Presidential 1916–1952, name series, Box 30, Dwight D. Eisenhower Presidential Library.

295 **"Chance hit"**: Churchill, *Closing the Ring*, p. 225.

295 **"spectacularly successful," "Although regraded"**: Saunders, "The Bari Incident," pp. 36–39.

296 **"curiosity aroused," "even in the late," "a polite"**: Glenn Infield, "Disaster at Bari," *American Heritage*, vol. XXII, no. 6 (Oct. 1971): p. 105.

297 **"talk of the war"**: *The Record* (Bergen County, NJ), May 2002.

298 **"not correct," "had not considered"**: Nicholas Spark interviews with S. F. Alexander, April 4, 1987, NSP.

299 **"one thousand deaths"**: Infield, *Disaster at Bari*, p. 177.

299 **Disputed by Italian historians**: Author interviews with Drs. Vito Antonio Leuzzi and Pasquale Trizio in Bari, Italy, October 2018.

299 **Explosion of SS *Charles Henderson***: Ibid.

300 **"a time bomb"**: Ibids

300 **Cleanup operation, two thousand mustard gas canisters**: Author interview with Francesco Morra, Rome, Oct. 2018; also, Francesco Morra, *Top Secret: Bari 2 Dicembre 1943: La Vera Storia della Pearl Harbor del Mediterraneo* (Roma: Castelvecchi, 2014), p. 113.

301 **"one of the best"**: Infield, *Disaster at Bari,* book jacket.

301 **"produced no information," "Had the mustard"**: Aikens, *Nurses in Battledress*, pp. 92–93.

302 **"It came as," "cover-up"**: Author interviews with George Southern, with the assistance of his son, historian Paul Southern, June and July 2018.

302 **"deadly cocktail"**: Southern, *Poisonous Inferno*, book jacket.

303 **"content to be"**: Ibid., p. 50.

303 **"The cover-up meant," "It made me"**: Author interviews with George Southern, with the assistance of his son, historian Paul Southern, June and July 2018.

303 **Bert Stevens background**: Southern, *Poisonous Inferno*, pp. 23, 98, and especially 154–58; Perera and Thomas, "Britain's Victims of Mustard-gas Disaster."

304 **A1, "fit for further service"**: Southern, *Poisonous Inferno*, p. 155.

304 ***mustard gas***: Ibid., p. 157; Perera and Thomas, "Britain's Victims of Mustard-gas Disaster."

304–5 **"Did at any time," "He never volunteered"**: Ibid., pp. 156–57.

305 **Bert Stevens pension backdated**: Alan Baker, Department of Health and Social Security, Friars House, to Michael McAloon, Ministry of Defence, March 6, 1986, Pension file, TNA: PIN 15/5071; also Perera and Thomas, "Britain's Victims of Mustard-gas Disaster."

305 **"special exercise":** Malcolm Beaumont, War Pensions Policy, Department of Health and Social Security to Mr. J. Nicol, Terry Resource and Advice group, July 3, 1991, Pensions file, TNA: PIN 15/5071 and 15/5217.

306 **"As it has turned out":** Southern, *Poisonous Inferno*, p. 158.

306 **"All the records":** Nicholas Spark interview with S. F. Alexander, March 31, 1987, NSP.

306 **"Should we frame":** Infield, *Disaster at Bari*, p. 248.

307 **sixty thousand affected servicemen:** Pechura and Rall, *Veterans at Risk*, pp. v–x.

307 **"There can be no question":** Karen Freeman, "The VA's Sorry, the Army's Silent," *Bulletin of the Atomic Scientists*, vol. 49, no. 2 (March 1993), p. 39.

308 **VA later identified five hundred Bari victims:** Jeanne B. Fites, Deputy Under Secretary of Defense, Requirements and Resources, to Hon. Porter Goss, House of Representatives, Pension file, in Congressional Hearing on Experiments with Human Test Subjects, Briefing Book Sept. 28, 1994, retrieved from https:// www.esd.whs.mil/Portals/54/Documents/FOID/Reading%20Room/Personnel _Related/12-F-0895_Chemical_Weapons_Exposure_Project_Section-B2_1993 _Binder2_Part2_Redacted.pdf.

308 **"[We] have heard":** Constance M. Pechura to Warren Brandenstein, May 26, 1992, cited in Gerald Reminick, *Nightmare in Bari: The World War II Liberty Ship Poison Gas Disaster and Cover-Up* (Palo Alto, CA: Glencannon Press, 2001), p. 193.

308 **"Extraordinary" experiments:** Pechura and Rall, *Veterans at Risk*.

308–9 **"Patch tests," "chamber tests," "man-break tests":** Ibid., pp. 31–41.

309 **Howard Skipper, mock "bombings":** Laszlo, *The Cure of Childhood Leukemia*, p. 201.

309 **"A terrible weapon":** Ibid.

309 **"Was injured":** Glenn Jenkins to Constance M. Pechura, Jan. 31, 1992, veterans testimony, National Academy of Sciences, cited in Smith, *Toxic Exposures*, p. 128.

310 **CWS test project in Panama:** John Lindsay-Poland, *Emperors in the Jungle: The Hidden History of the U.S. in Panama* (Durham, NC: Duke University Press, 2003), pp. 44, 45, 49–57; Smith, *Toxic Exposures*, pp. 55–56; Pechura and Rall, *Veterans at Risk*, pp. 157–59.

311 **"were convinced," "It was a war":** Pechura and Rall, *Veterans at Risk*, pp. 68–69.

311 **"The laboratory":** Smith, *Toxic Exposures*, p. 114.

313 **"I find it morally":** "Cancer Body to Probe Claims that Scientist Killed Subjects," Inter Press Service, Dec. 3, 2002.

313 **"belated justice," "a written confession":** Aponte-Vázquez, *The Unsolved Case of Dr. Cornelius P. Rhoads*, p. 15.

313 **"Few people":** Douglass Starr, "Revisiting a 1930s Scandal, ACR to Rename Prize," *Science*, vol. 300, issue 5619 (April 25, 2003): p. 574.

313 **"incredibly racist":** Ibid.

313–14 **"If we are going to tar," "due appropriate credit":** Eric T. Rosenthal, "The Rhoads Not Taken: The Tainting of the Cornelius P. Rhoads Memorial Award," *Oncology Times*, vol. 25, issue 17 (Sept. 10, 2003).

314 **"Dr. Rhoads' ties":** "About Us" brochure, "Engineering Discovery: The Story of SKI," retrieved from https://www.mskcc.org/about.

314 **"the modern age":** Lunardini, "The Birth of a Notion," p. 21.

315 **"perfect topic":** Author interview with Nicholas Spark, July 2018, and Nicholas Spark letter to the author, Aug. 8, 2018.

315 **"Historical novel," "sort out":** *Tucson* [AZ] *Citizen*, June 26, 1987; Author interview with Nicholas Spark, July 2018, and Nicholas Spark letter to the author, Aug. 8, 2018.

316 **"The idea that somehow":** Ibid.

316 **"Speak truth to power":** Ibid.

316 **"Dr. Alexander is on":** Nicholas Spark letter to the author, Aug. 8, 2018.

316 **"Not believing":** Ibid.

316 **spark essay:** Nicholas T. Spark, " 'For the Benefit of My Patients. . .': The Debacle at Bari: Government Responsibility Versus the Right to Know," 11th Grade, Historical Essay, NSP.

317 **"With his name":** Ibid.

318 **"Thus, 44 years":** *American Medical News*, Oct. 9, 1987.

319 **"a catalyst":** Press release from the Office of Senator Dennis DeConcini, Hart Senate Office Building, Washington, DC, May 19, 1988, NSP.

319 **"Without his early":** Ibid.; Certificate of Appreciation presented by Quinn H. Becker, Lieutenant General, U.S. Army, The Surgeon General, Department of the Army, April 7, 1988, SFAP.

319 **"for Washington":** *Arizona Daily Star,* May 21, 1988.

319 **"This [award]":** *The Record* (Bergen County, NJ), May 29, 1988.

319 **"I'm very gratified":** *Mohave Daily Miner,* May 20, 1988.

320 **"I think Churchill":** *The Record* (Bergen County, NJ), May 29, 1988.

320 **"Tucson Teenager":** *Arizona Daily Star,* May 21, 1988.

320 **"The Father of Chemotherapy":** Hon. Marge Roukema of New Jersey, In Tribute to Dr. Stewart F. Alexander, *Congressional Record*, vol. 134, no. 150 (Oct. 20, 1988).

320 **"who sifted through":** Hirsch, "An Anniversary for Cancer Chemotherapy."

Archives and Libraries

Churchill Archives Center, Cambridge, UK
Eisenhower Presidential Library, Abilene, KS
Franklin D. Roosevelt Presidential Library and Museum, Hyde Park, NY
George Southern, Private Archive
Houghton Library, Harvard University, Cambridge, MA
Imperial War Museum, London, UK
Library of Congress, Washington, DC
Memorial Sloan Kettering Cancer Center Archive, NY, NY
National Archives and Personnel Records Center, St. Louis, MO
National Archives and Records Administration, College Park, MD
National Archives of the United Kingdom, Richmond, UK
National Library of Medicine, Bethesda, MD
Navy Bureau of Medicine and Surgery, Falls Church, VA
Nicholas Spark Papers, Private Archive, Los Angeles, CA
Rauner Special Collections Library, Dartmouth College, Hanover, NH
Rockefeller Archive Center, Sleepy Hollow, NY
Stewart F. Alexander Papers, Private Family Archive
Ufficio Storico Marina Militare, Rome, Italy
US Army Center of Military History, Washington, DC
US Merchant Marine Academy Library, Kings Point, NY
US Naval Institute, Annapolis, MD

Select Bibliography

Aikens, Gwladys M. Rees. *Nurses in Battledress: The World War II Story of a Member of the Q.A. Reserves.* Halifax: Nimbus Publishing, 1998.

Ambrose, Stephen E. *Eisenhower: Soldier, General of the Army, President-Elect, 1890–1952,* vol. 1. New York: Simon & Schuster, 1983.

———. *The Supreme Commander: The War Years of General Dwight D. Eisenhower.* New York: Anchor Books, 1969.

Aponte-Vázquez, Pedro. *The Unsolved Case of Dr. Cornelius P. Rhoads: An Indictment.* San Juan: Publicaciones René 2004.

Atkinson, Rick. *An Army at Dawn: The War in North Africa, 1942–1943.* New York: Henry Holt, 2002.

———. *The Day of the Battle: The War in Sicily and Italy, 1943–1944.* New York: Henry Holt, 2007.

Boyd, Thomas Alvin. *Charles F. Kettering: A Biography.* Washington DC: Beard Books, 1957.

Brophy, Leo P., and George J. B. Fisher. *United States Army in World War II: The Technical Services. The Chemical Warfare Service: Organizing for War.* Washington, DC: Center of Military History, 1989.

———, Wyndham D. Miles, and Rexmond C. Cochrane. *United States Army in World War II: The Technical Services. The Chemical Warfare Service: From Laboratory to Field.* Washington, DC: Center of Military History, 1988.

Browning, Robert M., Jr. *U.S. Merchant Vessel War Casualties of World War II.* Annapolis, MD: Naval Institute Press, 1996.

Butcher, Harry C. *My Three Years with Eisenhower: The Personal Diary of Captain Harry C. Butcher, USNR, Naval Aide to General Eisenhower, 1942 to 1945.* New York: Simon & Schuster, 1946.

Casey, Robert J. *This Is Where I Came In.* New York: Bobbs-Merrill, 1945.

Churchill, Edward D. *Surgeon to Soldiers: Diary and Records of the Surgical Consultant, Allied Force Headquarters, World War II.* Philadelphia: J. B. Lippincott, 1972.

Churchill, Winston S. *Churchill: The Power of Words,* ed. Martin Gilbert. New York: DaCapo Press, 2013.

———. *The Second World War, Volume V: Closing the Ring.* Boston: Houghton Mifflin, 1951.

Cocks, E. M. Somers. *Kia-Kaha: Life at 3 New Zealand General Hospital 1940–1946.* Christchurch, NZ: Caxton Press, 1958.

Corner, George W. *A History of the Rockefeller Institute, 1901–1953: Origins and Growth.* New York City: The Rockefeller Press, 1964.

Cowdrey, Albert E. *Fighting for Life: American Military Medicine in World War II.* New York: Free Press, 1994.

DePastino, Todd. *Bill Mauldin: A Life Up Front.* New York: W. W. Norton, 2008.

DeVita, Vincent T., Jr., and Elizabeth DeVita-Raeburn. *The Death of Cancer: After Fifty Years on the Front Lines of Medicine, A Pioneering Oncologist Reveals Why the War on Cancer Is Winnable—And How We Can Get There.* New York: Farrar, Straus and Giroux, 2015.

Eisenhower, Dwight D. *Crusade in Europe.* London: William Heinemann, 1948.

Elphick, Peter. *Liberty: The Ships That Won the War.* Annapolis MD: Naval Institute Press, 2001.

Faguet, Guy B., MD. *The War on Cancer: An Anatomy of Failure, A Blueprint for the Future.* Dordrecht: Springer, 2005.

Faith, Thomas Ian. "Under a Green Sea: The U.S. Chemical Warfare Service 1917–1929." PhD diss., George Washington University, 2008; Ann Arbor, MI: University Microfilms, 2008.

———. *Behind the Gas Mask: The U.S. Chemical Warfare Service in War and Peace.* Urbana: University of Illinois Press, 2012.

Farber, David. *Sloan Rules: Alfred P. Sloan and the Triumph of General Motors.* Chicago: University of Chicago Press, 2002.

Frankenburg, Frances R., ed. *Human Medical Experimentation: From Smallpox Vaccines to Secret Government Programs.* Santa Barbara, CA: Greenwood, 2017.

Freireich, Emil J., and Noreen A. Lemak. *Milestones in Leukemia Research and Therapy.* Baltimore: Johns Hopkins University Press, 1991.

———. *The Conquest of Cancer: A Distant Goal.* Dordrecht: Springer, 2015.

Harris, Robert, and Jeremy Paxman. *A Higher Form of Killing: The Secret Story of Chemical and Biological Warfare.* New York: Hill and Wang, 1982.

Hastings, Max. *Winston's War: Churchill 1940–1945.* New York: Vintage, 2009.

Hersh, Seymour M. *Chemical and Biological Warfare: America's Hidden Arsenal.* New York: Bobbs-Merrill, 1968.

Hindley, Meredith. *Destination Casablanca: Exile, Espionage, and the Battle for North Africa in World War II*. New York: Public Affairs, 2017.

Infield, Glenn B. *Disaster at Bari*. New York: Macmillan, 1971.

———. *Secrets of the SS*. New York: Military Heritage Press, 1981.

Karig, Walter, Comm., Lt. Earl Burton, and Lt. Stephen L. Freeland. *Battle Report: The Atlantic War*. New York: Farrar & Rinehart, 1946.

Kleber, Brooks E., and Dale Birdsell. *The Chemical Warfare Service: Chemicals in Combat. USAWWII*. Washington DC: United States Army, 1966.

Kutcher, Gerald. *Contested Medicine: Cancer Research and the Military*. Chicago: University of Chicago Press, 2009.

Lamb, Richard. *War in Italy 1943–1945: A Brutal Story*. New York: Da Capo Press, 1993.

Laszlo, John, MD. *The Cure of Childhood Leukemia: Into the Age of Miracles*. New Brunswick, NJ: Rutgers University Press, 1996.

Lederer, Susan E. *Subjected to Science: Human Experimentation in America Before the Second Word War*. Baltimore, MD: Johns Hopkins University Press, 1995.

Lesch, John E. *The First Miracle Drugs: How the Sulfa Drugs Transformed Medicine*. Oxford: Oxford University Press, 2007.

Leslie, Stuart W. *Boss Kettering: Wizard of General Motors*. New York: Columbia University Press, 1983.

Manchester, William, and Paul Reid. *The Last Lion: Winston Spencer Churchill, Defender of the Realm, 1940–1965*. New York: Little, Brown, 2012.

Meyers, Morton A., MD. *Happy Accidents: Serendipity in Major Medical Breakthroughs in the Twentieth Century*. New York: Arcade, 2007.

Mikolashek, Jon B. *General Mark Clark: Commander of U.S. Fifth Army and Liberator of Rome*. Philadelphia: Casemate, 2013.

Moore, Arthur R., Capt. *"A Careless Word . . . A Needless Sinking": A History of the Staggering Losses Suffered by the U.S. Merchant Marine, both in Ships and Personnel, during World War II*. Kings Point, NY: American Merchant Marine Museum at the U.S. Merchant Marine Academy, 1983.

Morison, Samuel Eliot. *Sicily–Salerno–Anzio, January 1943–June 1944*. Boston: Little, Brown, 1962.

Morra, Francesco. *Top Secret: Bari 2 Dicembre 1943: La Vera Storia della Pearl Harbor del Mediterraneo*. Roma: Castelvecchi, 2014.

Mukherjee, Siddhartha. *The Emperor of All Maladies: A Biography of Cancer*. New York: Scribner, 2010.

Orange, Vincent. *Coningham: A Biography of Air Marshal Sir Arthur Coningham*. Washington, DC: Center for Air Force History, 1992.

Oren, Dan A. *Joining the Club: A History of Jews and Yale*. New Haven, CT: Yale University Press, 1985.

Patterson, James T. *The Dread Disease: Cancer and Modern American Culture.* Cambridge: Harvard University Press, 1987.

Pechura, Constance M., and David P. Rall, eds. *Veterans at Risk: The Health Effects of Mustard Gas and Lewisite.* Washington, DC: National Academy Press, 1993.

Pyle, Ernie. *Brave Men.* Lincoln, NE: University of Nebraska Press, 2001.

Reminick, Gerald. *Nightmare in Bari: The World War II Liberty Ship Poison Gas Disaster and Cover-Up.* Palo Alto, CA: Glencannon Press, 2001.

Rettig, Richard A. *Cancer Crusade: The Story of the National Cancer Act of 1971.* New York: Authors Choice Press, 1977.

Rhoads, Cornelius P., ed. *Antimetabolites and Cancer.* Washington, DC: American Association for the Advancement of Science, 1955.

Scislowski, Stanley. *Not All of Us Were Brave.* Toronto: Dundurn Press, 1997.

Sieff, Marcus. *Don't Ask the Price: The Memoirs of the President of Marks & Spencer.* London: George Weidenfeld & Nicholson, 1987.

Smith, Susan L. *Toxic Exposures: Mustard Gas and the Health Consequences of World War II in the United States.* New Brunswick, NJ: Rutgers University Press, 2017.

Southern, George. *Poisonous Inferno: World War II Tragedy at Bari Harbour.* Shrewsbury, England: Airlife Publishing, 2002.

Spiers, Edward M. *Chemical Warfare.* New York: Palgrave Macmillan, 1986.

Tucker, Jonathan B. *War of Nerves: Chemical Warfare from World War I to Al-Qaeda.* New York: Anchor Books, 2006.

Turner, Henry Ashby, Jr. *General Motors and the Nazis: The Struggle for Control of Opel, Europe's Biggest Carmaker.* New Haven, CT: Yale University Press, 2005.

Vilensky, Joel A. *Dew of Death: The Story of Lewisite, America's World War I Weapon of Mass Destruction.* Bloomington: Indiana University Press, 2005.

Weatherall, M. *In Search of a Cure: A History of Pharmaceutical Discovery.* Oxford: Oxford University Press, 1990.

Wiltse, Charles M. *United States Army in the Second World War, The Technical Services: The Medical Department: Medical Service in the Mediterranean and Minor Theaters.* Washington, DC: Office of the Chief of Military History, 1965.

Illustration Credits

Bari Harbor. Photograph taken by George Kaye. New Zealand. Department of Internal Affairs. War History Branch: Photographs relating to World War 1914–1918, World War 1939–1945, occupation of Japan, Korean War, and Malayan Emergency. Ref: DA-04528-F. Alexander Turnbull Library, Wellington, New Zealand. /records/22698031.

Unloading Cargo, Bari. New Zealand, Sherman tank, being unloaded in Bari, Italy, during World War 2. New Zealand. Department of Internal Affairs. War History Branch: Photographs relating to World War 1914–1918, World War 1939–1945, occupation of Japan, Korean War, and Malayan Emergency. Ref: DA-04503-F. Alexander Turnbull Library, Wellington, New Zealand. /records/22758990.

Unloading Tank, Bari. Kaye, George Frederick, 1914–2004. New Zealand. Department of Internal Affairs. War History Branch: Photographs relating to World War 1914–1918, World War 1939–1945, occupation of Japan, Korean War, and Malayan Emergency. Ref: DA-04487-F. Alexander Turnbull Library, Wellington, New Zealand. /records/22894737.

Nighttime Bombing, Bari. US Army Signal Corps, courtesy of NARA.

Smoking Ships, Bari. US Army Signal Corps, courtesy of US Army Heritage Center.

Ships in Flames, Bari. US Army Signal Corps, courtesy of US Army Heritage Center.

Man in Boat, Bari. US Army Signal Corps, courtesy of NARA and SD Cinematografica.

Smoldering Ruins, Bari. US Army Signal Corps, courtesy of US Army Heritage Center.

Sunken Ship. Bull, George Robert, 1910–1996. Sunken ship in Bari Harbour, Italy, World War II. Photograph taken by George Bull. New Zealand. Department of Internal Affairs. War History Branch: Photographs relating to World War 1914–1918, World War 1939–1945, occupation of Japan, Korean War, and Malayan Emergency. Ref: DA-06498-F. Alexander Turnbull Library, Wellington, New Zealand. /records/22733939.

Churchill and Eisenhower, Algiers. Imperial War Museum © IWM (NA 3286).

Lt. Col. Stewart F. Alexander. Stewart F. Alexander Papers.

Lt. Col. Bernice "Bunny" Wilbur. Library of Congress.

Col. Cornelius "Dusty" Rhoads. Courtesy of the US National Library of Medicine.

Churchill with Eisenhower. Library of Congress, Prints and Photographs Division, NYWT&S Collection, LC-DIG-ppmsca-04649.

Mustard Gas Victim. Stewart F. Alexander Papers.

Telegram (No Mention of Mustard Gas). Stewart F. Alexander Papers.

Sloan and Kettering Announce Plans. Courtesy of Memorial Sloan Kettering Cancer Center.

Rhoads and Chemotherapists at Sloan Kettering. Courtesy of Memorial Sloan Kettering Cancer Center.

Sloan Kettering Institute Lobby. Courtesy of Memorial Sloan Kettering Cancer Center.

Babe Ruth at Memorial Hospital. Courtesy of Memorial Sloan Kettering Cancer Center. Babe Ruth™ owned and licensed by the Family of Babe Ruth and the Babe Ruth League, Inc., c/o Luminary Group LLC, www.BabeRuth.com.

Children on Leukemia Ward, Memorial Hospital. Courtesy of Memorial Sloan Kettering Cancer Center.

Alexander Family Practice, New Jersey. Stewart F. Alexander Papers.

Alexander with Nicholas Spark and Senators. Stewart F. Alexander Papers.

Index